THE LYMPHOCYTE

IMMUNOLOGY SERIES

Edited by NOEL ROSE
Professor and Chairman
Department of Immunology and Microbiology
Wayne State University
Detroit, Michigan

1. Mechanisms in Allergy: Reagin-Mediated Hypersensitivity
   Edited by Lawrence Goodfriend, Alec Sehon, and Robert P. Orange
2. Immunopathology: Methods and Techniques
   Edited by Theodore P. Zacharia and Sidney S. Breese, Jr.
3. Immunity and Cancer in Man: An Introduction
   Edited by Arnold E. Reif
4. *Bordetella pertussis:* Immunological and Other Biological Activities
   J. J. Munoz and R. K. Bergman
5. The Lymphocyte: Structure and Function, Parts I and II
   Edited by John J. Marchalonis

Other Volumes in Preparation

THE LYMPHOCYTE

STRUCTURE AND FUNCTION

PART I

Edited by

John J. Marchalonis

The Walter and Eliza Hall Institute of Medical Research
Royal Melbourne Hospital
Victoria, Australia

MARCEL DEKKER, INC. New York and Basel

Library of Congress Cataloging in Publication Data
Main entry under title:

The Lymphocyte : structure and function.

(Immunology series ; v. 5)
Includes indexes.
1. Lymphocytes. I. Marchalonis, John J., 1940-
II. Series.
QP95.5.L94 599'.01'13 77-2415
ISBN 0-8247-6418-8

MARCEL DEKKER, INC.

270 Madison Avenue, New York, New York 10016

Current Printing (last digit):
10 9 8 7 6 5 4 3 2 1

PRINTED IN THE UNITED STATES OF AMERICA

PREFACE

Lymphocytes are small round cells of undistinguished appearance which are found in the blood of all vertebrates. Although various activities have been proposed for these cells, it is now clear that they function in immune recognition and facilitate the elimination of infectious agents, grafts, and tumors. These cells, which are morphologically so homogeneous, can be functionally differentiated into two broad categories, thymus-derived lymphocytes (T cells) and bone-marrow derived lymphocytes (B cells), and these categories can be further subdivided on the basis of biological properties and surface markers. Lymphocyte biology is an exciting and rapidly growing area of research in which immunologists, cell biologists, membrane biochemists, and molecular biologists are making important contributions. In assembling this volume I invited young scientists who are all actively engaged "at the bench" in order to capture the excitement of this challenging area of biology as well as to delineate general principles of lymphocyte structure and function.

John J. Marchalonis

CONTRIBUTORS TO PART I

NICHOLAS COHEN
Division of Immunology, Department of Microbiology, University of Rochester School of Medicine and Dentistry, Rochester, New York

MARC FELDMAN
I.C.R.F. Tumour Immunology Unit, Department of Zoology, University College London, London, England

JAMES W. GODING
Cellular Immunology Unit, The Walter and Eliza Hall Institute of Medical Research, Royal Melbourne Hospital, Victoria, Australia

CHRISTOPHER S. HENNEY
The Johns Hopkins University School of Medicine, Baltimore, Maryland

P. W. KINCADE*
Cancer Research Unit, The Walter and Eliza Hall Institute of Medical Research, Royal Melbourne Hospital, Victoria, Australia

T. E. MANDEL
Electron Microscopy Laboratory, The Walter and Eliza Hall Institute of Medical Research, Royal Melbourne Hospital, Victoria, Australia

J. F. A. P. MILLER
Experimental Pathology Unit, The Walter and Eliza Hall Institute of Medical Research, Royal Melbourne Hospital, Victoria, Australia

RICHARD G. MILLER
Ontario Cancer Institute, Toronto, Ontario, Canada, and Department of Medical Biophysics, University of Toronto, Toronto, Ontario, Canada

*Present address: Laboratories of Developmental Hematopoiesis, Sloan-Kettering Institute for Cancer Research, New York, New York.

GRAHAM F. MITCHELL*
The Basel Institute for Immunology, Basel, Switzerland

M. A. S. MOORE†
Cancer Research Unit, The Walter and Eliza Hall Institute of Medical Research, Royal Melbourne Hospital, Victoria, Australia

ROBERT A. PRENDERGAST
The Johns Hopkins University School of Medicine, Baltimore, Maryland

J. SPRENT‡
The Basel Institute for Immunology, Basel, Switzerland

*Present address: Experimental Pathology Unit, The Walter and Eliza Hall Institute of Medical Research, Royal Melbourne Hospital, Victoria, Australia.
†Present address: Laboratories of Developmental Hematopoiesis, Sloan-Kettering Institute for Cancer Research, New York, New York.
‡Present address: Department of Pathology, School of Medicine, University of Pennsylvania, Philadelphia, Pennsylvania.

CONTENTS

SECTION IV: IMMUNE FUNCTIONS OF LYMPHOCYTES

Author and subject indexes will appear at the end of Part II

CONTENTS OF PART II

Introduction: Lymphocytes—Past, Present, and Future

J. F. A. P. Miller

Experimental Pathology Unit
The Walter and Eliza Hall Institute of Medical Research
Royal Melbourne Hospital
Victoria, Australia

In the last 15 years, our knowledge of the origin, structure, and function of lymphocytes has increased considerably. This increase is certainly evident from the subject matter described in the chapters in this book.

We owe to Gowans the first clear demonstration of the immunologic function of lymphocytes. Contrary to what had been held for 50 years, small lymphocytes were shown not to be short-lived "end" cells but rather to be mobile and recirculating cells, able to transform to larger cells and to initiate immune responses after appropriate antigenic stimulation [1]. Other investigators rejected the idea, prevalent among immunologists prior to 1960, that the thymus had become redundant during evolution. On the contrary, this organ was shown to be essential for the production of those lymphocytes, now called T cells, responsible for cellular immunity (cellular resistance to infection, delayed-type hypersensitivity, allograft rejection, and other properties) [2]. Other lymphocytes (B cells) were found to be the precursors of antibody-forming cells and to arise independently of the thymus, being derived from the bursa in birds and from the bone marrow or fetal liver in other species (chapter 3). Research is now being directed toward finding when and where during ontogeny the stem cell becomes committed to the T- or B-cell pathway and what humoral influences might play a role in these differentiation processes.

Two lines of experimentation have added strong support for Burnet's clonal selection theory. One was the demonstration that immunoglobulin molecules are incorporated in the cell membrane of B lymphocytes and act as receptors for antigen. The other was the finding that a particular B cell can bind, via such molecules, only one of many antigenic determinants available [3]. The identity of the analogous antigen-binding receptor on T lymphocytes is still the subject of much controversy. Simplicity and logic dictate that the T-cell receptor for antigen should be similar to the surface immunoglobulin of B cells. There is, in fact, experimental evidence for an IgM-like molecule on normal T lymphocytes and on some T lymphomas (chapter 10). Some investigators, however, have failed to find immunoglobulin molecules on normal T cells and have suggested that the antigen-binding receptor on these cells is quite different from immunoglobulin. Since uncertainty prevails, it is premature to be dogmatic about this issue. It is hoped that immunochemists will standardize their reagents and techniques of cell purification and of biochemical extraction to solve this fundamental problem.

Although lymphocytes are very heterogeneous in their origin, function, life-span and immunologic task, in vivo and in vitro methods are now available to achieve enrichment of selected cell populations. These methods have been made possible by our increased knowledge of the physiology of lymphocytes (e.g., their different homing properties) (chapter 2) and of their physicochemical characteristics. Cells can be separated according to density, charge (chapter 5), and surface components (chapter 11). Many surface antigens have been identified by immunologic methods, and these antigens have given us yet another means of approaching the identification and purification of lymphocyte subsets, whether these represent cells of the same lineage but at different stages of differentiation or cells that belong to separate populations with different immunologic functions. The task of the future is to identify the exact function of these surface antigens and their possible role as binding sites for specific molecules, as homing devices, or as recognition structures involved in cell interactions.

Operationally, receptors may be defined as structures able to recognize specific molecules and to "translate," through defined connections, the information received from such a recognition event to other cellular components responsible for initiating a biologically significant effect. The plasma membrane, the boundary between the cell's internal and external milieu, holds the key to the understanding of how the cell "interprets" the various molecular influences that impinge upon it. Investigations of membrane structure and function are thus of immense importance if we are to gain an insight into the processes that control various facets of cell behavior, differentiation, and development. Many chapters in this book clearly illustrate this and describe the new technology now available for the functional study of cell membrane components, e.g., electron microscope investigations with freeze-fracture techniques (chapter 1), physicochemical procedures of isolating membrane fragments and relevant membrane components (chapter 10), the use of membrane-binding molecules, such as lectins, to study changes in conformational states (chapter 12) and so on (see sec. V). It has already become clear that receptors are not fixed but are, instead, mobile in the plane of the lymphocyte surface membrane (chapter 15). When cross linked by antigens or by mitogens, such as lectins (chapter 12), varying degrees of aggregation, patch formation, capping, and even shedding of receptors may occur. Such perturbations were found to be associated with alterations in membrane permeability and in intracellular levels of constituents, such as Ca^{2+} and cyclic nucleotides. This association, in turn, has been related to alterations in metabolic activity of the cell. Investigations of this type may enable us to determine what signals are essential to activate the cells and the early biochemical events that follow. The difference between a state of tolerance and immunity should soon be explicable in molecular terms at the level of the individual cell.

Investigations of the structure and function of the many constituents of the lymphocyte membrane are likely to yield information useful in other cellular systems. Methods derived from such studies should be applicable in such areas as parasitology, pregnancy, and cancer. For example, the mechanism by which parasites interact with host cells prior to penetration might be explored on a molecular scale at the level of the membranes involved, by use of the tools developed for studies of lymphocyte membrane receptors. Likewise, similar techniques might provide some insight into the interactions that occur between spermatozoa and ovum during the early stages of fertilization. Furthermore, since there is considerable evidence that changes in cell membrane behavior accompany the origin of malignancy, cancer research may benefit from the introduction of methods derived from lymphocyte membrane studies.

Genetic factors have a profound influence in immune responses [4]. Two groups of unigenic, autosomal, dominant control systems have been identified in the last 10 years (chapter 9). One is the allotype-linked specific immune response (Ir) gene group. These genes are expressed via B cells and control the structure of the specific immunoglobulin receptor and therefore its ability to effectively bind a particular antigenic determinant. The other is a series of genes linked to the species' major histocompatibility complex (H-linked Ir genes). These genes are expressed either at the level of some structure required for antigen to trigger T cells or at the level of some component involved in the cooperation that occurs between T and B cells (or T cells and macrophages). It is known that many T-cell functions in mice are restricted by the H-2 gene complex [5], and there is evidence that H-2 gene complex-associated components are involved in the effective operation of the T-cell receptor for antigen and therefore in determining whether the cell will respond in a given situation [6]. It is hoped therefore that future studies of the role of the major histocompatibility complex will help elucidate the identity of the T-cell receptor and define the requirements for T-cell triggering.

The influence of Ir genes is likely to be relevant, not so much in the overall response to complex antigens (e.g., bacterial or viral) in which multiple antigenic determinants are involved, but rather in the response to low concentrations of poorly immunogenic molecules, for example, tumor-specific antigens. Evidently, Ir genes must have been selected for survival value during evolution, and the many instances of an association between histocompatibility type and susceptibility to disease (chapter 9) support this notion. Unfortunately, we do not understand the pathogenetic mechanisms that underlie such relationships, and it is to be hoped that new techniques will be developed to elucidate these mechanisms. Only then might we be able to predict susceptibility to disease with a greater degree of certainty.

In the last seven years, it has become evident that T cells may become involved in controlling a wide variety of cellular and humoral immune responses by producing quantitative and qualitative modifications [7]. Evidence has been obtained to show that cooperative interactions occur between T cells and macrophages, between T and B cells, and possibly among T cells themselves. Antigen-activated T cells are known to release several factors that may be specific or nonspecific with respect to the antigenic determinants concerned. "Lymphokines" are essentially nonspecific effectors of cellular immunity responsible for various effects on monocytes, macrophages, and polymorphonuclear leukocytes. They may recruit leukocytes that produce the inflammatory lesions of delayed-type hypersensitivity, and they may enhance the microbicidal activity of macrophages important for cellular resistance to infection. It was largely as a result of the work of Mackaness [8] that evidence has accumulated to show that sensitized T lymphocytes release factors that "activate" macrophages to kill some intracellular bacteria. A similar mechanism plays a role in resistance to some viruses. The situation with other infectious agents is not clear, but T-cell deprivation does augment susceptibility to some protozoan and metazoan parasites and to some fungi. In view of this point, it is essential to investigate, in these systems, the possible involvement of T cells and macrophages and their role in protective immunity. Although the feeling has been expressed that immunology was born from the demand for protection against infectious disease and that essentially what was needed has been provided, it may be worthwhile pointing out that a recent World Health Organization survey [9] estimates that approximately 200 million people are infected with schistosomes, 300 million with filariae and other helminths, 250 million with malaria, and 1,000 million with a variety of intestinal parasites. Furthermore, of the immunologic methods available, none can satisfactorily halt the spread of gonococcal and syphilitic infections.

In many humoral immune responses, T and B lymphocytes work together, not separately, as part of a network in which collaborative and feedback loops determine the outcome [7]. Both facilitation and suppression of antibody production have been observed, but the exact mechanism involved is not known. A vast amount of in vitro work has been done in an attempt to determine this mechanism (chapter 8). As a result, certain antigen-specific T-cell factors have been implicated as mediators. One such factor is claimed to be IgT, a T cell-derived immunoglobulin with a capacity for binding to macrophages. Another is a nonimmunoglobulin, antigen-specific product coded by genes that, in mice, lie close to the K end of the histocompatibility complex (chapter 9). It is sometimes difficult to relate in vitro events to the in vivo situation. Thus, IgG responses are much more T-cell dependent than are IgM responses, and most investigators who have used in vitro systems to generate such T-cell factors have confined their observations to IgM responses. Furthermore, germinal center formation, which is a characteristic marker of effective T- and B-cell cooperation in vivo, has not been reproduced in any in vitro model. Other theories of T- and B-cell cooperation have invoked the operation of nonspecific T-cell factors. Since the fundamental function of T cells is cellular immunity, and since nonspecific factors are instrumental in many T cell-mediated responses and often act through macrophages, it is not unreasonable to assume that similar nonspecific factors indirectly influence B-cell responsiveness [7]. T cells and macrophages may thus exert a crucial role by removing excess antigen from the immediate microenvironment of the B cell and therefore prevent B-cell paralysis (chapter 6). This belief is in accordance with the observed correlations among antigen persistence, susceptibility of potential IgG or high-affinity antibody-forming cell precursors to paralysis, and absence of a T-cell influence. Whatever may be the mechanism of T- and B-cell interaction, it is clear that the existence of a dual system of interacting cell types allows more precise multilevel regulation of antibody production of crucial importance in the development of immunologic memory and immunologic tolerance.

The evidence for interaction among subsets of T cells is not as convincing as that for T and B cells. T cell-dependent suppression may be an example of one form of T-T interaction. It is not, however, clear whether suppressor T cells exist as distinct cellular entities or whether T cells from tolerant (or suppressed) animals are not responding because they are coated with an excess of antigen-antibody complexes, some of which could "leak" onto other T cells, thus preventing the latter from responding. It is probable that the mechanism of T cell-dependent suppression will become elucidated in the next few years. Another, but more controversial, form of T-T interaction may operate via "transfer factor" (TF). This phenomenon has been observed in the human but has not been reproduced unequivocally in any other animal species. It appears that human TF is a dialyzable component of molecular weight less than 10,000 daltons that acts essentially as an *initiator* of cellular immunity, converting naive lymphocytes (presumably

T cells) to an antigen-responsive state [10]. These lymphocytes can now behave as the original sensitized lymphocytes from which TF was extracted. It is now 20 years since the phenomenon was first described in the human species, and there have been reports of spectacular success in controlling infections with TF. In view of this success, it is imperative to attempt to reproduce the TF phenomenon in an animal model, not only to determine critically whether such a factor that regulates T cell-mediated immunity is universal, but also to explore precisely its mechanism of action.

It is evident that a deeper understanding of the mechanisms by which T and B cells interact will pave the way for practical methods of manipulating selectively different sets of lymphocytes and their responses. This procedure may eventually be applicable in clinical medicine for use in various infectious diseases, vaccinating procedures, anergic states, immune deficiency diseases, allergic conditions, autoimmune diseases, cancer, and transplantation of tissues or organs.

Progress in immunophylogenetic studies is described in chapter 4. The capacity to develop specific transplantation immunity, concomitantly with some degree of immunologic memory, appears to have been demonstrated in two phyla of advanced invertebrates: annelid worms and echinoderms [11]. In the annelids, adoptive transfer of such immunity has been achieved with coelomocytes (cells akin to leukocytes), not with serum. In lower invertebrates, there is evidence for an ability to recognize alien cells but not for the diversification of effector functions, nor for memory. Thus, for example, a hyperplastic proliferative contact reaction is seen in coelenterates and tunicates. It has been suggested that two separate sets of recognition patterns might have evolved. One would be akin to immunoglobulin (though not necessarily identical) and would be responsible for enabling the T cells of higher vertebrates to be activated by a multiplicity of antigens to perform the functions of cellular immunity. The other would be a more primitive recognition molecule that would enable T cells to recognize, on other cells of the same species, the major histocompatibility antigens of that species and to react by blast transformation and proliferation in the "mixed lymphocyte reaction." It remains a challenge to the immunophylogeneticist to clarify the evolutionary relationships among such recognition molecules, immunoglobulins, and cell surface (histocompatibility) antigens.

Burnet has often stressed that one of the most important functions of lymphocytes is to maintain the genetic integrity of the body [12]. The discovery that neonatal thymectomy (which impairs T cell-mediated immunity) renders animals more susceptible to the oncogenic activity of certain viruses [13] certainly supports the notion that T cells constantly scan other cells and eliminate those with altered antigenicity. More recently, identical observations have been made in "athymic nude" mice [14]. T cells may thus constitute part of what Burnet termed an "immunological surveillance" mechanism [12], the function of which is to eliminate antigenically distinct clones of cells before they can multiply and spread. In 1909, Ehrlich [15] clearly stated the same notion when he wrote: "I am convinced that during development and growth malignant cells arise extremely frequently, but in the majority of people they remain latent due to the protective action of the host. I am also convinced that this natural immunity is not due to the presence of antimicrobial bodies, but is determined purely by cellular factors. These may be weakened in older age groups in which cancer is more prevalent."

References

1. J. L. Gowans, and D. D. McGregor, Progr. Allergy **9**, 1 (1965).
2. J. F. A. P. Miller and D. Osoba, Physiol. Rev. **47**, 437 (1967).
3. G. L. Ada, Transplant. Rev. **5**, 105 (1970).
4. B. Benacerraf and H. O. McDevitt, Science **175**, 273 (1972).
5. R. M. Zinkernagel, Nature (London) **251**, 230 (1974).
6. J. F. A. P. Miller, M. A. Vadas, A. Whitelaw, and J. Gamble, Proc. Nat. Acad. Sci. U.S.A., **73**, 2486 (1974).
7. J. F. A. P. Miller, Ann. N. Y. Acad. Sci. **249**, 9 (1975).
8. G. B. Mackaness, Sem. Hematol. **7**, 172 (1970).
9. W. H. O. Working Paper, 30 May (1974), World Health Organization, Geneva, Switzerland.
10. H. S. Lawrence, Advan. Immunol. **11**, 195 (1969).
11. W. H. Hildemann, Nature (London) **250**, 116 (1974).
12. F. M. Burnet, *Immunological Surveillance,* Pergamon Press, Sydney, 1970.
13. J. F. A. P. Miller, L. W. Law, and R. C. Ting, Proc. Soc. Exp. Biol. Med. **116**, 323 (1964).
14. A. C. Allison, J. N. Monga, and V. Hammond, Nature (London) **252**, 746 (1974).
15. P. Ehrlich, Nederlandsch Tijdschrift voor Genesskunde, Eerste Helft, No. 5 (1909).

SECTION I

General Properties of Lymphocytes

CHAPTER 1

The Ultrastructure of Mammalian Lymphocytes and Their Progeny

T. E. Mandel

Electron Microscopy Laboratory
The Walter and Eliza Hall Institute of Medical Research
Royal Melbourne Hospital
Victoria, Australia

I. Introduction

Lymphocytes were identified morphologically more than a century ago, and their widespread distribution throughout the body was soon clearly appreciated. It was also recognized that lymphopoiesis was concentrated in particular organs, notably the thymus, lymph nodes, spleen, Peyer's patches, and, in birds, the bursa of Fabricius. However, conventional morphologic examination, whether by light, phase, or electron microscopy, gave few if any clues as to the diverse functional, developmental, and antigenic patterns these cells are now known to express. For many years, the classification of lymphocytes was based either on their size or on their location, and, in the absence both of sophisticated marker techniques and of relevant immunologic theory, little could be stated about the interrelationships, migration streams, and precise functions of these ubiquitous cells.

In recent years, it has become clear that lymphocytes can be classified into two quite distinct developmental groups. These groups are, (a) the thymus-derived T lymphocytes, respnsible, in general, for cell-mediated immunity, and, (b) bone marrow, or bursa-derived, B lymphocytes, responsible for humoral immune phenomena. Collaboration between B and T cells in some forms of immune responsiveness is also well established. This knowledge, together with recent data on cell migration streams, allows one to approach the morphology of lymphocytes in a fresh light, and it is becoming possible to correlate the structural and functional aspects of these cells. In this chapter, in which we discuss the ultrastructure of mammalian T and B lymphocytes and their progeny, we shall emphasize these functional aspects. Since some aspects of lymphocyte physiology and function are best studied in the somewhat artificial models of lectin-stimulated lymphoid cells, and in neoplastic lines, these too will be considered briefly.

II. Lymphocyte Structure

Traditionally, lymphocytes have been classified as small, medium, and large on the basis of their size, nucleocytoplasmic ratios, and staining characteristics, but the distinction among these groups is largely arbitrary, and one group merges smoothly into the next. The resolution of the light microscope limits the amount of information which can be obtained from the examination of normal stained preparations of lymphoid cells, but with appropriate labeling technics much valuable information can be obtained when use is made of specific cell surface components as tags for particular lymphocyte groups. Such techniques have recently been adapted for electron microscopy. Since the light microscope structure of lymphoid cells has recently been reviewed in detail by Yoffey and Courtice [1] and by Elves [2], who give a comprehensive bibliography of the relevant literature, it will not be discussed in this chapter.

In the past 15 to 20 years, the electron microscope has been used with increasing frequency for the study of cellular fine structure, and the use of aldehyde primary fixation instead of the older osmium fixatives, of stable cross-linked plastics as embedding media, and of more reliable staining techniques have all contributed to a clearer and more incisive picture of lymphocyte structure.

An electron micrograph of a typical small lymphocyte is shown in Fig. 1. These cells have a characteristic appearance in the electron

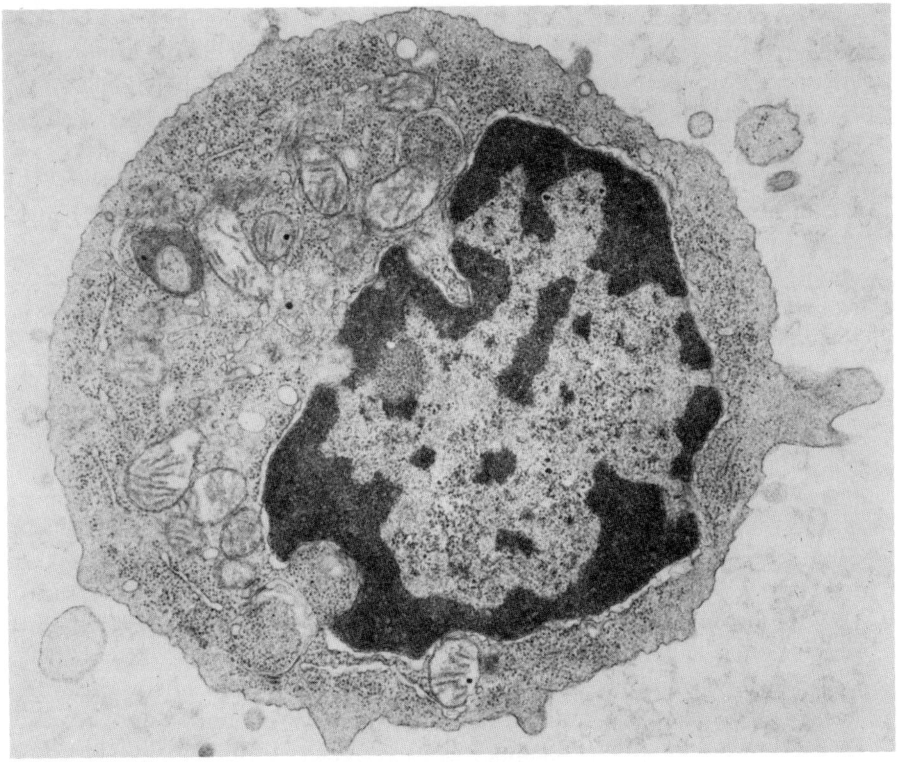

FIG. 1. Small lymphocyte from the thoracic duct lymph of an adult CBA mouse. This cell is typical of peripheral T cells but in this plane of section shows a relatively large amount of cytoplasm. The nucleus has heavily marginated chromatin, and a portion of the nucleolus is also visible. The cytoplasm contains numerous monoribosomes, very little rough-surfaced endoplasmic reticulum (RER), some large mitochondria, and a small Golgi region. Note the thin band of organelle-free cytoplasm just below the surface membrane. ×20,500.

microscope. Their nucleus is typically round or somewhat indented but may, on occasions, show a deep cleft. Nuclear blebs [3-5] have been described in a variety of situations, though their significance remains unclear. Small lymphocyte nuclear chromatin, particularly in aldehyde-fixed cells stained with uranyl salts, is dense and deeply staining and lies at the nuclear periphery. Nuclear pores are present and are generally free of dense chromatin. A nucleolus is usually seen in suitably sectioned cells. Heiniger et al. [6] demonstrated ultrastructural differences between thymic and peripheral (lymph node) small lymphocytes and showed that the former had a smaller mean nucleolar volume and represented a more uniform population with regard to the frequency distribution of nucleolar cross-sectional diameter than did lymph node small lymphocytes. Since the majority of lymph node cells are T cells, these findings may reflect a difference between intrathymic and peripheral T cells. More recently, Suter et al. [7] showed that complement receptor lymphocytes (CRL), identified as those B cells which could be separated from the spleen and lymph nodes by binding antigen-antibody-complement complexes, could be distinguished morphologically from non-CRL by the presence in their nuclei of large and complex nuclear bodies. In both of these studies, however, it is possible that only a subpopulation of cells within a group was being identified.

In the electron microscope, the cytoplasm of small lymphocytes is usually sparse and contains relatively few organelles (Fig. 1). Characteristically, a few large mitochondria, a small Golgi zone that contains a pair of centrioles, numerous free ribosomes, and a few small vesicles and lysosome-like bodies are present. Generally, rough-surfaced endoplasmic reticulum (RER) is sparse or absent. A great variety of ribosomal patterns are, however, present among cells identified as small lymphocytes, and Feldman and Nordquist [8] classified such cells into various groups on this basis. Suter et al. [7] also distinguished CRL by the presence of a pale cytoplasmic matrix that contained relatively few ribosomes but more numerous coated vesicles than were found in the non-CRL.

Small lymphocytes also contain a few microtubules and a narrow submembranous zone of microfibrils. The demonstration of both of these structures requires optimal fixation and staining, and microtubules in particular tend to disappear if cells are fixed in the cold and are frequently not seen in tissues fixed solely with osmium. Usually, numerous fine processes extend from the cell periphery, and, on occasions, a uropod may be seen. The cell processes contain fine microfibrils (Fig. 2) which form a dense network from which other organelles are usually excluded.

Lamelin et al. [9] and Matter et al. [10] used sophisticated cell surface labeling studies to clearly define the light and electron microscope structure of T and B cells. Ultrastructurally [10], T and B cells were examined for the presence on the surface of the former of the alloantigen θ and the heteroantigen "mouse specific lymphocyte antigen" (MSLA) [11] and, on the latter of "mouse-specific bone-marrow derived lymphocyte antigen" (MBLA) [12] and surface immunoglobulin (SIg). Matter et al. [10] showed that, in general, T small lymphocytes, identified by their possession of θ and MSLA, had a dense cytoplasm and a better developed microfibril system than did cells identified as B small lymphocytes by the presence of MBLA and SIg. Recently, the scanning electron microscope has also been used to distinguish human T cells from B cells [13-15]. B cells generally had a more irregular outline with numerous microvilli than did T cells, which had a much smoother surface.

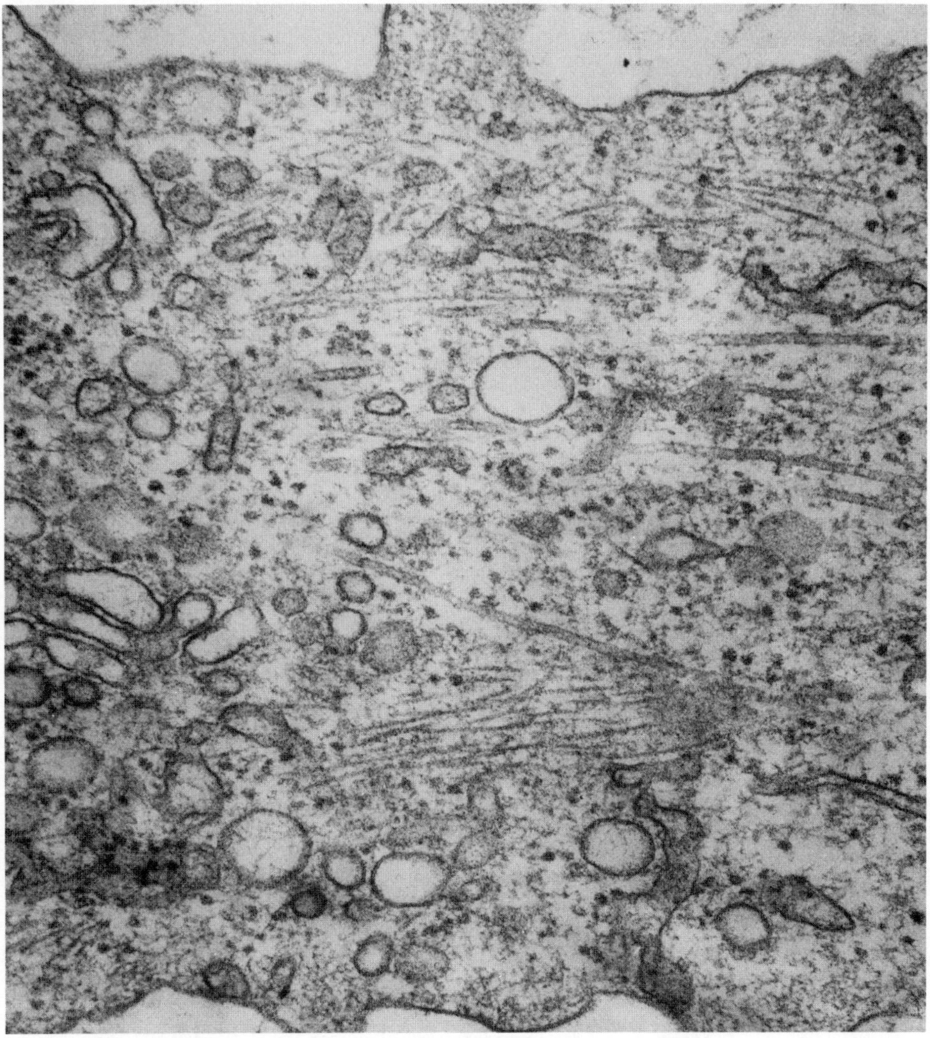

FIG. 2. Portion of a uropod of an "activated," cortisone-resistant T lymphocyte that shows the fine fibrillar network just below the surface membrane, bundles of large filaments scattered through the cytoplasm, and some elongated microtubules. ×60,000.

As in the light microscope, larger cells are also identified with the electron microscope and can be classified as medium and large lymphocytes and lymphoblasts. Again, the distinction between any two groups is blurred and arbitrary, and all intermediate forms exist. Zucker-Franklin [15] noted the great heterogeneity in the ultrastructural appearance of human thoracic duct lymphocytes and commented on the great variation in the size of the Golgi apparatus, the number of ribosomes, and the extent of development of RER and suggested that some lymphocytes were metabolically more active than others. She also noted the presence of bundles of microfibrils deep in the cytoplasm, structures previously noted by de Petris et al. [16] in monocytes.

In general, as lymphocytes increase in size, their nuclei become larger, the chromatin more dispersed, and the nuclear outline more irregular; in lymphoblasts particularly, large and sometimes multiple nucleoli are present (Fig. 3).

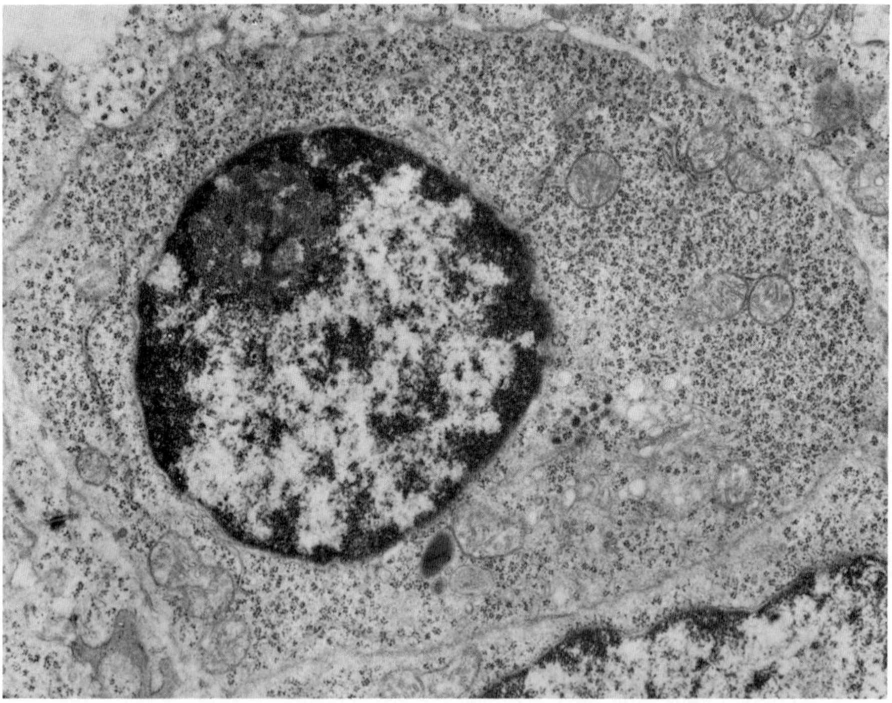

FIG. 3. Lymphoblast from the thymus of a 16-day (CBA × C57BL/6) F_1 mouse fetus. In this section, the nucleus is cut tangentially. Chromatin is relatively diffuse, and part of a large nucleolus is present. The copious cytoplasm is filled with numerous polyribosomes and contains a well-developed Golgi region and some mitochondria. The polysomes extend to the cell membrane (cf. Fig. 1). ×12,000

The cytoplasm of the larger cells contains more and often a greater concentration of organelles than are usually seen in small lymphocytes. With the light microscope, such features are not evident. Cytoplasmic basophilia can be interpreted ultrastructurally as being due to the concentration of ribosomes, either membrane associated or free mono- and polyribosomes. Generally, cells classified as lymphoblasts contain very large numbers of free ribosomes, whereas early plasmablasts are characterized by the development of RER. The morphologic distinction between large lymphocytes and lymphoblasts rests largely on nucleolar development and concentration of ribosomes, both of which are better developed in the blasts.

There are clearly a great many uncertainties inherent in a purely morphologic classification of lymphoid cells, whether based on optical or electron microscopy, and little can be said regarding the lineage or functional status of particular cells in the absence of functional or antigenic studies. However, studies that utilized such methods are now being reported [10,17-20], and more confident statements regarding the precise status of morphologically defined cells will be possible. Another morphologic problem still to be solved concerns the fine structure of prelymphoid stem cells. Although some studies have been reported which suggest that such stem cells have, indeed, been identified, the absence of unequivocal functional or antigenic markers results in uncertainty as to the true nature of these cells.

III. The B-cell System

A. Differentiation of B-lineage Cells

Both T and B cells can exist as typical lymphocytes of varying sizes, but their further differentiation reflects their differing functions. B cells differentiate ultimately into specialized, protein-producing and -secreting plasma cells, the ultrastructural features of which are characteristic of these functions [21,22]. The role of plasma cells in antibody production was first clearly enunciated by Fagraeus [23], and immunofluorescent studies [23-27] demonstrated the presence of antibody within them. Functional studies on isolated single cells by Nossal [28] proved that the cells actually produced and secreted specific antibody against the immunizing antigen. Such early studies on antibody production by single cells have been reviewed by Nossal and Makela [29].

The electron microscope has been used in the studies of B-cell progeny to answer three main questions. The high resolving power of the instrument was used, first, to characterize the morphology of antibody-forming cells (AFC), second, to establish the intracellular localization and production pathway of the antibody, and, third, to seek evidence for the mode of antibody secretion.

B. Ultrastructure of Antibody-forming Cells

The ultrastructure of plasma cells was first described by Braunsteiner et al. in 1953 [30], and subsequent early studies have been summarized by Bessis [31]. The ultrastructural features of these cells make them distinctive and readily recognizable in either lymphoid tissues or in cell suspensions [21,22]. In tissue sections, particularly from hyperimmunized animals, plasma cells occur in distinct groups composed of cells of somewhat varying morphology, which probably reflects the different degrees of maturity of the individual cells. The least mature cells of this series, referred to usually as plasmablasts, have a morphology similar to that of lymphoblasts. Ultrastructurally, however, they contain some flattened cisternae of RER in addition to numerous free polysomes (Fig. 4). As these cells mature, their RER increases in amount, and a mature plasma cell is filled with flattened parallel cisternae. Further maturation

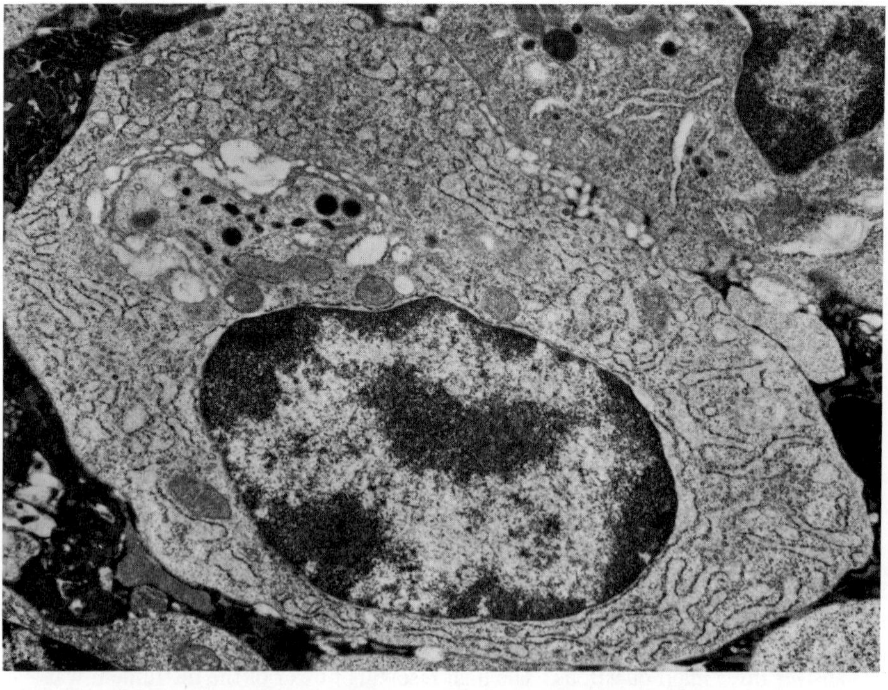

FIG. 4 Immature plasma cells from the spleen of a normal (unimmunized) CBA mouse. The cell contains numerous flattened cisternae of RER and a large Golgi zone. Dense vesicles are present around the Golgi region. The nucleus contains densely aggregated chromatin, but in this section the nucleolus is not visible. ×9,600

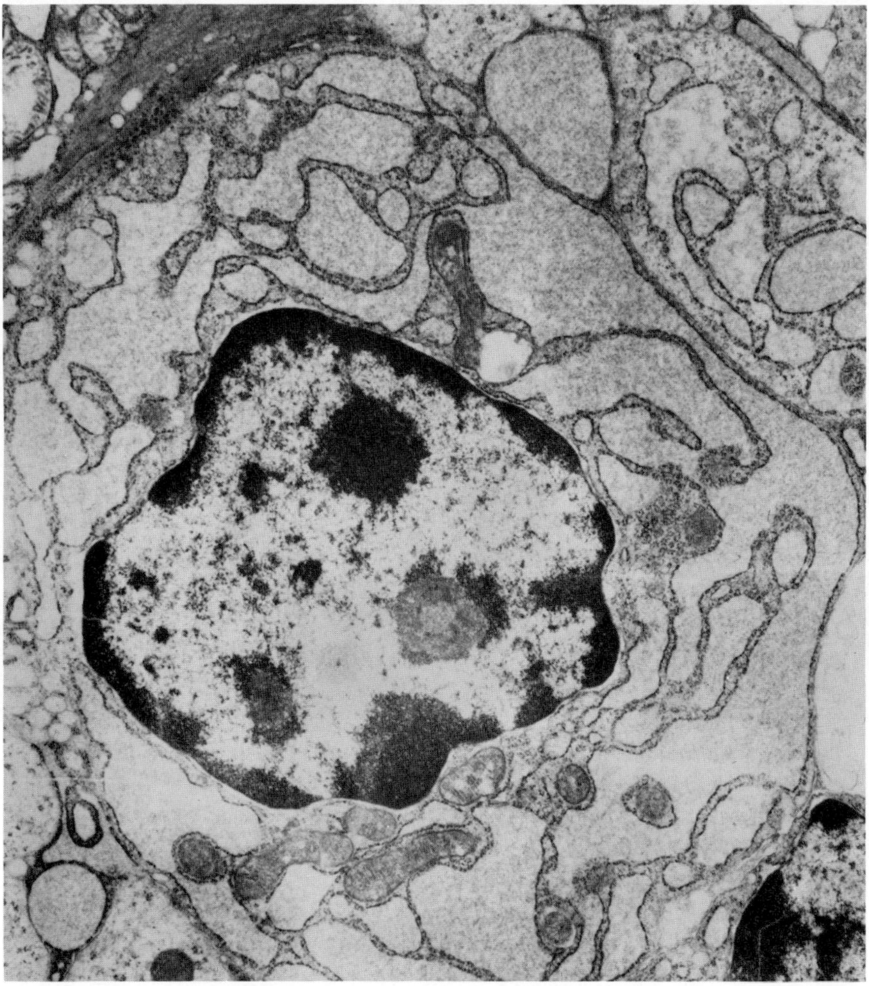

FIG. 5. A "mature" plasma cell with grossly dilated RER, which is filled with fine flocculent material, presumably immunoglobulin. X9,600

results in dilatation of the cisternae, which become filled with a finely floculent material (Fig. 5). At the same time, the number of free ribosomes decreases. In fully mature plasma cells, the RER may be widely dilated, rounded up, and filled with electron-dense material (Russell bodies) and, occasionally, crystals. The Golgi zone is also typically well developed (Fig. 6) and contains numerous cisternae, lamellae, and vesicles. A few small dense vacuoles may also be seen

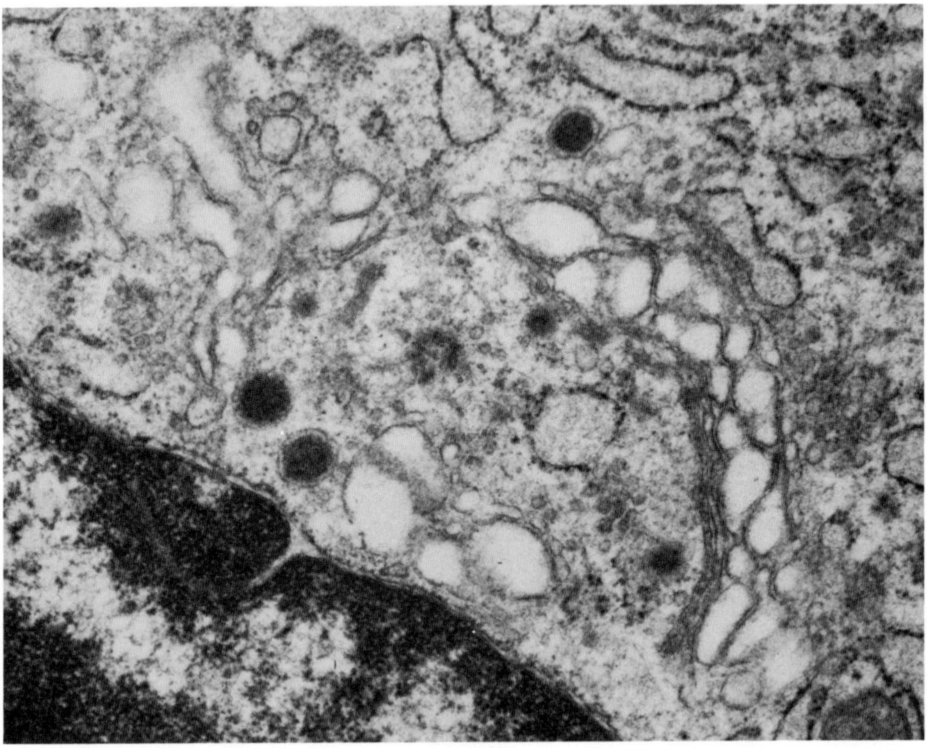

FIG. 6. Detail of the Golgi region of a relatively mature plasma cell that shows the well-developed vesicles and cisternae of this structure. Note the difference in the density of the contents of the RER and of the Golgi cisternae. ×32,000

associated with the Golgi. During maturation, the nucleus rounds up and becomes eccentrically displaced; its chromatin condenses into heavy blocks which form the classic "cartwheel" appearance typically seen in smeared and stained plasma cells in the light microscope. Immature cells also have a large and prominent nucleolus, which tends to become buried and lost in the condensing chromatin. While fully mature plasma cells are nondividing end cells, less mature members of the series can divide, and mitotic figures of these cells can be recognized in the electron microscope.

Although it was recognized as early as 1948 [23] that plasma cells were, indeed, concerned with antibody secretion, it was not known with any certainty whether cells without the typical structure of plasma cells could also produce antibodies. In recent years, therefore, ultrastructural and functional studies have been combined to positively identify AFC. These studies have generally been of two distinct types. AFC were either examined for the presence of antibody against an antigen which could be identified ultrastructurally, either directly [32,33] (e.g., ferritin), histochemically [34] [e.g., horseradish peroxidase (POX)], or by radioautography [35], or cells secreting antibody were indirectly identified by hemolytic plaque formation [36-43] or by rosette technics [43-45] and isolated and examined.

The role of plasma cells in antibody secretion is clearly beyond doubt, and both light [23,28,29,46] and electron microscope studies [30,31,36,47, 48] implicated these cells in this process. However, while the majority of active AFC were identified with the light microscope as mature plasma cells or their immediate precursors (reviewed in Ref. 29), many workers drew attention to actively secreting cells which resembled typical small lymphocytes. Indeed, Attardi et al. [49] identified about two thirds of active cells as small lymphocytes. Numerous studies have been reported describing the fine structure of AFC and have confirmed that cells without the morphologic features of typical plasma cells can, indeed, secrete antibody.

In the earliest of these studies, de Petris et al. [32] used rabbits hyperimmunized with ferritin and could only find antiferritin antibody in relatively well-developed plasma cells. In a subsequent study [33], they examined the time course of antibody appearance and were able to show specific labeling in immunized animals 48 hr after a booster injection but not before this time. The label was first found in cells identified as "blasts" and these cells were considered to be identical with cells variously referred to by other workers as "transitional cells" [23], "large lymphocytes" [29], "activated reticular cells" [50], "large pyroninophilic cells" [51], and "hemocytoblasts" [52,53]. At time points between 2 and 5 days after a booster injection, progressively more highly differentiated cells were labeled.

In somewhat similar studies in which the intracellular localization of antibody was taken as evidence for antibody production, Avrameas et al. [34,54,57] found that a variety of morphologically distinct cells were labeled. They used POX as the antigen and located anti-POX antibody by incubating lightly fixed cells with POX and revealed its presence histochemically. Antibody was first identified in "hemocytoblasts" [34] and later in immature and mature plasma cells. "Hemocytoblasts" were identified as large cells that contained a large electronlucent nucleus, an extensive and complex nucleolus, and a cytoplasm rich in free ribosomes but with a poorly developed RER. They subsequently showed [55] that, under their conditions of immunization, antibody was found in three types of cells: in typical plasma cells, in a few large lymphocytes or lymphoblasts, and in very abundant "modified" or "specialized" small lymphocytes which they called "lymphoplasmacytes." These latter cells could be induced to differentiate from a lymphoid precursor by an antigenic stimulus and were characteristically small, dense, circulating cells. By contrast, the more typical plasma cells, under their conditions of fixation, were identified as large, clear, fixed cells. Similar cells were found in rabbits, rats, mice, and guinea pigs [56,57]. They considered that the plasma cells and lymphoplasmacytes arose from different precursors and were not part of the same lineage [55]. Both cell types, however, were believed to produce 7S antibody. In recent studies, Miller et al. [58,59] used POX to investigate the appearance of anti-POX AFC in the popliteal lymph nodes of mice. The first AFC detected after a primary challenge appeared after 6 to 8 days and were all differentiated plasma cells [58]. By contrast, after secondary challenge, two populations of AFC were detected; a stable non-dividing population of mature plasma cells whose content of antibody increased 3 days after challenge and a new dividing population of cells whose numbers increased exponentially between 18 hr and 5 days and included "stimulated" lymphocytes and small lymphocytes in addition to plasma cells.

Bosman et al. [35] used radioiodinated antigens and radioautography to label lymph node cells from immunized animals and, in an electron microscope analysis, showed that 17% of the cells were labeled (cf. 2% of controls) and that 90% of the labeled cells were lymphocytes, blasts, or plasma cells. They noted that almost twice as many lymphocytes as plasma cells were marked by the isotope; the lymphocytes ranged in morphology from "mature monoribosomal" to "immature polyribosomal" cells. In a later study [60] using histochemistry and radioautography, they identified anti-POX-containing cells histochemically and used radioiodinated class-specific antisera to identify the immunoglobulin heavy-chain class. They showed that plasma cells accounted for five sixths of the POX-containing cells labeled with anti-γG in contrast to one tenth labeled with anti-γM. The remaining doubly labeled cells were lymphocytes.

In a different type of experimental approach, AFC were identified by either plaque formation (PFC) or by rosette formation (RFC). The earliest ultrastructural studies on isolated PFC were those of Bussard and Binet [36] who examined rabbit popliteal lymph node cells making direct (19S IgM) plaques in sheep red blood cell (sRBC) suspensions. They found that *all* PFC were typical plasma cells. Fitch et al. [37] showed that in spleen cells from rats immunized with sRBC, most direct PFC were plasma cells. Harris et al. [38] and Hummeler et al. [40] distinguished two categories of 19S PFC in rabbit lymph node cells; some cells were typical plasma cells, whereas others had the morphology of lymphocytes. When PFC were obtained from free floating cells from the blood or lymph, however, classic plasma cells could not usually be found [41,60-62]. The blastlike cells found in efferent lymph [62] could apparently transform into typical plasma cells when they were reinfused into an autologous, unstimulated lymph node, which suggested that plasma cell precursors were present as free floating forms which differentiated to mature plasma cells only in the lymphoid organs.

Cunningham et al. [39] examined efferent sheep lymph and lymph node AFC produced by immunization with *Salmonella muenchen* and detected the AFC by plaque formation in sensitized sheep erythrocyte monolayers. They also detected two morphologic forms of AFC; the majority resembled cells found in "normal" efferent lymph, and a minority, found only among the lymph node cells, were typical plasma cells. However, all intermediate forms between these two groups could be identified. Neher and Siegel [42] showed that 19S anti-sRBC plaque-forming cells, obtained from mouse spleen cell suspensions on Days 3 to 6 after primary immunization, had a developmental pattern that ranged from "immunoblasts" early in the response to mature plasma cells later. In contrast to studies that used lymph node cells, however [39], no lymphocytes were identified in this splenic plaque-forming population. Gudat et al. [43], who employed rosette and plaque formation, further analyzed spleen and lymph node AFC and showed that whereas in the lymph node population RFC were lymphocytes or plasma cells, in the spleen some RFC were also macrophages. Whereas most *RFC* (70-100%) were lymphoid, the majority of *PFC* were plasma cells. Among PFC, however, no difference in cell distribution could be shown between 19S and 7S producers.

In contrast to the situation in immunized animals, when "spontaneous" RFC from the spleens of nonimmunized mice were examined, no plasma cells were seen, and all RFC were either "inactive" monoribosomal small lymphocytes or macrophages [44]. It is unlikely, however, that all or even most of these lymphoid RFC were AFC; rather, they were probably antigen-binding cells.

It is clear therefore that the type of cell detected and identified as an AFC depends very greatly on several parameters, including the immunization history of the animal, the source of the cells, and on technical factors, such as the method of fixation and the sensitivity of the method of detection. The "lymphoplasmacytes" of Avrameas et al. [55], for example, appear to require a special form of fixation for their detection. The immediate source of AFC seems to determine their morphology; e.g., free circulating cells tend to be cytologically less differentiated than fixed tissue cells, though they may be on the same developmental pathway.

C. Subcellular Localization of Antibody

Immunofluorescent techniques clearly demonstrated the presence of intracellular antibody within antigenically stimulated [24,63] and neoplastic [64] lymphoid cells, but it required the resolving power of the electron microscope to visualize its precise subcellular localization. Because of its physical and immunogenic properties, ferritin has been widely used in ultrastructural studies both as an antigen per se and as a marker molecule, either directly to localize antiferritin antibodies or conjugated chemically to anti-immunoglobulins to detect the location of antibody. It was shown by de Petris et al. [32,33] that antiferritin antibody first appeared in the perinuclear space (PNS) of blastlike cells and subsequently in some, but not all, cisternae of the RER. The Golgi apparatus was labeled inconsistently, and ferritin could not be demonstrated in association with either ribosomes (free or membrane bound) or with the cell surface [32,33]. However, since ferritin is a very large molecule (mol wt approx. 650,000), its size, whether used alone or conjugated to Ig, may well impede its movement through a cell. It is therefore possible that not all Ig-containing sites may be labeled. In view of this problem, Leduc et al. [34] used the much smaller immunogenic enzyme, POX (mol wt 40,000) as a tracer and detected it cytochemically [65]. They confirmed the initial appearance of anti-POX antibody in the PNS of "hemocytoblasts" and noted its persistence in this site in immature, but not in mature, plasma cells [34]. They also showed the movement of antibody into some cisternae of RER and demonstrated its consistent presence in the lamellar portion of the Golgi apparatus in all stages of plasma cell differentiation. In mature plasma cells, they showed that antibody became concentrated either in large, spherical, intracisternal granules (Russell bodies) or that it apparently overflowed into all parts of the cytoplasm. When POX was used as a tracer conjugated chemically to human Ig to study the localization of anti-HIg antibodies in hyperimmunized rabbit lymph node cells, antibody activity was also noted on ribosomes in addition to its presence in the PNS, RER, and the Golgi zone [54]. It has also been claimed [55] that after an additional antigenic stimulus, AFCs are able to initiate a second cycle of antibody production, with antibody accumulating in the PNS even before previously formed material is secreted at the cell periphery.

Suzuki et al. [66] used POX-conjugated monospecific antisera to demonstrate the different intracellular localization of μ and K chains in a human lymphoblastoid cell line known to secrete IgA and free K chain. They claimed that K chains were present in the RER and its membrane, the external layer of the nuclear envelope, and on the ribosomes lining it and the RER. By contrast, the major chain site was on the clusters of cytoplasmic polysomes, although chains were also detected on the external layer of the nuclear envelope and on the ribosomes on the RER and the nuclear membrane.

Enzymatic studies take advantage of the lower molecular weight of POX and other immunogenic enzymes and of the great sensitivity of the cytochemical reaction used for their demonstration. Their small size facilitates diffusion through fixed cells, and their catalytic activity can be used to increase the amount of the reaction product. However, it is necessary to both beware of diffusion of the reaction product away from the site of the enzyme and to take into account the possible presence of endogenous enzymes.

Numerous studies that utilized biochemical and cell fractionation techniques have been reported dealing with the biosynthesis, intracellular transport, and secretion of immunoglobulins (e.g., see review References 67 and 68). Such questions have recently been investigated in the electron microscope. Studies referred to above on the localization of antibodies by cytochemistry and immunoelectron microscopy implied that a sequential intracellular transport of Ig occurs. Such studies, however, have not been able to critically define these intracellular pathways, since they deal, in the main, with the localization of completed antibody molecules. These restrictions can, however, be overcome with radioisotopic pulse labeling, in which the addition of precursor molecules can be followed during the synthesis of Ig molecules and can be related to their subcellular localization. Zagury et al. [69] used electron microscopic radioautography to follow the incorporation of a tritium-labeled amino acid (leucine) and tritium-labeled carbohydrate precursors (galactose and glucosamine) into the developing Ig chains in cell suspensions prepared from an immunoglobulin-secreting mouse myeloma. They showed that the polypeptide chain was synthesized in the region of the RER and that the appearance of the ^{3}H-labeled leucine Ig chain over the Golgi region occurred at times *after* its appearance in the RER, which suggested that the completed polypeptide chain was transported from the RER to the Golgi. The incorporation of glucosamine occurred both in the Golgi and in the RER, while [^{3}H] galactose was added only in the Golgi. The completed antibodies then left the Golgi to be secreted from the cell. These studies are in basic agreement with methodologically similar studies on the synthesis of proteins in other exportable protein-producing cells, such as those of the pancreas [70-73] and salivary gland [74]. The major difficulty with radioautographic studies lies in their inability to precisely localize the intracellular origin of the isotope responsible for the development of radioautographic silver grains, particularly when the origin may be from very small organelles, such as polyribosomes. Despite these difficulties, such studies correlate very well with biochemical data on Ig synthesis in subcellular fractions [75,76].

D. Ultrastructural Evidence for Antibody Secretion

The high resolving power of the electron microscope should be able to give some indication as to the mechanism of antibody release. Early ultrastructural studies on protein-secreting cells resulted in the classification of a variety of morphologically distinct forms of secretory activity, and Palay [77] grouped these into three types, referred to as "holocrine," "apocrine," and "merocrine." Other variations of these processes have also been described, but to date there is still no clear notion of the mechanism of antibody release from immunoglobulin-forming cells [69].

"Holocrine" secretion, in which a cell is lysed with the consequent release of its content of antibody, has been suggested as one mode of immunoglobulin secretion [34,60,78]. Lysed cells have been seen in the centers of hemolytic plaques [38,42], but it is unlikely that this is either the only form of secretion or even a normal mode in the usual course of antibody synthesis. The best evidence against this form of secretion comes from the work of Nossal et al. [79-81], who showed that single, living PFCs could be transferred from one red cell layer to another many times and over a prolonged period and continue to make fresh plaques. Indeed, they showed that final death of the cell, as shown by its lysis, did not lead to enhanced plaque formation.

A process similar to apocrine secretion, in which a segment of cytoplasm is pinched off, has also been suggested as a method of secretion by AFC. This process, referred to as clasmatosis or microclasmatosis, has been seen in microcinematographic [48] and in some ultrastructural studies [22,55,82,83] but has been refuted in others [42].

Merocrine secretion, in which the synthesized cell product is secreted via a storage granule, is the typical mode of release from protein-secreting cells, such as pancreatic acinar cells. Apart from "Russell body" plasma cells, which appear to be the end step of plasma cell differentiation, active AFC do not show marked evidence of storage of secretory product in such specialized structures. However, Leduc et al. [34] suggested that, in at least some instances, this form of secretion could occur, possibly via a transient connection between the RER and the cell surface. Other investigators have also noted such connections [21,22,34,84,85], but, although a close association was noted in about 60% of cells examined by Neher and Siegel [42], no active fusion or discontinuity of the adjacent membranes was seen by them.

Various authors have suggested that diffusion or some form of active transport across the surface membrane is responsible for the passage of intracellular antibody to the extracellular environment [42,86]. This possibility is, however, considered highly unlikely on thermodynamic grounds by Singer [87], since it would require a large amount of energy for a hydrophilic molecule to cross a hydrophobic lipid-based membrane.

In view of the demonstrated passage of antibody from the RER to the Golgi, it would seem unlikely that either diffusion into the cytoplasm or a movement back into the RER would precede secretion. Zagury et al. [69] consider that Ig-filled Golgi-derived vesicles migrate to the cell surface, where they fuse with the plasma membrane and discharge their contents by a mechanism similar to the discharge of secretory products from storage granules. This mechanism of "reverse pinocytosis" is attractive, particularly in view of the fact that it is difficult to demonstrate cell membrane-associated antibody in actively secreting AFC, as should be the case were the Ig molecules secreted directly through the plasma membrane. Zagury et al. [69], however, point out that there is little convincing morphologic evidence for this process in plasma cells.

E. Lectin-stimulated B Cells

A variety of plant lectins have been widely used over the past decade to study the activation of small lymphocytes, and the results of such studies were recently reviewed [88]. It has also been determined that not all lymphocytes respond to all lectins and, more importantly, that differential activation of T or B cells can be obtained with appropriate lectins and with different presentation to the T or B cells of the same lectin. Studies on human lymphocytes by Chessin et al. [89], Douglas et al. [90], and Barker et al. [91] suggested that they responded differently to phytohemagglutinin (PHA) and to pokeweek mitogen (PWM), and light and electron microscope analysis showed that whereas PHA-stimulated cells became blastlike, a proportion of PWM-activated cells assumed the morphology of plasma cells [88-89]. This finding has also been confirmed in the mouse, where T and B cells can be identified with more certainty. Soluble PHA and concanavalin A (con A) were shown to activate only T cells, whereas PWM activated both T and B cells [94-96]. In addition, PWM-activated cells have been shown to produce significant quantities of IgM in vitro [97] and to develop large quantities of RER [98].

F. Ultrastructure of Neoplastic B Cells

The various B cell neoplasms, including multiple myeloma and Waldenström's macroglobulinemia in man, and the spontaneous and induced plasma cell tumors of mice have been of enormous importance in immunology, particularly as a source of homogeneous, monoclonal, intact immunoglobulins and free chains. Some of the voluminous literature on mouse myelomas was recently reviewed by Potter [68], who deals in detail with many features not relevant to this chapter. The fine structure of these cells has also been repeatedly studied, and all ultrastructural reports confirm the plasma cell-like nature of the majority of these tumors [99-110]. A great range of morphologic types was, however, noted; cells ranged in morphology from poorly differentiated, blastlike lymphocytic cells (Fig. 7) to well-differentiated plasma cells that had a structure virtually identical with that of normal, nonmalignant plasma cells (Fig. 8). As with normal AFC, even poorly differentiated cells

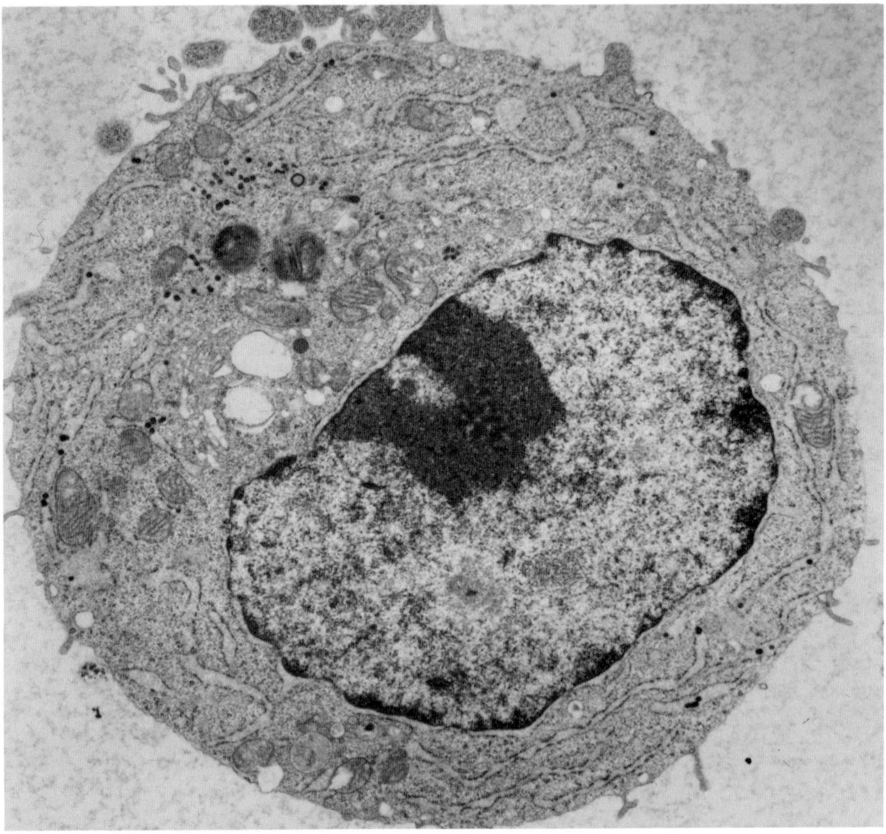

FIG. 7. A relatively poorly differentiated myeloma, MOPC 11. Note the very large size of the cell, the large nucleolus, and copious cytoplasm. The flattened cisternae of the RER contain numerous virus particles. ×8,000

may produce large amounts of immunoglobulin [105-109]. However, with progressive transplantation, morphologic changes may occur in the tumors, leading to blastlike "dedifferentiation" in tumors which were originally well differentiated, and such a change may be accompanied by a total or partial loss of Ig production [103,106,109]. Viruses have been reported consistently in all studies of murine myelomas, though both the number and type of virus may vary greatly [68,99-109]. In particular, intracisternal A-type particles are always seen (Fig. 9a), but intracytoplasmic (extracisternal) A-type (Fig. 9b) and extracellular and surface budding C-type particles are of variable occurrence (Fig. 10). In contrast to mouse tumors, however, virus particles have not been unequivocally identified in human material.

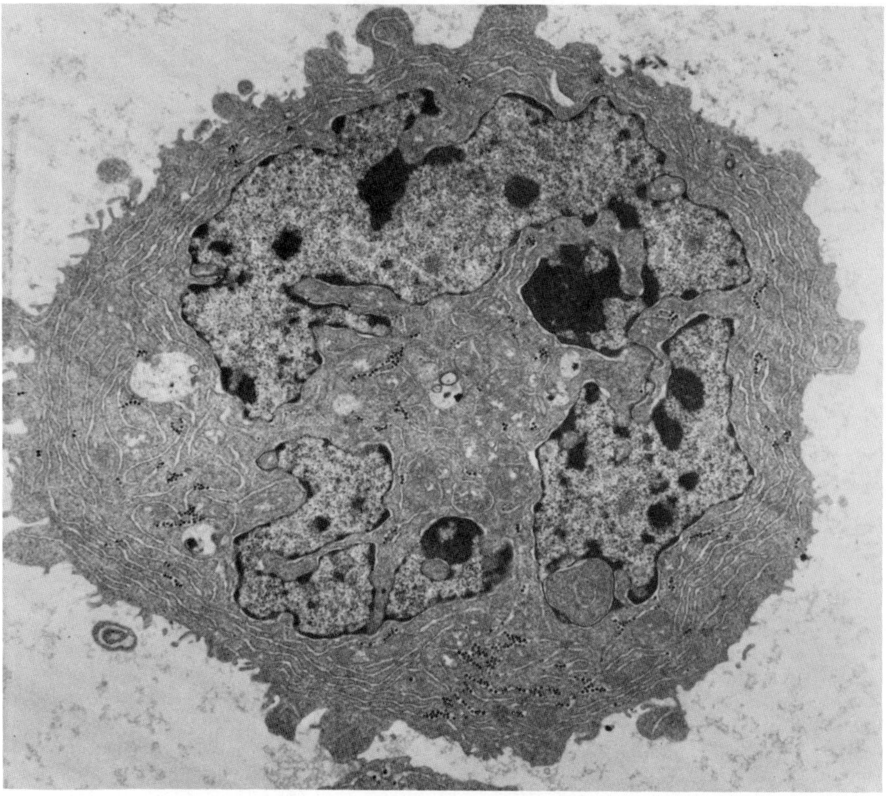

FIG. 8. A well-differentiated IgA-secreting murine myeloma, MOPC 315. The extensive cytoplasm contains large quantities of RER, which is filled with A-type virus particles. ×5,200

IV. The T-cell System

A. Differentiation of T Cells

Unlike B cells, many of which ultimately differentiate into AFC with a morphology that clearly reflects their protein-secreting function, T cells differentiate into cells which express their functions more subtly and show little specialized morphologic evidence of their complex role. There has been far less specific ultrastructural study of differentiated T cells per se, although, of course, most T cells from peripheral lymphoid organs of normal or specifically immunized animals are probably the progeny of previously antigenically stimulated cells. The relative dearth of ultrastructural data is somewhat paradoxical, since the

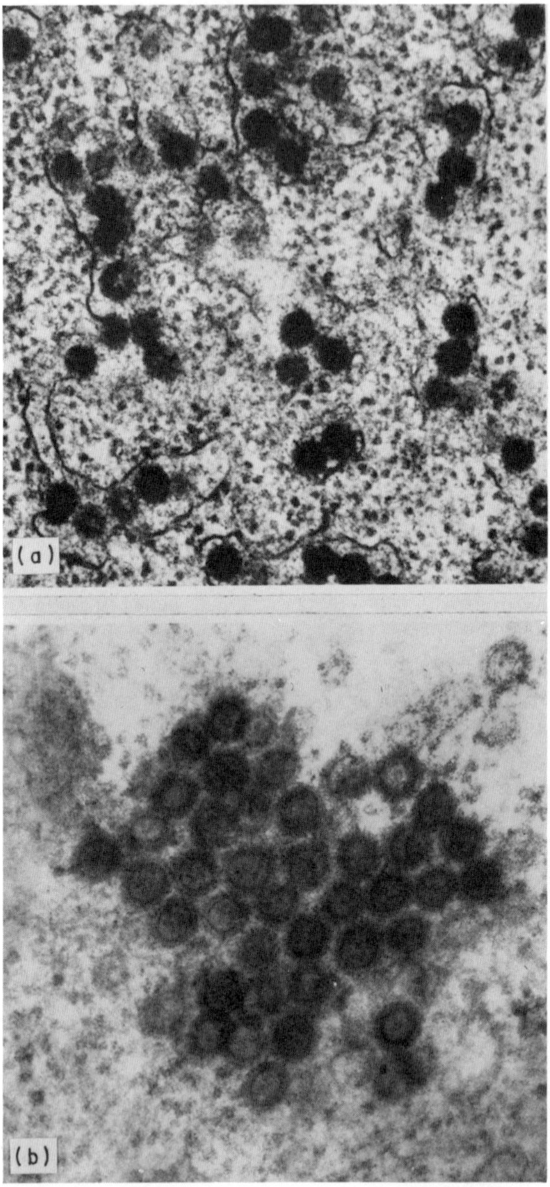

FIG. 9a. Detail of the cytoplasm of an IgG 2a-secreting murine myeloma, PIBU, that shows the RER filled with free and budding intracisternal A-type virus particles. ×65,000.

FIG. 9b. Portion of the cytoplasm of an in vivo passaged murine myeloma, HPC 89F, that shows a group of intracytoplasmic A-type virus particles. This myeloma produces IgG 2b. ×95,000

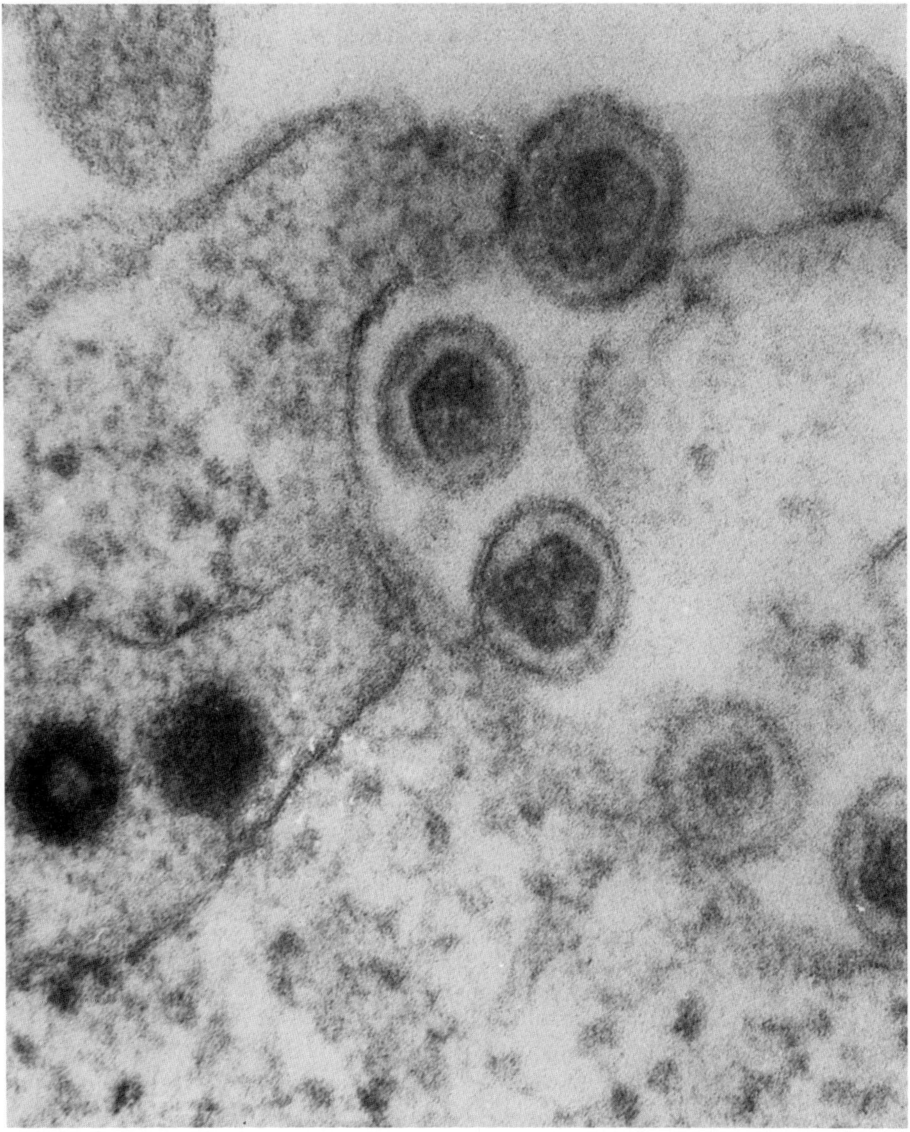

FIG. 10. Portion of an in vitro passaged myeloma cell line, HPC 108 (secreting K light chain), that shows extracellular C-type and intracisternal A-type virus particles. X140,000

initial studies on lectin (PHA) -stimulated cells clearly showed that small lymphocytes were not end cells, and it is now known that the cells that respond to a soluble form of this agent are, in fact, T cells. Furthermore, unlike mammalian B cells, the early stages of T-cell production in the thymus can be studied, since this inductive organ for T-cell development is readily identified and is accessible to experimental manipulation. To date, the B-cell inductive organ has not been clearly identified in mammals, though, of course, in birds the bursa of Fabricius has been extensively studied.

In the mouse, the species most widely studied, the earliest T-cell precursors enter the thymic anlage from the fetal liver on about the 11th day of gestation [110,111]. Over the next 2 to 3 days, these large basophilic blastlike cells gradually accumulate by migration into the thymus and begin to proliferate. Ultrastructurally, these basophilic cells are large and have the typical morphology of lymphoblasts, with copious dense cytoplasm filled with polyribsomes but relatively few other organelles and a large nucleus that contains prominent nucleoli (Fig. 3) [112]. The proliferation of these cells results in the production of typical small thymic cortical lymphocytes [112]. This process of differentiation has also been studied in vitro. Early undifferentiated fetal mouse thymus has been grown in organ culture. The blastlike cells differentiate into typical small lymphocytes [113]. The ultrastructure of the majority of the typical small thymic lymphocytes has been described [6,114], and, as a population, they can be distinguished from peripheral small lymphocytes [6], (Fig. 11). It is clear from a variety of other nonmorphologic studies that the intrathymic small lymphocytes can be subdivided into two populations; a major group accounts for about 90% of the total, being small, dense, and short lived, located predominantly in the cortex, and expressing the TL antigen, high levels of θ antigen but low levels of H-2 and being cortisone sensitive. The minor population, which appears to be the functionally active group, is also composed of small lymphocytes, though they are generally larger and less dense than the major group [115]. This minor population, located mainly in the thymic medulla, is cortisone resistant and differs antigenically in being TL negative and in expressing high levels of H-2 but low levels of θ antigen. It is usually stated that these cells are descendants of the major population, but the full story of their development is by no means clear. Ultrastructural studies have done little to clarify the situation, but, with the availability of precise markers for each subpopulation and with the use of suitable model systems, the problems of this early phase of T-cell differentiation should be resolved.

In addition to these problems, there are also the questions of the inductive stimuli responsible for the high rate of intrathymic mitotic activity and differentiation of the stem cells. These events are independent of antigenic stimulation and are probably under some as yet poorly understood thymic

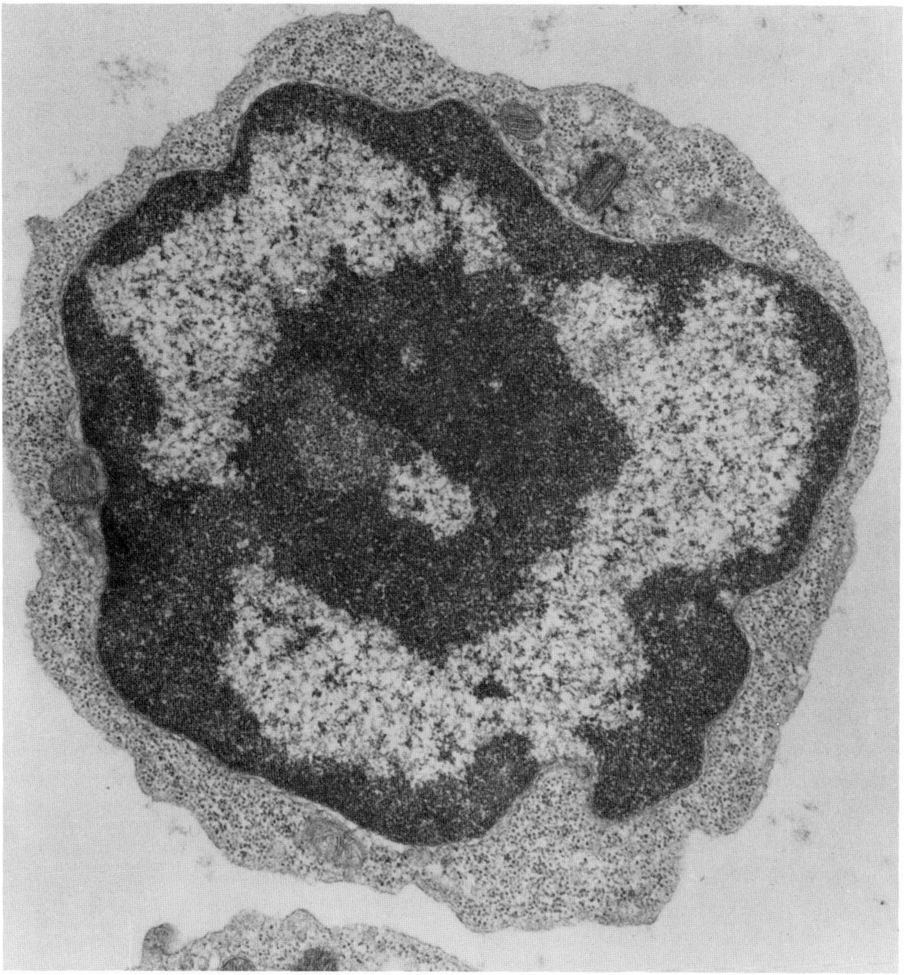

FIG. 11. A typical small lymphocyte from the thymus of a young adult CBA mouse. When compared with Fig. 1, this cell shows less cytoplasm which contains fewer organelles and lacks the conspicuous submembranous zone of microfibrils. The cytoplasm contains numerous monoribosomes but has few other organelles. ×21,250

epithelial cell influence. A close-range relationship between proliferating lymphocytes and epithelial cells in the thymic cortex of the guinea pig has been described [116], and the suggestion was made that the induction of mitotic activity was in some way due to close contact between thymocytes and cortical epithelial cells.

Once they leave the thymus, the thymus-derived T cells can apparently react with antigens and, in vitro, with other substances, such as PHA and con A and other lectins and undergo a second stage of differentiation and proliferation to form the functional population of T cells responsible for various helper and cell-mediated immune phenomena. The elegant studies of Sprent and Miller (Refs. 117-120: see also Sprent, chapter 2) have clearly established the functional, kinetic, and light microscope features of this antigen-dependent, second stage of T-cell differentiation. Electron microscope studies of thoracic duct lymphocytes obtained from semiallogeneic irradiated hosts injected with parental thoracic duct or thymus small lymphocytes showed that the parental cells responded to the foreign histocompatibility antigens of the host by undergoing blast transformation. The cells thus formed were large actively dividing cells with a cytoplasm filled with polyribsomes but with few other organelles. When such cells were reinfused into an irradiated syngeneic host, they could again be recovered from the thoracic duct but now with the morphology of typical small lymphocytes [121]. Matter et al. [10] suggested that "virgin" T cells (called by them "T-1" cells) were monoribosomal small lymphocytes with few cytoplasmic filaments, which, after appropriate antigenic stimulation, transformed into large blastlike "activated" "T-2" cells and developed a copious polyribosome-filled cytoplasm. These cells then differentiated into functionally active "T-3" small lymphocytes, characterized by a dense cytoplasm and a well-developed network of microfibrils and filaments. Such "differentiated" cells were frequently seen with prominent uropods and probably correspond to the cells described by McFarland et al. [122].

B. Ultrastructure of Cytotoxic Lymphocytes

The development of cytotoxic lymphocytes (CL) or killer cells has also been studied in the electron microscope. Abel et al. [123] immunized BALB/c mice with L cells of C3H origin and examined lymphoid cells from the hosts for killer activity on L-cell monolayer cultures. They showed that within 18 hr of exposure to the target L cells, large lymphoid cells that contained numerous ribosomes but little RER developed in the population of sensitized cells and attached to the target cells. The initial attachment was via broad processes (Fig. 12). A single, putative CL could attach to more than one

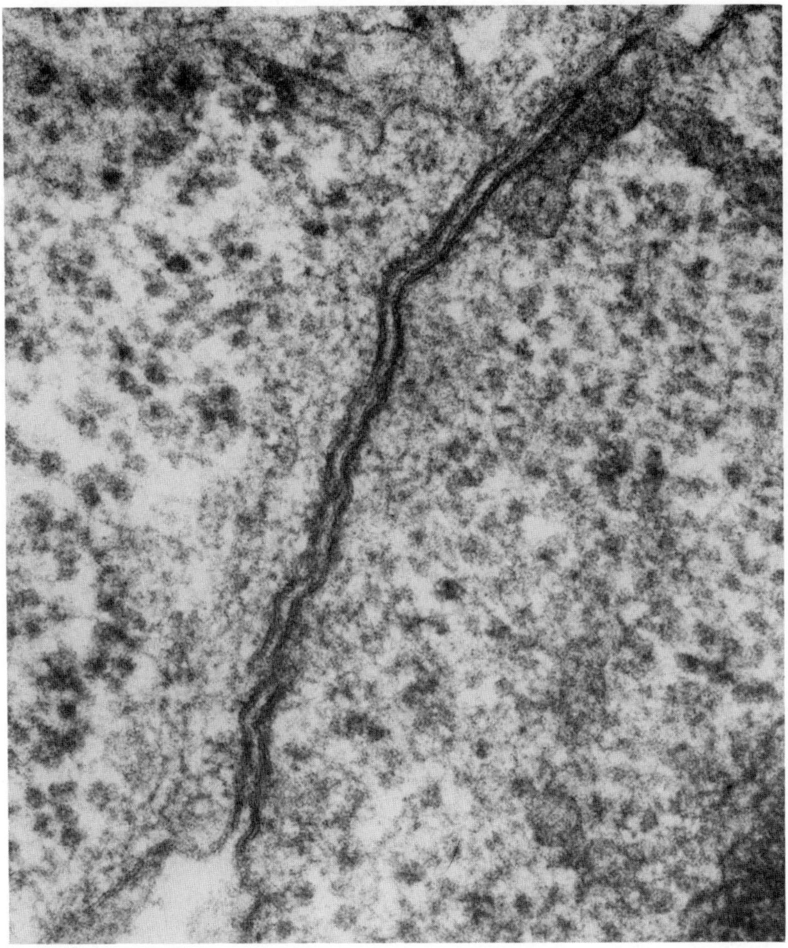

FIG. 12. Detail of the contact zone between a cortisone-resistant T cell (*below*) and an allogeneic (myeloma) target cell (*above*). Note the broad but simple contact between these cells. The surface membranes lie in parallel, separated by an electron lucid gap of 15 to 20 nm. ×104,000

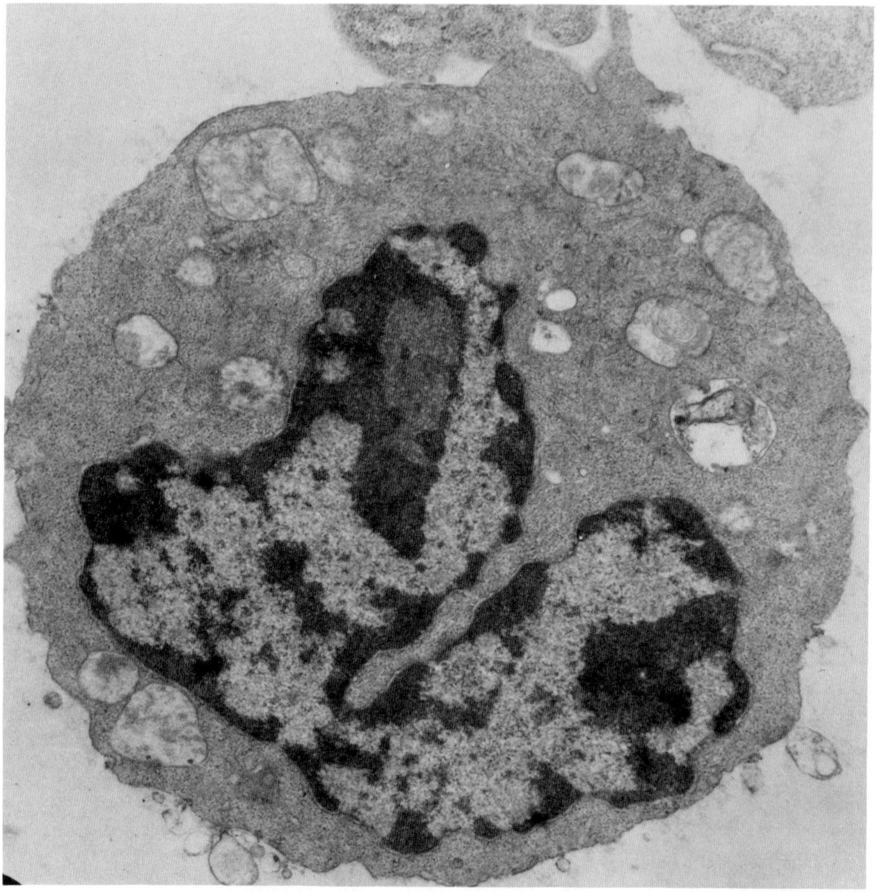

FIG. 13. An "activated" T cell after sensitization in vitro with allogeneic mitomycin C-treated spleen cells. When compared with Fig. 1, this cell is characterized by its larger size and its more active-looking cycoplasm. ×12,800

target cell. The contact rapidly became more complex, and prominent spikelike interdigitations were seen between the lymphoid cells and the L cells. Evidence of cell lysis followed, and Abel et al. [123] claimed that disruption of the lymphocyte surface membrane with cytoplasmic leakage was seen in addition to target cell damage. Sellin et al. [124] suggested that intercellular communication occurred between sensitized lymphoid cells and appropriate target cells by demonstrating the transfer of fluorescein from either cell type to the other. In an ultrastructural study of contact-induced cell lysis, Koren et al. [125] used equidensitometry to analyze electron micrographs of the contact

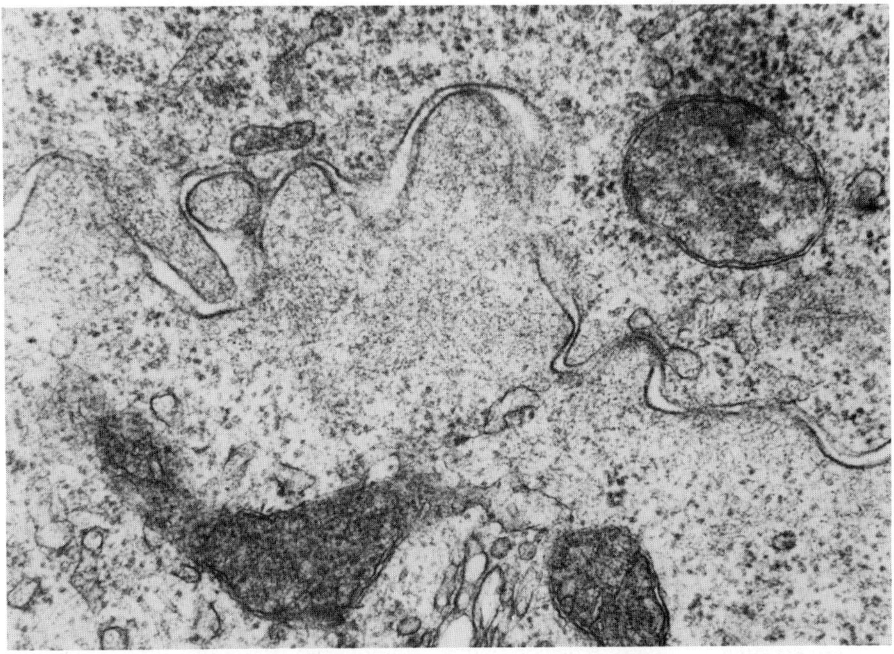

FIG. 14. Detail of the contact between an activated ("killer") T cell (*below*) and an allogeneic target cell (*above*). When compared with Fig. 12, this contract shows far greater complexity and is characterized by large processes which appear to burrow into the target cell. Although there appears to be fusion of the adjoining cell membranes, tilting in a goniometer stage shows that the surface membranes actually preserve their integrity. Note the well-developed microfibrillar network just below the surface of the "killer" cell. ×41,600

zones and also suggested that intercellular communication was present between CL and target cells. They noted the apparent disruption of the *target* cell membrane but noted that the CL surface membrane apparently remained intact. A totally in vitro system was developed by Wagner [126,127] to study both the development of CL and their functional capacity. With this system, defined cell populations can be analyzed, and either total thymus cells or cortisone-resistant thymus cells have been used as a source of CL. With this system, Mandel et al. [128] studied the ultrastructure of developing CL. They showed that over a period of 6 days, a proportion of the relatively small lymphocytes present in the cortisone-resistant thymus population developed into large blastlike cells similar to those described by Abel et al. [123] (Fig. 13). When such cells were added to a ^{51}Cr-labeled population of mouse myeloma cells, the sensitized CL formed complex junctions with the target cells (Fig. 14). The CL sent interdigitating processes into the cytoplasm of the TC, and, in a standard electron microscope examination, there appeared to be membrane disruption between the CL and target cell at such contact regions. However, when such junctions were examined in a goniometer stage capable of being tilted so that the membrane could be oriented parallel to the electron beam, the integrity of both the target cell and the killer cell membranes was evident. It would appear therefore that at least the initial lysis of the target cell occurs via small disruptions of the surface membrane rather than through the production of large and readily visible tear. The contacts necessary for killing are, however, energy dependent, and the morphology of the contact region of the CL suggests that an active rearrangement of the lymphocyte membrane is necessary after initial contact with an appropriate target cell [128]. The submembranous region of the CL at such contact zones is filled with microfibrils, and the killing can be inhibited by cytochalasin B, a drug known to inhibit microfibril function [128-130].

References

1. J. M. Yoffey and F. C. Courtice, *Lymphatics, Lymph and the Lymphomyeloid Complex,* Academic Press, London and New York, 1970.
2. M. W. Elves, *The Lymphocytes,* 2nd edit., Lloyd-Luke Ltd., London, 1972.
3. P. H. Sebuwufu, Nature (London) **212**, 1382 (1966).
4. G. F. Smith and P. T. O'Hara, Nature (London) **215**, 773 (1967).
5. J. Toro and I. Olah, Nature (London) **212**, 315 (1966).
6. M. J. Heiniger, H. Riedwye, H. Giger, B. Sordat, and M. Cottier, Blood **30**, 288 (1967).
7. E. R. Suter, H. Probst, and P. Dukor, Eur. J. Immunol. **2**, 189 (1972).
8. J. D. Feldman and R. E. Nordquist, Lab. Invest. **16**, 564 (1967).
9. J. P. Lamelin, B. Lisowska-Berstein, A. Matter, J. E. Ryser, and P. Vassalli, J. Exp. Med. **136**, 984 (1972).
10. A. Matter, B. Lisowska-Bernstein, J. E. Ryser, J. P. Lamelin, and P. Vassalli, J. Exp. Med. **136**, 1008 (1972).
11. N. U. Shigeno, U. Hammerling, C. Arpels, E. A. Boyse, and J. L. Old, Lancet 2, 320 (1968).
12. M. C. Raff, S. Nase, and N. A. Mitchison, Nature (London) **230**, 50 (1971).
13. A. Polliak, N. Lampen, B. D. Clarkson, E. de Harven, Z. Bentwich, F. P. Siegel, and H. G. Kunkel, J. Exp. Med. **138**, 607 (1973).
14. P. S. Lin, H. G Cooper, and H. H. Wortis, N. Engl. J. Med. **289**, 548 (1973).
15. D. Zucker-Franklin, J. Ultrastruct. Res. **9**, 325 (1963).
16. S. de Petris, G. Karlsbad, and B. A. Pernis, J. Ultrastruct. Res. **7**, 39 (1962).

17. U. Hammerling, T. Aoki, E. de Harven, E. A. Boyse, and L. J. Old, J. Exp. Med. **128**, 1461 (1968).
18. U. Hammerling, T. Aoki, H. A. Wood, L. J. Old, E. A. Boyse, and E. de Harven, Nature (London) **223**, 1158 (1969).
19. T. Aoki, U. Hammerling, E. de Harven, E. A. Boyse, and L. J. Old, J. Exp. Med. **130**, 979 (1969).
20. T. Aoki, M. A. Wood, L. J. Old, E. A. Boyse, E. de Harven, M. P. Lardis, and C. W. Stackpole, Virology **45**, 858 (1971).
21. H. Z. Movat and N. V. P. Fedorko, Exp. Mol. Pathol. **1**, 535 (1962).
22. A. Weinstock, Anat. Rec. **162**, 289 (1968).
23. A. Fagraeus, Acta Med. Scand. Suppl. **204**, 1 (1948).
24. E. H. Leduc, A. H. Coons, and J. M. Connolly, J. Exp. Med. **102**, 61 (1955).
25. L. G. Ortegan and R. E. Mellors, J. Exp. Med. **106**, 627 (1957).
26. J. J. Vazquez, Lab. Invest. **10**, 1110 (1961).
27. P. Urso and T. Mankinoden, J. Immunol. **90**, 897 (1963).
28. G. J. V. Nossal, Brit. J. Exp. Pathol. **39**, 544 (1958).
29. G. J. V. Nossal and O. Makela, Annu. Rev. Microbiol. **16**, 53 (1962).
30. H. Braunsteiner, K. Fellinger, and F. Pakesch, Blood **8**, 916.
31. M. C. Bessis, Lab. Invest. **10**, 1040 (1961).
32. S. DePetris, G. Karlsbad, and B. Pernis, J. Exp. Med. **117**, 849 (1963).
33. S. DePetris and G. Karlsbad, J. Cell Biol. **26**, 759 (1965).
34. E. H. Leduc, S. Avrameas, and M. Boutielle, J. Exp. Med. **127**, 109 (1968).
35. C. Bosman, J. D. Feldman, and E. Pick, J. Exp. Med. **129**, 1029 (1969).
36. A. E. Bussard and J. L. Binet, Nature (London) **205**, 675 (1965).
37. F. W. Fitch, D. A. Rowley, and S. Coulthard, Nature (London) **207**, 994 (1965).
38. T. N. Harris, K. Hummeler, and S. Harris, J. Exp. Med. **123**, 161 (1966).
39. A. J. Cunningham, J. B. Smith, and E. H. Mercer, J. Exp. Med. **124**, 701 (1966).
40. K. Hummeler, S. Harris, and T. N. Harris, Fed. Proc. **25**, 1734 (1966).
41. K. Hummeler, T. N. Harris, N. Tomassini, M. Hechtel, and M. B. Farber, J. Exp. Med. **124**, 255 (1966).
42. G. H. Neher and B. V. Siegel, Int. Arch. Allergy Appl. Immunol. **39**, 133 (1970).
43. F. G. Gudat, T. N. Harris, S. Harris, and K. Hummeler, J. Exp. Med. **130**, 448 (1970).
44. F. Reyes and J. F. Bach, Cell. Immunol. **2**, 182 (1971).
45. U. Storb, W. Bauer, R. Storb, T. M. Fliedner, and R. S. Weiser, J. Immunol. **102**, 1474 (1969).
46. O. Makela and G. J. V. Nossal, J. Immunol. **87**, 447 (1961).
47. W. Bernhard and N. Granboulan, in *Cellular Aspects of Immunity, Ciba Foundation Symposium* (G. E. W. Wolstenholme and M. O'Connor, eds.), J. & A. Churchill, Ltd., London, 1960, p. 92.
48. J. P. Thiery, in *Cellular Aspects of Immunity* (G. E. W. Wolstenholme and M. O'Connor, eds.), J. & A. Churchill, Ltd., London, 1960, p. 50.

49. G. Attardi, M. Cohn, K. Horibata, and E. J. Lennox, Bacteriol. Rev. **23**, 213 (1959).
50. A. H. E. Marshall and R. G. White, Brit. J. Exp. Pathol. **31**, 157 (1950).
51. J. L. Gowans, D. D. McGregor, and D. M. Cowen, Nature (London) **196**, 651 (1962).
52. A. Fagraeus, in *Ciba Foundation Symposium Cellular Aspects of Immunity*, J. & A. Churchill, Ltd., London, 1960, p. 3.
53. H. J. Wellensiek and A. H. Coons, J. Exp. Med. **119**, 685 (1964).
54. S. Avrameas and M. Boutielle, Exp. Cell Res. **53**, 116 (1968).
55. S. Avrameas and E. H. Leduc, J. Exp. Med. **131**, 1137 (1970).
56. S. Avrameas, H. R. P. Miller, and E. Leduc, Immunology **20**, 85 (1971).
57. W. D. Kuhlmann and S. Avrameas, Cell. Immunol. **4**, 425 (1972).
58. H. R. P. Miller, S. Avrameas, and T. Ternynck, Amer. J. Pathol. **71**, 239 (1973).
59. H. P. R. Miller, S. Avrameas, and T. Ternynck, Amer. J. Pathol. **71**, 261 (1973).
60. C. Bosman and J. D. Feldman, Cell. Immunol. **1**, 31 (1970).
61. J. G. Hall, B. Morris, G. D. Moreno, and M. C. Bessis, J. Exp. Med. **125**, 91 (1967).
62. M. S. C. Birbeck and J. G. Hall, Nature (London) **214**, 183 (1967).
63. A. H. Coons, E. M. Ledre, and J. M. Connolly, J. Exp. Med. **102**, 49 (1955).
64. R. A. Rifkind, E. F. Osserman, K. C. Hsu, and C. Morgan, J. Exp. Med. **116**, 423 (1962).
65. R. C. Grahma, Jr. and M. J. Karnovsky, J. Histochem. Cytochem. **14**, 291 (1966).
66. I. Suzuki, M. Takahaski, M. Kamai, and T. Yamamoto, J. Immunol. **104**, 907 (1970).
67. T. A. Waldmann and W. Strober, Progr. Allergy **13**, 1 (1969).
68. M. Potter, Physiol. Rev. **52**, 631 (1972).
69. D. Zagury, J. W. Uhr, J. D. Jamieson, and G. E. Palade, J. Cell. Biol. **46**, 52 (1970).
70. J. D. Jamieson and G. E. Palade, J. Cell Biol. **34**, 577 (1967).
71. J. D. Jamieson and G. E. Palade, J. Cell Biol. **34**, 597 (1967).
72. J. D. Jamieson and G. E. Palade, J. Cell Biol. **39**, 580 (1968).
73. J. D. Jamieson and G. E. Palade, J. Cell Biol. **39**, 587 (1968).
74. J. D. Castle, J. D. Jamieson, and G. E. Palade, J. Cell Biol. **53**, 290 (1972).
75. I. Schenkein and J. W. Uhr, J. Cell Biol. **46**, 42 (1970).
76. A. L. Shapiro, M. D. Scharff, J. V. Maizel, and J. W. Uhr, Proc. Nat. Acad. Sci. USA **56**, 216 (1966).
77. S. L. Palay, in *Frontiers in Cytology* (S. L. Palay, ed.), Yale University Press, New Haven, 1958, p. 305.
78. L. G. Ortega and R. E. Mellors, J. Exp. Med. **106**, 627 (1957).
79. G. J. V. Nossal, A. E. Bussard, H. Lewis, and J. C. Mazie, in *Developmental Aspects of Antibody Formation and Structure* (J. Sterzl and I. Riha, eds.), Czechoslovak Acedemy of Science, Prague, 1970, p. 655.

80. G. J. V. Nossal, A. E. Bussard, H. Lewis, and J. C. Mazie, J. Exp. Med. **131**, 894 (1970).
81. G. J. V. Nossal, N. L. Warner, and H. Lewis, Cell. Immunol. **2**, 41 (1971).
82. S. S. Han, I. H. Han, and A. G. Johnston, Proc. Soc. Exp. Biol. Med. **121**, 782 (1966).
83. R. D. Moore, V. R. Numae, and M. D. Schoenberg, Exp. Mol. Pathol. **4**, 370 (1965).
84. G. H. Neher and B. V. Siegel, Vox Sang. **14**, 63 (1968).
85. G. D. Sorenson, Lab. Invest. **13**, 196 (1964).
86. E. Helmreich, M. Kern, and H. N. Eisen, J. Biol. Chem. **263**, 464 (1961).
87. S. J. Singer, Advan. Immunol. (1974), in press.
88. G. Moller, ed., Transplant Rev., "Lymphocyte Activation by Mitogens" **11** (1972).
89. L. N. Chessin, J. Borjeson, P. Welsh, S. D. Douglas, and H. L. Cooper, J. Exp. Med. **124**, 873 (1966).
90. S. D. Douglas, P. F. Hoffman, J. Borjeson, and L. N. Chessin, J. Immunol. **98**, 17 (1967).
91. B. E. Barker, M. E. Lutzner, and P. Farves, in *Proceedings of the Third Leucocyte Culture Conference,* (W. O. Rieke, ed.), Appleton-Century-Crofts, New York, 1969, p. 587.
92. S. D. Douglas, J. Borjeson, and L. N. Chessin, J. Immunol. **99**, 340 (1967).
93. S. D. Douglas and H. H. Fudenberg, Exp. Cell. Res. **54**, 277 (1969).
94. G. Janossy and M. F. Greaves, Clin. Exp. Immunol. **9**, 483 (1971).
95. G. Janossy and M. F. Greaves, Clin. Exp. Immunol. **10**, 525 (1972).
96. M. F. Greaves, S. Bauminger, and G. Janossy, Clin. Exp. Immunol. **10**, 537 (1972).
97. R. M. E. Parkhouse, G. Janossy, and M. F. Greaves, Nature [New Biol.] **235**, 21 (1972).
98. M. F. Greaves and G. Janossy, Transplant Rev. **11**, 87 (1972).
99. A. E. Howatson and E. A. McCulloch, Nature (London) **181**, 1213 (1958).
100. D. F. Parsons, E. B. Darden, Jr., D. L. Lindsley, G. T. Pratt, and M. P. Edwards, J. Biophys. Biochem. Cytol. **9**, 353 (1960).
101. A. J. Dalton, M. Potter, and R. M. Merwin, J. Nat. Cancer Inst. **26**, 1221 (1961).
102. E. L. Kuff, N. A. Wivel, and K. K. Lueders, Cancer Res. **28**, 2137 (1968).
103. A. J. Dalton, M. Potter, and R. M. Merwin, J. Nat. Cancer Inst. **40**, 1375 (1968).
104. P. Ebbesen, T. Schiodt, and H. E. Christensen, Cancer Res. **29**, 1851 (1969).
105. K. Sarkar and G. Tolnai, Cancer Res. **29**, 1904 (1969).
106. P. Ebbesen and M. H. Nielsen, Acta Microbiol. Scand. **B78**, 390 (1970).
107. J. P. Watson, R. S. Sarkar, and M. Cohn, Proc. Nat. Acad. Sci. USA **66**, 344 (1970).
108. E. L. Kuff, K. K. Lueders, H. L. Ozer, and N. A. Wivel, Proc. Nat. Acad. Sci. USA **69**, 218 (1972).

109. T. Mandel, A. Abbot, N. L. Warner, and A. W. Harris, unpublished results.
110. M. A. S. Moore and J. J. T. Owen, J. Exp. Med. **126**, 715 (1967).
111. J. J. T. Owen and M. A. Ritter, J. Exp. Med. **129**, 431 (1969).
112. T. Mandel, Z. Zellforsch, **106**, 498 (1970).
113. T. Mandel and P. J. Russell, Immunology **21**, 659 (1971).
114. R. G. Murray, A. Murray, and A. Pizzo, Anat. Rec. **151**, 17 (1965).
115. S. Konda, E. Stockert, and R. T. Smith, Cell. Immunol. **7**, 275 (1973).
116. T. Mandel, Aust. J. Exp. Biol. Med. Sci. **47**, 153 (1969).
117. J. Sprent and J. F. A. P. Miller, Cell. Immunol. **2**, 171 (1971).
118. J. Sprent and J. F. A. P. Miller, Cell. Immunol. **2**, 469 (1971).
119. J. Sprent and J. F. A. P. Miller, Cell. Immunol. **3**, 361 (1972).
120. J. Sprent and J. F. A. P. Miller, Cell. Immunol. **3**, 385 (1972).
121. T. Mandel, J. Sprent, and J. F. A. P. Miller, unpublished data.
122. W. McFarland, D. H. Heilman, and J. F. Moorhead, J. Exp. Med. **124**, 851 (1966).
123. M. E. Abel, J. C. Lee, and W. Rosenau, Amer. J. Pathol. **60**, 421 (1970).
124. D. Sellin, D. F. H. Wallach, and H. Fischer, Eur. J. Immunol. **1**, 453 (1971).
125. H. S. Koren, W. Ax, and E. Freund-Noelbert, Eur. J. Immunol. **3**, 32 (1973).
126. H. Wagner, Eur. J. Immunol. **1**, 498 (1971).
127. H. Wagner and M. Feldmann, Cell. Immunol. **3**, 405 (1972).
128. T. Mandel, A. Abbot, H. Wagner, and M. Rollinghoff, in preparation.
129. J. L. Cerottini and K. T. Brunner, Nature [New Biol.] **237**, 272 (1972).
130. N. K. Wessels, B. S. Spooner, J. F. Ash, N. V. Bradley, M. A. Ludeuna, E. L. Taylor, J. T. Wrenn, and K. M. Yaunda, Science **171**, 135 (1971).

CHAPTER 2

Recirculating Lymphocytes

J. Sprent*

The Basel Institute for Immunology
Basel, Switzerland

Gowans and his colleagues defined recirculating lymphocytes as long-lived cells which migrate continuously between the bloodstream and the central lymphatics via the lymph nodes [1]. The pool of recirculating lymphocytes was originally envisaged as a population of small lymphocytes homogeneous with respect to both morphology and function. It is now known, however, that there are two distinct classes of lymphocytes, *namely,* thymus-derived (T) lymphocytes and bursa- or bone marrow-derived (B) lymphocytes [2-5]. T lymphocytes are believed to control cell-mediated immune responses, such as allograft rejection, graft-versus-host reactions, and delayed-type hypersensitivity; they also collaborate with B lymphocytes in antibody responses to certain (T-dependent) antigens. B lymphocytes appear to function simply as the

*Present address: Department of Pathology, School of Medicine, University of Pennsylvania, Philadelphia, Pennsylvania.

precursors of antibody-forming cells. In view of this information, it becomes necessary to consider the origin, life-span, and migration of lymphocytes in terms of these two cell types.

A prerequisite for any study of T and B lymphocytes is the availability of markers for distinguishing these cells. At present, such markers are most clearly defined in the mouse, and this chapter is based largely on work performed on this species. In the mouse, T lymphocytes are characterized by their surface membrane content of the θ antigen; B lymphocytes, by contrast, are θ negative and, unlike T lymphocytes, express a high density of surface immunoglobulin and will bind immune complexes via receptors for the Fc portion of antibody. T and B lymphocytes also differ by a number of other criteria, one of the most interesting of which is the expression of the Ly antigens. For example, Ly-1, 2, and 3 antigens are found only on T cells whereas Ly-4 is restricted to B cells [5a,5b].

I. The Cells of the Recirculating Lymphocyte Pool

Information on the properties of recirculating lymphocytes has come largely from studies that employed thoracic duct lymphocytes (TDL). This cell population consists almost entirely of typical small lymphocytes; the few remaining cells (2-5%) are large lymphocytes [1]. Evidence now to be considered indicates that TDL comprise a mixed population of long-lived recirculating T and B lymphocytes.

A. T Lymphocytes

1. Origin

Although the origin of lymphocytes has long been controversial, it is now considered that a large proportion arise in the thymus. The thymus in all vertebrates, like the bursa of Fabricius in birds, is termed a primary lymphoid organ [6,7]. These organs differ from secondary lymphoid organs, e.g., the spleen and lymph nodes (LN), in three main respects. First, primary lymphoid organs are comprised of cells derived not only from mesoderm (lymphocytes) but also from endoderm (the epithelial cell component). Second, lymphopoiesis in these organs is intense, independent of antigenic stimulation, and prominent before the time of birth. Third, primary lymphoid organs rarely show the cytologic hallmarks of an immune response (although in hyperimmune states they may contain appreciable numbers of antibody-forming cells [8]). An organ with these characteristics is clearly suited for being a center for lymphocyte formation and dissemination.

Evidence that lymphocytes migrate from the thymus to the secondary lymphoid organs has come from four approaches:

1. It is well accepted that mitotic activity in the thymus is far higher than in other lymphoid organs [9,10]. The rate of cell death within the thymus, however, is controversial: some workers have maintained that most cells die in situ [11,12]; others, by contrast, reported that pyknotic (dead) cells were comparatively rare and concluded therefore that many cells must leave the thymus [9,13,14]. This controversy appears to stem in part from the widely divergent views on the duration of pyknosis [15].

2. Direct evidence that some lymphocytes migrate from the thymus to the peripheral lymphoid organs arose from studies that involved intrathymic injection of radioactive cell markers. Studies with the guinea pig [16], hamster [17], calf [18], mouse [19], and rat [20] all showed that intrathymic injection of tritiated thymidine ([^{3}H]TdR) was followed soon afterward by the appearance of labeled cells in the spleen, lymph nodes, and intestines. Migration of labeled cells to these regions was found to be particularly prominent in neonatal animals. Whether more cells are released from the thymus of the neonate than of the adult, however, has yet to be proved.

Lymphocytes in the thymic parenchyma are considered to enter the thymic vessels by first passing into thin-walled lymphocyte-packed channels in the interlobular septae. In the guinea pig, these channels are claimed to be directly connected with lymphatic vessels [21,22]; in rats, by contrast, they are held to be blind structures, the lymphocytes within them entering the circulation by penetrating the walls of capillary blood vessels [23,24].

3. Studies on the cell content of the thymic vessels corroborate the above histologic evidence that lymphocytes leave the thymus via veins and lymphatics.

Exit of cells into veins is supported by reports that absolute and differential lymphocyte counts in blood from thymic veins of the rat [15,25] and the guinea pig [26] are higher than in the thymic artery or in venous blood from other regions.

Experiments of Williams et al. [27] suggest that lymphocytes leave the thymus of the calf via both veins and lymphatics. These authors raised an alloantiserum against bovine thymus cells and found that, after appropriate absorption, it stained 3 to 8% of lymphocytes from thymic vein blood, thymic lymph and thymic LN. These cells were considered to have arisen from the thymus, since the antiserum, although staining most thymus cells, stained less than 1% of lymphocytes from arterial blood or thoracic duct lymph. Exit of thymic lymphocytes via lymphatics was also claimed by Kotani et al. [21] who observed that removal of the right lobe of the guinea pig thymus was followed by a 50% reduction in the number of lymphocytes that emerged per hour from the right lymphatic duct.

4. There are many reports that lymphocytes migrate from chromosomally

marked syngeneic thymus grafts placed under the kidney capsule of thymus-deprived mice, i.e., neonatally thymectomized (NTx) mice or adult thymectomized, irradiated, and marrow-protected (TxBM) mice (reviewed in Refs. 7, 28, and 29). Within the first 2 weeks of grafting, most of the cells in mitosis in the grafts were found to be of donor origin. Subsequently, however, the dividing cells were predominantly derived from the host. From about the 15th day, cells with the graft marker appeared in peripheral blood and reached 90% after 30 to 50 days. This proportion gradually fell at later stages in association with a reciprocal increase in cells of donor origin.

These studies were interpreted as indicating that precursor cells from bone marrow continually enter the thymus, are "processed" there, and then migrate into the circulation as T cells [29]. This concept, also proposed by other workers [7], is consistent with evidence that lymphopoiesis in the thymus depends upon a supply of blood-borne stem cells that originate from the bone marrow or, in the embryo, from the yolk sac [30,31]. It has been suggested that the thymic epithelium exerts an inductive influence on the differentiation of these cells to T lymphocytes [32]. Such differentiation might be controlled by locally acting humoral factors produced by the epithelial cells [33]. Evidence that bone marrow cells, incubated in vitro with thymus extracts, assume some of the surface membrane characteristics of T cells [34] is consistent with this view. It should be stressed, however, that despite concerted efforts [34a] it has yet to be proved that cells treated with thymic extracts manifest the *functional* properties of mature T lymphocytes. The precise mechanism of action of thymic "hormones" is thus far from clear. On this point it may be mentioned that Stutman [34b] has postulated that certain cells are functionally immature on leaving the thymus but subsequently attain immunocompetence in the periphery under thymic hormonal control.

There is compelling evidence that a large proportion of recirculating lymphocytes are thymus dependent. Miller et al. [35] observed that the output of TDL from NTx mice was greatly reduced in comparison with sham-operated mice. More recently, TDL outputs were also found to be reduced in TxBM mice and in congenitally athymic nude (*nu/nu*) mice [36]. The lowered lymphocyte outputs observed in these mice were shown to be due to a specific reduction in numbers of lymphocytes expressing the θ antigen; in normal mice, this antigen is present on nearly all thymus cells and on a proportion of peripheral lymphocytes [3]. Decreased levels of recirculating lymphocytes after perinatal thymectomy have also been observed in other species, including rats [37,38] (also TxBM rats [39]), guinea pigs [40], and sheep [41].

Although the above evidence indicates that a proportion of recirculating lymphocytes are thymus dependent, it does not prove that they are thymus derived. Direct evidence on this point arose from studies based on the observation that the reduction in the size of the recirculating lymphocyte pool (RLP) of NTx mice could be prevented by injecting these (parental strain) mice soon after birth with large numbers of F_1 hybrid thymus cells [42]; most of the TDL collected from these "thymus-reconstituted" mice were shown to carry not only the θ antigen but also the alloantigens that characterized the donor thymus cells. This experiment gave direct support to the contention, based largely on circumstantial evidence, that the θ antigen is a specific marker for T cells [3]. According to this criterion, approximately 85% of TDL, 80% of LN cells, and 35% of spleen cells are T lymphocytes.[1] As will be considered below and in Sec. II, it is probable that most, though not all, of these cells form part of the RLP.

Until recently it was generally assumed that despite their manifold functions, T cells are a homogeneous population differing only in their antigenic specificity. The development of the Ly surface markers by Cantor and Boyse [5a] now suggests, however, that T cells comprise a number of different subpopulations. Approximately 30% of T (θ-positive) cells in spleen and LN express Ly-1 but not Ly-2 or Ly-3 antigens (Ly-1^+ cells) [5a]. Another 50% display all three antigens (Ly-123^+ cells), while a minority (5-10%) express Ly-2 and Ly-3 but not Ly-1 (Ly-23^+ cells). The function of these cells is currently under intensive investigation. At present it is considered that Ly-1^+ cells control delayed-type hypersensitivity reactions [42a], act as helper cells for collaborative antibody responses [5a,42c] and respond in mixed-lymphocyte culture [5a]. The Ly-23^+ subpopulation, by contrast, is able to manifest cell-mediated lympholysis [5a] and contains specific "suppressor" cells which inhibit antibody production [42c,42d]. The function of Ly-123^+ cells has yet to be elucidated.

The distribution of Ly antigens on T cells from thoracic duct lymph closely resembles that on splenic and LN T cells [42e]. Thus the subdivision of T cells considered above would appear to apply to recirculating T cells.

2. *Migration*

a. Recirculation from Blood to Lymph. Studies in a variety of species, including the rat [43-45], mouse [36], guinea pig [46], sheep [47], dog [47], calf [47,48], and man [49], have shown that lymphocyte outputs from chronic thoracic duct fistulas decline rapidly during the first 1 to 2 weeks of drainage before reaching a low plateau. Gowans [44,50] made the important discovery that the decline in TDL outputs from rats could be prevented by reinfusing the collected cells intravenously. He also observed that when the cells were radioactively labeled in vitro with [^{3}H]adenosine before injection, labeled cells appeared rapidly in the lymph; other workers reported similar findings with TDL labeled in vivo with [^{3}H]TdR [51,52]. These experiments provided the first unequivocal evidence that lymphocytes recirculate continuously between blood and lymph. Lymphocyte recirculation has since been demonstrated in other species, including the mouse [36], sheep [53], and man [54]; it appears to be very limited in the pig [55].

It was mentioned above that, in mice, approximately 85% of TDL collected within the first day of cannulation are θ positive, i.e., are T cells [36, 56]. In recent studies, this proportion was found to decrease with more prolonged drainage and after 4 days reached a plateau of 40 to 50% [36]. When the output of θ positive cells was considered in absolute terms, it was clear that T cells were mobilized very rapidly through the fistulas, most of the cells being removed within 5 days; in fact, of the total numbers of θ positive cells collected over this period, more than 60% were recovered during the first 24 hr. This finding was consistent with observations on the time taken for radioisotopically labeled TDL to enter thoracic duct lymph of rats [39,57,58] or mice [36] after intravenous injection. With TDL collected soon after establishing the fistulas, i.e., lymphocytes which in the mouse, and also in the rat, consist predominantly of T cells, most of the transferred cells were recovered from the lymph within 1 to 2 days of injection; maximum cell numbers were found at 18 to 24 hr.

b. Sites of Recirculation. Conditions which induce a decrease in the size of the RLP are associated with a striking depletion of lymphocytes from discrete regions of the lymphoid tissues, namely, the periarteriolar lymphocyte sheath (PALS) of the spleen, the LN paracortex, and the interfollicular areas of Peyer's patches. Conditions that cause such depletion include chronic thoracic duct drainage (CTDD) [1,36], neonatal thymectomy [59], congenital thymic aplasia [60], treatment with antilymphocyte serum (ALS) [61], extracorporeal irradiation of the blood [62], and attachment of ^{32}P-impregnated strips to the spleen [63]. Cell labeling studies have indicated that migration to the above areas is a property of T cells, but not of B cells [36,59]; these areas have therefore been termed "thymus dependent" [59].

Entry to the T-dependent areas of the LN occurs through the walls of postcapillary venules, specialized small vessels lined by cuboidal or columnar endothelium [1,36,38,57]. Opinions vary as to whether lymphocytes leave these vessels by passing through the cytoplasm of the endothelial cells [64] or by migrating between them [65]. Once cells enter the paracortical areas of the LN, they migrate to the medullary sinus and thus gain access to the efferent lymphatic vessel. The precise route of migration from the paracortex to the medullary sinus has not yet been established.

Whereas the capacity to migrate to normal (unstimulated) LN is restricted to lymphocytes, localization of cells in the spleen appears to be largely nonspecific; this presumably reflects the lack of direct arteriovenous anastomoses in this organ [66]. Lymphocytes, along with other blood-borne cells, gain rapid entry to the marginal zone and to the red pulp venous sinusoids which represent the termination of the splenic artery. Lymphocytes, but not other cells, migrate soon afterward to the peripheral white pulp; the T cells present then move to the PALS [1,36,38,57,67]. The route by which T cells leave the spleen from the PALS is not clearly understood. The lymphatic supply to the spleen, at least in most species, is very limited [66], and most cells probably leave via the splenic vein. This was shown clearly by Ford [68,69] in his experiments on isolated perfused spleens from rats. Mitchell [70] described "bridging channels (pseudolymphatics)" between the PALS and the red pulp venous sinuses of the rat and the mouse. She proposed that lymphocytes reach the veins from the PALS via these channels.

Studies with the γ-emitting isotope ^{51}Cr have provided useful information on the homing properties of circulating T cells. When ^{51}Cr-labeled TDL or LN cells from normal mice [36,71] or rats [72] were injected intravenously, measurement of radioactivity levels in the recipients indicated that a high proportion (25-40%) of the injected cells lodged in the spleen soon after injection, e.g., by 1 hr in some studies; thereafter, cell numbers (radioactive counts) rapidly decreased until a plateau was reached after 24 hr. Homing to LN, by contrast, did not reach maximum levels until 24 hr after injection. However, of the cells which eventually reached the LN, more than 50% localized in the nodes within 1 to 4 hr of injection.[2] Whereas T cells take an average of 18 hr or more to recirculate from blood to lymph through the LN, their mean transit time through the spleen is only about 6 hr [68]. It would seem likely therefore that the slow increase in LN counts observed between 4 and 24 hr is caused by the gradual increase in the LN of cells which initially home to and then migrate through the spleen.

LN homing therefore probably consists of two components: "primary" migration, rapid accumulation of cells which enter LN directly from the circulation soon after injection; and "secondary" migration, gradual accumulation of cells which reach LN only after temporary sequestration in other organs, particularly the spleen. It may be added that, since primary migration of T cells to LN is complete within a few hours of injection, their slow tempo of recirculation from blood to lymph (compared to rapid migration through the spleen) is probably a reflection of the time taken for the cells to traverse rather than to enter the LN. Arguing on different grounds, Ford and Simmonds [58] reached a similar conclusion.

Whether the Ly phenotype of T cells affects their migratory properties has yet to be investigated. Studies on the homing patterns of T cells pretreated with the appropriate anti-Ly antisera might answer this question.

3. Lifespan

Until recently, small lymphocytes were considered to have an average life-span of only a few days [74]. The first clear evidence that some lymphocytes are long-lived cells came from the studies of Otteson in man [75]. He observed that, in patients injected with ^{32}P, most of the peripheral blood cells which became labeled retained their radioactivity for 100 days or more. Otteson's findings were subsequently confirmed by other workers who observed radiation-induced "lethal" chromosomal abnormalities in peripheral blood lymphocytes (PBL) of patients given therapeutic irradiation as long as 10 years previously [76,77].

Everett and his colleagues [78,79] studied the life-span of lymphocytes in rats by determining the rate at which cells in various tissues became labeled during a 10-day course of repeated injections of [^{3}H] TdR. They arbitrarily defined cells which became labeled in less than 5 days as "short-lived" and the remainder as "long-lived." According to their definition, nearly all thymus cells were short-lived, whereas 90% of TDL were long-lived; cells from other regions consisted of a mixture of short- and long-lived cells. Other workers approached the question of lymphocyte longevity more directly by studying the rate of cell labeling during many months of continuous intravenous infusion of [^{3}H] TdR [80,81]. With this method, some PBL of rats were found to have a life-span of 9 months or more.

Quantitative information on the life-span of recirculating lymphocytes arose from the studies of Caffrey et al. [52], who injected rats repeatedly with [^{3}H] TdR for 2 weeks and then studied the decline in percentage labeling of TDL. From this approach, they concluded that TDL consist of 90% long-lived cells and 10% short-lived cells. A recent reappraisal of these experiments, however, contends that the TDL studied by Caffrey et al. probably did not consist of two populations but of only a single population of long-lived cells (see Ref. 82). Indeed, studies in mice on the rate at which TDL become labeled during three times daily injections of [^{3}H] TdR have failed to find any evidence for the existence of short-lived small lymphocytes in this population [82]. The rate of cell labeling in these experiments was directly proportional to the time over which the isotope was administered. The injections were continued for up to 8 weeks in some mice, and at this time approximately 40% of TDL were labeled. From this finding, it was concluded that if cell labeling had continued at the same rate, 100% of the cells would have been labeled after about 4 to 6 months. It might be added that the linearity of labeling observed in these studies suggests that, with respect to their Ly phenotype, the three subclasses of T cells in thoracic duct lymph all have a long (though not necessarily identical) lifespan.

Sprent and Basten [82] sought direct information on the life-span of recirculating T cells by pulsing mice repeatedly with [^{3}H] TdR for 6 weeks and then estimating the proportion of T cells in thoracic duct lymph which were labeled at this time. By using a double-labeling technique in which T cells were defined as cells which did not bind ^{131}I-labeled immune complexes (a marker for B cells), they established that 38% of the T cells present showed nuclear (^{3}H) labeling. From this finding, they concluded that if the cells had continued to label at the same rate, their average life-span would have been of the order of 4 months.

The above data suggest that T cells in the RLP of the adult mouse remain in interphase for an average of 4 to 6 months. This interval might represent the average life-span of the cells, i.e., the time between the entry of the cells into the pool and their death. Conversely, the T-cell pool might become autonomous of the thymus in adult life, the cells in the pool surviving indefinitely but entering mitosis on an average of once every 4 to 6 months. To distinguish between these possibilities, three points should be considered:

1. The size of the RLP in mice decreases steadily with age: at 1 year, it was found to be 50% lower than the maximum level reached at about 2 months of age [83].
2. Adult thymectomy accentuates the decline in the pool size: in mice thymectomized at 7 weeks of age, TDL outputs measured 1 year later were approximately 80% lower than at 1 week post-thymectomy [83].
3. Within the first 2 months of adult thymectomy, the turnover of cells in the RLP is similar to that in nonthymectomized mice: in mice thymectomized at 6 weeks of age, and, 4 weeks later, given multiple injections of [^{3}H]TdR for 30 days, the rate of labeling of TDL was similar to that in nonthymectomized mice [82].

These data suggest that, in the adult, the turnover of T cells in the RLP is only partly dependent on the presence of the thymus. In other words, a large proportion of the recently divided cells that enter the pool are probably derived from precursors that reside outside the thymus. It is possible that these precursors lie within the RLP itself. If so, the above data, taken together, might imply that recirculating T cells, although not having an indefinite life-span, survive for 1 year or more but enter mitosis at rare intervals. This possibility is consistent with the thesis considered in Sec. II that the RLP consists of memory cells which are temporarily withdrawn from the circulation at intervals to respond to specific antigen.

The above discussion emphasizes that the average interval between one phase of DNA synthesis and the next may underestimate the true life-span of lymphocytes. This definition, nevertheless, is convenient, and, bearing in mind its essential inaccuracy, it will be retained for the remainder of this chapter.

Studies on the identity of recently divided cells that enter the lymph during CTDD have provided additional information on the rate at which T cells enter the pool. In mice, the absolute output of recently divided small and large lymphocytes remained constant during a 9-day period of CTDD, except for a transient increase observed at 1 to 2 days [82]; this was established by allowing mice to drain lymph for various intervals, pulsing these mice with [^{3}H]TdR for a period of 24 hr, and then measuring the total numbers of labeled cells that entered the lymph over the next 6 hr. The output of labeled cells over this period at the end of the third day of drainage consisted of 7×10^5 small lymphocytes and 6×10^5 large lymphocytes of which 28 and 8%, respectively, were θ positive. From this finding, it can be calculated that the daily output of θ positive cells at this stage comprised a total of 8×10^5 small lymphocytes and 2×10^5 large lymphocytes. Although the identity of the recently divided cells that entered the lymph was not investigated at other stages of drainage, the fact that the total output of labeled cells did not alter appreciably at other times suggests that the above values are probably representative of the normal entry of T cells into the pool.

It was mentioned previously that outputs of θ positive lymphocytes reached a low plateau after 5 days of CTDD. During this time, a total of 1.5 to 2×10^8 θ positive cells were collected [36]. From the above data, it is evident that only a minority (5×10^6) of these cells had entered mitosis during the 5-day collection period. The figure of 1.5 to 2×10^8 θ positive lymphocytes can thus be regarded as a rough estimate for the size of the pool of long-lived recirculating T cells in adult mice. On this point, mention should be made of work on the calf by Cronkite and his associates [84,85]. These workers observed that the cellularity of the lymph declined in a biphasic fashion during extracorporeal irradiation of the blood or thoracic duct lymph. One cell component was mobilized very rapidly (half time = 1.2 days) and was calculated to comprise a total of 4.8×10^9 small lymphocytes/kg of body weight. The identity of these cells was not established, although it would seem highly likely that they were T cells. In this respect, it may be mentioned that on a body weight basis, the T-cell pool in mice can be calculated to be 6 to 8×10^9/kg, i.e., surprisingly close to the above figure.

B. B Lymphocytes

1. Origin

B cells, like T cells, are considered ultimately to arise from hematopoietic stem cells [86]. While the thymus appears to provide the sole environment for the differentiation of stem cells into T cells, the site of the inductive environment that governs B-cell differentiation is less clearly understood. In birds, strong evidence suggests that this environment lies in the bursa of Fabricius; thus, chickens bursectomized at or before hatching have very few lymphocytes that express surface Ig [87] or receptors for the Fc portion of antibody [5]. The origin of B cells in mammals, however, has proved difficult to define. Since the bursa is lacking in mammals, concerted efforts have been made to define the "bursal analog." Various organs have been accorded this status, in particular, the gut-associated lymphoid tissues or parts thereof [88,89]. Direct evidence that lymphocytes with the characteristics of B cells are produced in such tissues, however, is lacking.

In the fetus, there is strong evidence that B cells arise in the liver. Ig-synthesizing cells can first be detected in the liver at about 14 days of gestation [90,91]. These cells are probably lymphoid precursors, since they are larger than normal B lymphocytes, release Ig (7S IgM) at a rapid rate, but do not express detectable Ig on their surface. When cultured in vitro, however, they rapidly differentiate into typical Ig-positive small lymphocytes [92]. Cells with easily detectable surface Ig first appear in the liver at about 16 days of gestation [93]. These cells appear slightly later in the spleen but cannot be found in the bone marrow until around the time of birth.

Many studies have demonstrated a very rapid turnover of small lymphocytes in the adult bone marrow of various species (reviewed in Ref. 94). In mice [95] and rats [79], for example, more than 80% of marrow lymphocytes become labeled after repeated intraperitoneal injections of [^{3}H]TdR for 3 to 4 days. Most marrow small lymphocytes in mice appear to be B cells at various stages of differentiation. In this species, approximately 25% of marrow cells are small lymphocytes [94,95]. Of the latter, 50% show varying amounts of surface Ig [96], but virtually none are θ positive [3]. Osmond and Nossal [95] studied the turnover of Ig-positive cells in mice given repeated intraperitoneal injections of [^{3}H]TdR. Within 1.5 days of starting the injections, 40% of total marrow small lymphocytes, but only 1% of Ig-positive cells, were labeled; by 3.5 days, however, labeling of Ig-positive cells reached 60%. From these and other data, the authors argued persuasively that small lymphocytes in marrow are initially Ig negative but then rapidly express increasing amounts of surface Ig. Support for this notion comes from evidence that Ig-negative marrow small lymphocytes labeled with [^{3}H]TdR in vitro become Ig positive soon after intravenous injection (i.e., when recovered from the spleen) or when cultured in vitro [97].

Of the Ig-positive cells in marrow, 10% have been defined as "precursor" (pre-B) cells [98,99]. Pre-B cells are larger than other B cells and take longer to differentiate into antibody-forming cells in the presence of antigen. They are present in spleen and in marrow but are not found in LN. Although this distribution also corresponds to that of pluripotential stem cells, pre-B cells can be distinguished from stem cells by their antigen specificity.

Studies in *nu/nu* mice showed that approximately 20% of small lymphocytes in the spleen, but only 5% in LN, were labeled after repeated injection of [^{3}H]TdR for 5 days [100-102]. Since more than 80% of marrow lymphocytes were labeled at this stage, these data suggest that many B cells might originate in the bone marrow and then migrate to organs such as the spleen. Studies of Brahim and Osmond [103,104] in the guinea pig support this view: they observed that after marrow cells were labeled in situ; i.e., after intramyeloid injection of [^{3}H]TdR, labeled lymphocytes appeared shortly afterward in spleen and, to a lesser extent, in LN. Similar findings have been reported by other workers [105]. Direct evidence on the identity of these cells will be required, however, before such studies can be said to prove conclusively that B cells in the peripheral lymphoid tissues are bone marrow derived.

While the above evidence clearly suggests that a proportion of B cells in the secondary lymphoid organs originate in the marrow,[3] there is as yet no definite information on whether B cells also arise in other regions, e.g., the gut-associated lymphoid tissues. Moreover, it should be pointed out that in such organs as the spleen, it is by no means certain that the B cells present are all of exogenous origin. Indeed, the observation that pre-B cells occur not only in marrow but also in spleen might suggest that a proportion of the B cells in this organ arise in situ. This emphasizes the difficulty of interpreting observations of rapid cell labeling in a particular organ after parenteral injection of isotope. Thus, such labeling might indicate formation of cells in situ from precursor cells, immigration of newly formed cells from other organs, or division in situ (or in other organs) of long-lived cells responding to antigen.

2. *Migration*

For reasons not clearly apparent, many workers have assumed that the majority of B cells in the secondary lymphoid organs are sessile. Evidence detailed below suggests in fact that, like T cells, most mature B cells form part of the RLP.

a. Recirculation from Blood to Lymph. TDL collected within the first day of establishing thoracic duct fistulas in normal mice [36,56] or rats [107] consist of 15 to 20% small B lymphocytes. Studies on the identity of TDL from athymic (*nu/nu*) mice and TxBM mice showed that these cell populations contained a far higher proportion of B lymphocytes, i.e., 97 and 73%, respectively [36]. In absolute terms, however, the thoracic duct output of B cells from these mice was similar to that from normal (euthymic) mice. (Henceforth in this chapter, NTx, TxBM, and *nu/nu* mice will be referred to collectively as "B" mice.)

During CTDD of normal mice, the proportion of B cells in the lymph increased gradually from 15% on the first day of drainage to a plateau of 40 to 50% on the fourth day [36]. Since the total output of TDL fell rapidly during this time, it was evident that the mobilization of B cells into the fistulas was extremely slow. In fact, it was calculated that, even after drainage for 8 days, the output of B cells per unit time was only two- to threefold less than that measured on the first day. CTDD of "B" mice gave similar findings.

It was mentioned previously that, in calves, extracorporeal irradiation of the blood or lymph caused the cellularity of the lymph to decline in a biphasic fashion [85]. The slowly mobilizable component was calculated to have a half-time release of more than 25 days. It would seem probable that B cells accounted for this component, although this has yet to be proved.

A priori, the slow decline in B cell numbers during CTDD could indicate either that thoracic duct B lymphocytes are long-lived cells which recirculate from blood to lymph or that lymph-borne B cells are nonrecirculating cells with a rapid turnover. Direct evidence that B cells do recirculate has come from studies in which populations of thoracic duct B cells were radioisotopically labeled, injected intravenously, and the thoracic duct lymph of the recipients monitored for the appearance of labeled cells. With this approach in rats, Howard [39] observed that about 20% of the injected cells (TDL from TxBM rats) appeared in the lymph within 48 hr; this value compared to a recovery of 33% for cell populations that consisted predominantly of T cells, i.e., TDL from normal rats. In similar studies in mice [36], only 10% or less of B cells injected intravenously appeared in thoracic duct lymph within 72 hr; this figure compared to a 50% recovery of normal TDL collected over 48 hr. These studies suggest, therefore, that although B cells do recirculate, on the average, they do so more slowly than do T cells, particularly in mice. (Evidence that B cells in thoracic duct lymph are long-lived cells will be considered in Sec. I.B.2.b.)

Further direct evidence that B cells recirculate has come from studies on the migratory properties of cells that carry immunologic memory. Strober [108] observed that when TDL from hapten-primed rats were passaged from blood to lymph through irradiated hosts, they retained their capacity to mount a secondary response to the hapten on further transfer.

To calculate the size of the recirculating pool of B cells is difficult. CTDD of *nu/nu* mice for 10 days yielded a total of 1.6×10^8 TDL [36]; of these TDL, more than 90% were long-lived small B lymphocytes [82]. To regard this as an estimate for the size of the B-cell pool would be unwise for two reasons. First, the mobilization of long-lived cells into the lymph in this study was still continuing when drainage was arbitrarily terminated at 10 days. Second, it could be argued that most of the B cells that appear in the lymph during chronic drainage are mobilized only as a result of the cell depletion induced during the first few days of drainage. The above data imply nevertheless that the vast majority of B cells in the secondary lymphoid organs have at least the *potential* to recirculate.

b. Sites of Recirculation. Certain areas in the lymphoid tissues of "B" mice show normal concentrations of small lymphocytes. These areas include the peripheral region of the splenic white pulp; the superficial cortex, primary follicles, germinal centers, and medullary region of the LN; and the follicles of Peyer's patches [59,60]. Cell populations enriched for B cells, e.g., spleen cells from "B" mice, were found to home specifically to these regions after intravenous injection [67,109]. These areas were therefore termed "thymus independent." Because they have since been shown to be traversed by circulating B cells, e.g., TDL from "B" mice [36] or rats [110], these areas can now be referred to as "B-cell dependent."

Thoracic duct B cells labeled with $[^3H]$uridine ($[^3H]$UdR) and injected intravenously can be detected in the spleen and LN soon after injection [36]. In the spleen, the cells localize initially in the red pulp and the marginal zone; by 4 hr, however, they are situated predominantly in the white pulp, particularly the peripheral regions. In LN, B cells can first be detected in the walls of the postcapillary venules, particularly in regions where these vessels pass close to the primary follicles. Soon afterward, the cells appear to migrate to the primary follicles and the other B-dependent areas. As with T cells, however, their subsequent route to the medullary sinus and the efferent lymphatics is obscure. In mice, only rare B cells have been found to enter germinal centers; in chickens, by contrast, homing of B (bursal) cells to germinal centers is claimed to be considerable [111].

Although CTDD induces a rapid depletion of cells from the T-dependent areas, depletion from the B-dependent areas occurs only very slowly. In fact, in mice, it was found to be prominent only after drainage for 10 days or more [36].

Further information on the homing properties of B cells arose from studies with cells labeled with ^{51}Cr. Like T cells, ^{51}Cr-labeled B cells (TDL from "B" mice) localized in large numbers in the spleen soon after injection [36]. Homing of B cells to LN, by contrast, was three- to fourfold less than that of T cells, even at 24 hr postinjection; levels were very low at 4 hr and reached maximum levels after about 24 hr. This spleen-seeking propensity of B cells is consistent with the fact that, unlike T cells, B cells exist at a much higher concentration in the spleen (50%) than LN (25%).

Evidence has already been considered that in mice, and to a lesser extent in rats, B cells, unlike T cells, appear only very slowly in the central lymph after intravenous injection. The simplest explanation here might be that after entering LN, B cells subsequently take longer than T cells to traverse the nodes. This explanation fails to take into consideration the above evidence that B cells are restricted in their capacity to reach LN. The reverse explanation has therefore to be considered, namely, that once B cells gain entry to LN, they then migrate through the nodes rapidly. Although the first possibility has yet to be excluded, the second is favored by the following points:

1. Although fewer B cells than T cells were recovered from lymph within 48 to 72 hr of intravenous injection, the time between cell injection and the stage at which maximal cell outputs were first observed was quite similar for both cell types, i.e., about 24 hr [36,39,112].

2. As with T cells, maximal localization of ^{51}Cr-labeled B cells in LN of mice occurred at about 24 hr postinjection [36]; the fact that localization was no higher at 48 than at 24 hr suggests therefore that there was no "damming up" of cells in the nodes during this time.

3. In mice, prior splenectomy of recipients of B cells, a procedure which hastened the arrival of the cells in LN, caused a parallel increase in the rate at which they appeared in the lymph [36].

Taken together, these points suggest that, at least in mice, T and B cells probably traverse LN at a similar rate; if so, it might explain why the proportions of T and B cells in LN and TDL are quite similar. It can thus be argued that B cells recirculate from blood to lymph, not less rapidly, but less frequently than T cells. According to this view, B cells would spend much of their time circulating from arterial to venous blood through the spleen and recirculate (enter lymphatics) only on the rare occasions when they randomly enter LN rather than the spleen. This raises the possibility that the slow depletion of the B-dependent areas of the LN during CTDD reflects, not slow mobilization of cells resident in these areas, but continual replenishment of the areas with lymphocytes gradually mobilized from other organs, e.g., the spleen. Direct information on this point is clearly needed.

The speed at which B cells migrate through the spleen is not known. Studies on the in vitro perfusion of isolated rat spleens suggest indirectly that it may be comparatively rapid. Ford [69] observed that after continuous perfusion of spleens for 6 hr, the cells in the perfusate gave high antibody responses on adoptive transfer; i.e., there was no evidence that B cells had been selectively trapped in the spleen during this time. This finding is relevant to the observation that in recipients of ^{51}Cr-labeled cells, the redistribution of counts from the spleen to LN between 4 and 24 hr (secondary migration) was much less marked in recipients of B cells than of T cells [36]. In view of Ford's data, this observation could be interpreted as follows: T and B cells both home to and migrate through the spleen within a few hours of intravenous injection; the B cells that emerge from the spleen then preferentially reenter the spleen rather than the LN; the T cells, by contrast, are trapped predominantly by the LN. Thus, a state of equilibrium would eventually be reached where the spleen was enriched for B cells and the LN for T cells.

Alternatively, it could be argued that B-cell migration through the spleen is slow. This view is favored by Ford [113], who believes that it would explain, firstly, the restricted secondary migration of B cells from the spleen to other organs and, secondly, the high B/T ratio in the spleen. As mentioned previously, both of these observations can be explained as reflecting an innate restriction in the capacity of B cells to enter LN, i.e., to penetrate the walls of postcapillary venules. In this respect, it may be mentioned that although splenectomy in mice increases localization of radiolabeled B cells in LN, it does not increase localization to the level found with T cells [36]. The poor LN-seeking ability of B cells in this species is therefore probably not simply a reflection of trapping by the spleen. Perhaps the most compelling evidence that B-cell migration through the spleen is slow comes from the report that, in rats, radiolabeled B cells injected intravenously take as long as 18 hours to migrate en masse to the peripheral regions of the white pulp [113a]. Clearly the only direct method for settling this important question is to measure the time taken for purified B cells to migrate through isolated spleens perfused in vitro.

3. Life-span

Although it has been suggested on circumstantial grounds that B lymphocytes are predominantly short-lived cells [114], there is now clear evidence that some B cells in the secondary lymphoid organs have a long life-span. Parrot and de Sousa [109] investigated the homing properties of long-lived lymphocytes from the spleen and LN of normal mice repeatedly injected with [^{3}H]TdR for 28 days; the cells were taken from the mice 3 days after the last injection of isotope to allow disappearance of short-lived cells. Autoradiography indicated that the labeled cells homed not only to the T-dependent areas but also to the B-dependent areas. Bianco et al. [115] used an approach similar to that described above to label long-lived cells in LN and observed that a proportion of these cells expressed receptors for complement, a marker for B cells. Firm evidence that most B cells in LN are long-lived has come from the studies of Röpke and Hougen [100-102]. As mentioned previously, these workers found that less than 5% of small lymphocytes from LN of *nu/nu* mice were labeled after a 5-day course of [^{3}H]TdR injections; by 30 days, 35 to 40% were labeled.

It was mentioned earlier that TDL from normal mice became labeled in a linear rather than a biphasic fashion during repeated injection of [^{3}H]TdR [82]. This finding strongly suggested that both the B cells and the T cells in this population were long-lived. Direct evidence on the life-span of circulating B cells has come from studies on the turnover of TDL from "B" mice. With these mice, as with normal mice, three injections per day of [^{3}H]TdR caused a linear increase in labeling of thoracic duct small lymphocytes [82, 101]. The rate of cell labeling in "B" mice, however, occurred more rapidly than in normal mice: whereas in normal mice only 12% of small TDL were labeled after administration of the isotope for 2 weeks, approximately 30% of such cells were labeled at this time in *nu/nu* and TxBM mice. If labeling in the "B" mice had continued in a linear fashion, 100% of the cells would have been labeled after about 7 weeks.

Howard [39] studied the labeling of TDL from TxBM rats infused continuously with [^{3}H]TdR for 7 days. Of the small lymphocytes present, nearly all of which carried a marker specific for B cells, 10 to 11% were labeled; this figure compared to 3 to 11% labeling of small TDL from normal rats.

It would be unwise to assume that studies on B cells in "B" animals necessarily provide relevant information on the properties of B cells that exist in a normal physiologic environment. For example, it could be argued that the life-span of B cells is under the control of T cells. To answer this objection, Sprent and Basten [82] studied the identity of TDL from normal mice which were labeled at the end of a 6-week course of three injections per day of [^{3}H]TdR. The results showed that, of the cells identified in the lymph at this time as small B lymphocytes, 80% were labeled. If a single population of B cells had been present, i.e., as was found in "B" mice, 100% of the cells would therefore have been labeled after 7 to 8 weeks.

The above data indicate that the average life-span of B cells, both in normal and in "B" mice, is only slightly less than that of T cells. This finding, together with the fact that B cells comprise only a small proportion of normal TDL, probably explains why the labeling pattern of TDL from normal mice repeatedly injected with [^{3}H]TdR showed evidence of only a single cell population.

During CTDD of *nu/nu* mice, the output of recently divided small lymphocytes decreased from about 10^6 cells/24 hr on the first day of drainage to 1 to 2 $\times$ 10^5 cells/24 hr on subsequent days [82]. It is difficult to explain this observation. As suggested elsewhere [82], it is possible that CTDD removes precursor cells from which recently divided B lymphocytes are generated. Conversely, B cells might vary in their susceptibility to mobilization, recently divided lymphocytes entering the lymph more readily than cells generated earlier. According to the second possibility, many of the B cells that appear in the lymph after several days of CTDD would have a life-span considerably in excess of 7 weeks. There is clearly a need for further work in this area.

While it is generally accepted that most large lymphocytes in thoracic duct lymph have a very rapid turnover [57,82,116], the existence of a population of short-lived small lymphocytes is controversial. As mentioned earlier, Everett and his coworkers maintained that about 10% of small TDL from normal rats were short-lived, a claim questioned by other workers who have argued that these studies failed to show definite evidence for the presence of a short-lived population. Recent evidence of Strober [117] strongly suggests, however, that some short-lived B cells do exist in thoracic duct lymph. He observed that when rats were injected repeatedly with very high doses of [^{3}H]TdR for 48 hr (which destroys cells with a rapid turnover), the capacity of their TDL to mount a primary adoptive immune response to ferritin was abolished.

With respect to cell labeling kinetics, studies in mice have failed to find any evidence for the existence of short-lived small lymphocytes in lymph. For B cells, this finding applied even during prolonged thoracic duct drainage of *nu/nu* mice [82], i.e., in a situation where the reduction in the number of long-lived cells in the lymph presumably would have facilitated the detection of any short-lived cells present. Thus, in mice at least, if short-lived small lymphocytes do exist in lymph, they must be present in very small numbers.

II. Formation of the Recirculating Lymphocyte Pool

Despite firm evidence that recirculating lymphocytes are derived from the thymus and the bursa or its equivalent, the factors that control the entry of these cells into the RLP are poorly understood. There would appear to be two main possibilities: firstly, cells continually leave the primary lymphoid organs and directly enter the RLP as potentially long-lived cells, and, secondly, cells leaving the primary lymphoid organs must undergo a phase of "maturation" in the secondary lymphoid organs, e.g., by contact with antigen, before they can enter the RLP.

A. T Lymphocytes

Lymphocytes in the mouse thymus comprise two subpopulations.[4] The majority (more than 90%) are found in the cortex and are characterized by their high surface membrane content of θ antigen, low content of H-2 antigen, and are cortisone sensitive and TL positive [118-125]. The remainder occupy the medulla and have less θ antigen, more H-2 antigen, and are cortisone resistant and TL negative. Cortical and medullary thymus cells also show subtle differences in size and electrophoretic mobility [126]. Cortical cells proliferate more rapidly than do medullary cells: Shortman and Jackson [127] showed that during repeated administration of [^{3}H]TdR, nearly all small cortical (high θ) cells were labeled within 3 days, whereas only 30% of small medullary (low θ) lymphocytes were labeled at this stage. The interrelationship between the cells of the cortex and the medulla is controversial; while some workers claim that the medullary cells are derived from cortical cells [10,23, 25,128-130], others maintain that the two cell types probably develop by quite separate pathways of differentiation [122,127]. Both cell types appear to arise by sequential division from large lymphocytes [127].

Medullary (cortisone-resistant) thymus cells share many of the properties of peripheral T cells. They have a similar content of θ and H-2 antigen [118,121-123], are heterogeneous with respect to the expression of Ly 1,2 and 3 antigens [5a], are an excellent source of "helper" cells in collaborative antibody responses [129,131], respond well to phytohemagglutinin (PHA) and in mixed lymphocyte cultures (MLC) [132], and home to LN and to spleen after intravenous injection [133]. Cortical thymus cells, by contrast, are presumed to be immunoincompetent, express the Ly-123$^+$ phenotype [5a] and home predominantly to the spleen rather than to LN after intravenous injection [134]. However, in spite of this bulk of information on the properties of these two types of thymus cells, direct evidence on the identity of the cells which migrate from the thymus under normal physiologic conditions has not yet been obtained.

A small proportion of thymus lymphocytes appear to have the *potential* to form long-lived recirculating cells: when thymus cells from mice were labeled in vitro and injected intravenously, 1 to 2% were recovered from thoracic duct lymph within 48 hr [135]; in similar experiments in rats, a 10% recovery was reported [136]. Evidence for the potential longevity of these cells came from the observation that when rats were cannulated 2 weeks after injection of labeled thymus cells, the small percentage of TDL labeled at this time was similar to that found within 1 day of cell injection [78].

Although there is no direct evidence on the identity of the cells in the thymus which have the capacity to recirculate, it would seem almost certain that they are from the medulla, particularly since medullary cells are able to home to LN, a property held to be specific for recirculating lymphocytes [71]. Can we therefore conclude that the pool of recirculating T cells is built up from cells that join the pool directly from the medulla? Three points in particular militate against this view:

1. Cell migration from the thymus appears to be considerable. Williams et al. [27] calculated that the number of lymphocytes with the characteristics of thymus cells that emerged from the thymic veins and lymphatics of the calf was sufficient to replace the entire RLP every 4½ days. Fewer cells were found to migrate from the rat thymus: on the basis of the number of labeled cells found in the spleen after intrathymic injection of [^{3}H]TdR, Weissman [20] calculated that the RLP could be repopulated from the thymus every 30 to 60 days. Since the average life-span of recirculating T cells, at least in the mouse, is of the order of many months, the above data suggest that comparatively few of the cells that migrate from the thymus directly enter the RLP. Indeed, it has been observed that only extremely small numbers of labeled cells migrate into thoracic duct lymph of rats after intrathymic injection of [^{3}H]TdR [137,137a]. (TDL were not examined in the above studies of Williams et al. and Weissman.)

2. Elliott [138] reported that in "B" mice grafted with a chromosomally marked thymus, 80 to 90% of the cells in the graft which responded to PHA in vitro carried the graft marker; this result was observed even at 6 months postgrafting, i.e., at a time when most of the cells in the graft

were shown in other studies [7,28] to be of host origin. Since the PHA-responsive cells in the graft were proved to be cortisone resistant, these data strongly suggest that, at least in this experimental model, most of the immunocompetent (medullary) cells do not leave the thymus. Davies and his colleagues [28] had shown previously that in "B" mice that carried thymus grafts for 6 months, the majority of the PHA-responsive cells in the peripheral blood at this time were of host origin. This finding clearly raises the possibility that the cells which normally migrate from the thymus are not derived from the competent (PHA-responsive) population of the medulla. Recent work of Weissman et al. [138a] supports this notion. These workers observed that egress of labeled cells from the thymus after in situ labeling was abolished when hydrocortisone was administered parenterally 1 day before labeling.

3. The number of lymphocytes that migrate from the thymus under germfree conditions is unknown. Studies in germfree mice [139], pigs [140], and chickens [141], however, have shown no apparent diminution in thymic lymphopoiesis. This finding suggests, but does not prove, that the release of cells from the thymus is largely antigen independent. However, antigen does appear to play a role in determining the size of the RLP: TDL outputs measured over 1 or 2 days were found to be more than five times lower in germfree mice than in conventional mice [142].

In view of these points, it becomes necessary to consider the alternative possibility, namely, that entry of thymic cells into the RLP is controlled by extrathymic factors, e.g., the presence of antigen. According to this possibility, the secondary lymphoid organs should contain not only long-lived recirculating T cells but also considerable numbers of short-lived immature nonrecirculating T cells. The existence of the latter is supported by the following three lines of evidence.

1. Thymectomy in adult life is known to cause only a very slow reduction in the size of the RLP [83]. In recent studies, however, Waksal et al. [143] reported that in 10-week-old mice thymectomized at 4 to 6 weeks of age, "the spleen showed massive depletion of lymphocytes, while the lymph nodes remained normal." This finding is consistent with the report of Raff and Cantor [144] that adult thymectomy caused an early fall in the number of θ positive cells in the spleen, but not in LN, blood, or thoracic duct lymph. Also, with respect to this point, Bach et al. [145] claimed that within 1 week of adult thymectomy (but not sham thymectomy), there was a marked reduction in the number of T cells in the spleen capable of forming rosettes with sheep erythrocytes; T rosette-forming cells in the spleen were found to be more sensitive to anti-θ serum and more resistant to treatment with ALS in vivo than those in LN [146].

Recent studies of Cantor and Boyse [5a] suggest that most of these "short-lived" T cells bear the Ly-123$^+$ phenotype, i.e., like the cells of the thymic cortex. These workers reported that, in the spleen, the proportion of Ly-123$^+$ cells fell sharply soon after adult thymectomy, whereas proportions of Ly-1$^+$ and Ly-23$^+$ cells increased.

2. Olsson and Claesson [147] investigated the θ-antigen content of cells in the spleen and LN of mice given repeated injections of [^{3}H]TdR for 6 days. On the basis of differential sensitivity to anti-θ serum in the presence of complement, they concluded that short-lived (labeled) T cells were more common in spleen than LN and that short-lived T cells expressed a higher concentration of θ antigen than did long-lived (unlabeled) T cells. Whether short-lived T cells of high θ content were deficient in adult thymectomized mice was not investigated.

3. Cantor, Asofsky, and Tigelaar [144,148-151] provided evidence that the capacity of cells to produce splenomegaly in neonatal F_1 mice was optimal only when the cell suspension to be tested contained two different types of T (θ-positive) lymphocytes; these lymphocytes were termed "T_1" and "T_2" cells. T_1 cells were regarded as the "precursor" cells in graft-versus-host (GVH) reactions, while T_2 cells acted as "amplifiers." T_1 cells were found in thymus and spleen but not in thoracic duct lymph. In the thymus, T_1 cells were cortisone sensitive and TL positive; in the spleen, they were resistant to ALS, and their number decreased within a few weeks of adult thymectomy. T_2 cells, by contrast, were found in blood, LN, and thoracic duct lymph but not in thymus; the number of T_2 cells was greatly reduced in ALS-treated mice but not in adult thymectomized mice. T_1 cells were therefore regarded as short-lived nonrecirculating lymphocytes, whereas T_2 cells were long-lived and resided in the RLP. Synergy between subpopulations of T cells has since been reported for the mixed lymphocyte reaction (MLR) [152] and the generation of cytotoxic lymphocytes (CL) [152,153].

Taken together, the above points provide strong, if circumstantial, evidence that there exists in spleen a population of short-lived nonrecirculating T cells of recent thymic origin. The function of these cells is debatable. Raff and Cantor [144] postulated that T_1 and T_2 cells belong to the same lineage, T_1 being driven to T_2 by contact with antigen. As mentioned above, Cantor and Asofsky [149] maintained that, at least with respect to the GVH reaction, T_2 cells functioned simply to amplify the response of T_1 cells. The experiments that purported to demonstrate this point, however, are by no means conclusive. Neither does this proposal explain why TDL, even from mice thymectomized several weeks previously, i.e., cells that presumably contain only T_2 and not T_1 lymphocytes, are, nevertheless, most effective at producing GVH reactions [112]. Furthermore, Wagner [153, 154] recently provided clear evidence that in the synergistic response between thymus and LN cells which leads to the generation of CL in vitro, most of the CL are derived from LN, not from thymus; thus, according to the classification of Cantor et al., the CL generated here were predominantly of T_2 rather than of T_1 origin. Finally, on this point, it is difficult a priori to visualize the RLP as being composed of cells whose function is simply to amplify the response of short-lived precursor T cells present in other organs. The alternative possibility is that T_2 cells are not "amplifiers" but are fully immunocompetent in their own right, their relationship with T_1 cells being genealogic, not functional. This explanation, in fact, is a restatement of an earlier suggestion of Miller and Mitchell [83] that "lymphocytes which emigrate from the thymus are short-lived cells and can establish a progeny of long-lived recirculating cells only if they interact with antigens in the appropriate environment of the secondary lymphoid tissues."

In accord with the suggestion of Miller and Mitchell, and in line with the evidence considered above, T-cell differentiation, in general, might proceed as follows (see Fig. 1): T cells are continually released from the thymus, their release being antigen independent. These cells are virgin (T_v) lymphocytes which have yet to encounter specific antigen. The properties and surface membrane characteristics of T_v cells are more akin to those of the cells of the thymic cortex than of the medulla (though this does not exclude the possibility that the cells peripheralize through the medulla). T_v cells change their surface membrane characteristics soon after leaving the thymus. The cells at this stage fail to recirculate and home predominantly to the spleen, where they soon die unless they encounter specific antigen. If they do meet antigen, however, they mount a "primary response" to the antigen; this encounter determines that some of the responding cells are driven to form long-lived recirculating memory (T_m) lymphocytes.

According to this notion, most, perhaps all, recirculating T cells are memory cells, and any response they mount, in effect, represents a secondary response; the reduced levels of recirculating lymphocytes in germfree mice would reflect a deficiency of memory cells, a consequence of low exposure to antigen. When the RLP of the conventional animal reached its maximum size, i.e., in the adult, the cells present would presumably have a sufficient range of specificity to mediate a response to most environmental antigens subsequently encountered. The RLP might thus gradually become autonomous of the thymus and, perhaps by a feedback mechanism, account for thymic atrophy in the adult. If this hypothesis were true, the turnover of cells in the RLP of the adult would simply reflect division of cells already present in the pool which were responding to antigens they had previously encountered; this explanation would account for the observation mentioned in Sec. I that the turnover of recirculating lymphocytes is not detectably influenced by thymectomy in adult life.

Verification of the above hypothesis[5] will depend on demonstrating

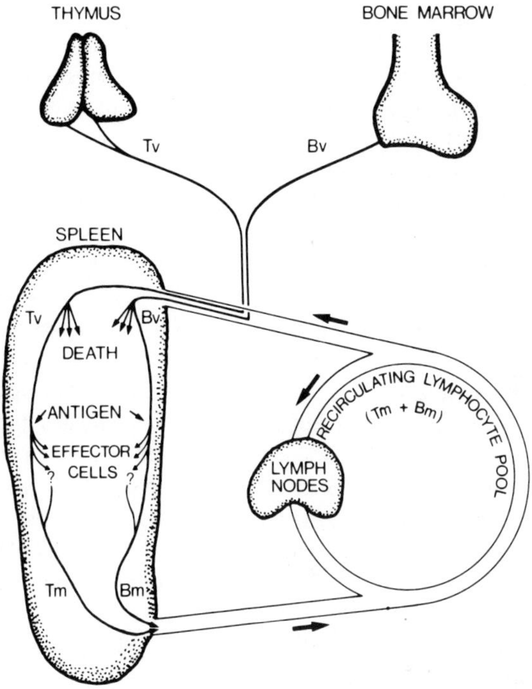

FIG. 1. A schematic representation of the proposed formation of the recirculating lymphocyte pool (RLP). Virgin (v) lymphocytes are envisaged as migrating in large numbers from the primary lymphoid organs, the thymus releasing T_v lymphocytes and the bone marrow (and perhaps other organs) B_v lymphocytes. Virgin cells do not recirculate from blood to lymph and migrate predominantly to the spleen where they soon die unless they meet specific antigen. Virgin cells encountering specific antigen mount a "primary" response to the antigen and differentiate into effector cells and memory (m) cells. Memory T (T_m) and B (B_m) cells join the RLP to become long-lived recirculating lymphocytes. According to this scheme the RLP of normal animals is comprised of a mixture of T_m and B_m lymphocytes carrying specificity for previously encountered antigens.

unequivocally that cell migration from the thymus is as extensive as some workers claim, that the cells that leave the thymus are predominantly nonrecirculating and short-lived, and that if such cells exist, they can be induced to form long-lived recirculating lymphocytes in the presence of antigen. This list, imposing as it is, serves to underline how little firm evidence is available on T-cell differentiation.

B. B Lymphocytes

Evidence mentioned earlier suggests that a large proportion of B cells in the secondary lymphoid organs originate in the bone marrow. The production of these cells is probably antigen independent, since the turnover of Ig-positive cells in the marrow of germfree mice is similar to that found in conventional mice [95]. Most marrow lymphocytes appear to be unable to recirculate: Strober and Dilley [155] observed that when marrow cells from rats were injected intravenously into irradiated rats, only 0.1% of the small lymphocytes present in the suspension appeared in thoracic duct lymph within 48 hr.

The studies of Brahim and Osmond [103,104] suggest that most of the cells which migrate from the marrow of the guinea pig to the secondary lymphoid organs are short-lived: they observed that after intramyeloid injection of [^{3}H]TdR, the labeled small lymphocytes which appeared shortly afterward in the spleen and LN disappeared within a few days; the authors considered it unlikely that this finding reflected extensive division of the cells with consequent loss of label. While the number of lymphocytes that migrate from the marrow has not been measured directly, it is probably considerable [94]. The number of newly formed (but potentially long-lived) B cells that enter thoracic duct lymph, by contrast, is quite small, i.e., approximately 10^6/day in *nu/nu* mice [82]. This point raises the possibility that the entry of B cells into the RLP as long-lived cells is governed by a selective process. Recent studies of Strober [117] are of particular relevance to this point.

Strober observed that the cells in thoracic duct lymph of rats which gave a primary response to ferritin were nonrecirculating cells with a rapid turnover. Thus, the cells which responded to this antigen on adoptive transfer could not be passaged from blood to lymph through an intermediate irradiated host and were not found in donors pretreated with high (suicidal) doses of [^{3}H]TdR for 48 hr. With TDL from primed rats, by contrast, the cells which mounted a secondary response to ferritin on transfer could recirculate and were present in donors treated with [^{3}H] TdR.[6]

Similar though not identical results were obtained by Strober and Dilley [155,157] with the hapten dinitrophenyl (DNP). With this antigen, as with ferritin, the secondary response was shown to be mediated by recirculating cells, whereas the cells that gave a primary response were unable to recirculate. However, whereas treatment with high doses of [^{3}H]TdR abolished the primary response of TDL to ferritin, this treatment had no effect on their response to DNP. The authors explained this discrepancy by postulating that the slower turnover of cells that responded in a "primary" situation to DNP reflected a degree of "environmental priming" to this antigen. Assessing their data as a whole, the authors proposed that nonrecirculating short-lived B cells are "virgin" (B_1) cells and that contact with antigen determines their differentiation into long-lived recirculating "memory" (B_2) cells. They suggested that partial differentiation of virgin cells along this pathway might occur in situations where contact with antigen was limited, e.g., with environmental priming of DNP-reactive cells.

Recent work of Schlegel et al. [158] and Schrader [159] complements the above findings. These workers observed that most of the cells from mouse spleen which mount a primary response to the hapten 4-hydroxy-3-iodo-5-nitrophenylacetic acid (NIP) differ in size, density, adherence properties, and electrophoretic mobility from the spleen cells of NIP-primed mice which give a secondary response to the hapten. There is also evidence that unprimed hapten-reactive B cells are much more susceptible to tolerance induction than are primed cells [160,161].

The concept of Strober and Dilley implies that the entry of B cells into the RLP is restricted to cells which have previously responded to antigen. The pool of recirculating B cells, like the T-cell pool, might thus consist predominantly or entirely of memory cells. According to this concept, germfree mice should have lower numbers of recirculating B cells than should normal mice. While this possibility has yet to be proved, it is, nevertheless, probably correct. As mentioned previously, TDL outputs from germfree mice were found to be reduced by more than fivefold in comparison with normal mice. The proportion of B cells in TDL from germfree mice was not investigated. However, since TDL from normal mice consist of 15 to 20% B cells, the proportion of B cells in germfree TDL would have to be close to 100% for the B-cell output from these mice *not* to be reduced. This would be a most unlikely finding in view of evidence that the proportions of B cells in spleen and LN of germfree mice are similar [162] or only slightly higher [96] than in normal mice.

In view of the evidence considered above, the differentiation of B cells might proceed as follows (see Fig. 1): B cells arise in the bone marrow (and perhaps also in other organs) by antigen-independent differentiation from stem cells; most marrow small lymphocytes consist of nonrecirculating virgin (B_v) cells with a rapid turnover.[7] B_v cells migrate rapidly from their sites of origin to the secondary lymphoid organs,[8] a few cells entering thoracic duct lymph, although not as members of the RLP. Most B_v cells soon die unless they meet antigen to which they are specifically reactive. Cells which do encounter antigen are driven to differentiation into memory (B_m) cells which enter the RLP as long-lived cells.

This scheme implies that memory cells reside within the RLP and are not sessile. How, then, can one explain the finding that CTDD for 5 days, although greatly reducing the primary response, has no effect on the secondary response

[165,166]? Most regimes used for antigen priming probably induce an overabundance of primed cells (see Ref. 166). Moreover, although CTDD mobilizes large numbers of long-lived B cells, it is by no means an efficient method for inducing B-cell depletion. Thus, to induce a detectable reduction in the secondary response, CTDD would probably have to be continued for a period of many weeks. One would, nevertheless, expect CTDD to cause a substantial reduction in the overall number of memory cells in the lymphoid tissues. Recent evidence of Strober and Dilley [157] supports this view: they demonstrated by adoptive transfer that the numbers of B memory cells in spleens of primed rats were reduced 25-fold when the spleens were taken from donors subjected to CTDD for 5 days.

Although it is argued above that, in most situations, memory cells reside in the RLP, there is evidence nevertheless that some memory cells may be sessile when generated under certain circumstances, e.g., in LN that drain the sites of local injection of antigen [167-169]. This might be a consequence of prolonged local retention of antigen. Studies of Smith et al. [170] emphasize, however, that most of the memory cells generated in this situation are not sessile but enter the circulation and disseminate to other regions.

The scheme for B-cell differentiation considered above is closely analogous to that proposed for T cells. It is perhaps useful to attempt to assess this general concept for T- and B-cell differentiation in terms of the evolutionary pressures which presumably shaped the immune system.

According to the clonal selection theory [171], the immune system probably evolved in response to two main pressures.

1. The necessity to have available sufficient clones of antigen-reactive cells to enable responses to be mounted against any antigen encountered. To guard against the risk of these cells being tolerized or otherwise inactivated in situations of unusual antigen presentation, a reserve mechanism would presumably be required to replace these cells. This mechanism could conceivably be controlled by specific chalones [172] released by each cell clone. It is, however, clearly difficult to envisage how such chalones could determine differentiation of T or B cells of the required specificity from stem cells. A simpler mechanism would be to rely on a continuous production of multiple clones of cells that collectively embrace all specificities. Since many of the antigens to which these cells were reactive would never be encountered, there would be no advantage in these cells being long-lived. Indeed, their longevity would be a distinct disadvantage, since it would rapidly lead to a state of overall lymphocyte excess. It can thus be argued that selective pressure would favor a system that involves a continuous nonantigen-dependent production of cells with a limited life-span.

2. The need for being able to mount an amplified response to antigens encountered previously. Of the enormous range of antigenic specificities that an animal might meet in a particular ecosystem, those antigens it did meet would, in all probability, be reencountered. For virgin cells to die after responding to an antigen would therefore be wasteful and inefficient. If these cells were to survive, however, i.e., as long-lived lymphocytes, they could then assist the short-lived virgin population to mount a more effective response upon subsequent exposure to the antigen. Would such memory cells be sessile? If they were, they would have to be present in very large numbers throughout the body to be able to effectively guard the various possible antigen entry sites. Alternatively, memory cells might be mobile and thus be able to migrate selectively to regions of antigen concentration. The advantages of the second possibility are obvious.

III. Factors That Control Lymphocyte Recirculation

Evidence is accumulating that lymphocyte migration is controlled by certain structures on the lymphocyte surface membrane. To date, comparatively little attention has been directed toward resolving the nature of these structures. This is perhaps surprising, since these structures probably play a critical role in enabling lymphocytes to encounter and then respond to antigen. For this reason, it is considered that although much of the evidence available on the factors that control lymphocyte migration is fragmentary and inconclusive, the essential importance of the subject warrants it being considered in some detail.

The most convincing demonstration that cell surface structures influence lymphocyte migration has come from studies of Woodruff and Gesner [72]. They observed that when ^{51}Cr-labeled TDL from normal rats were incubated in vitro with the proteolytic enzyme trypsin, their homing properties were radically altered. Within 1 to 4 hr of cell injection, the localization of radioactive counts in LN was about 50 times lower in recipients of trypsin-treated cells than in rats given untreated TDL. At later times, the counts in LN rapidly increased and reached control levels by 24 hr.[9] Homing of trypsin-treated cells to the spleen, by contrast, was increased at 1 to 4 hr after injection; it then fell rapidly and in parallel with a reciprocal increase in LN counts. Homing to all other organs examined was normal. Trypsin-treated TDL were reported to be able to recirculate from blood to lymph but with a "slight delay" compared with untreated cells.

Trypsin-treated TDL were shown by autoradiography to localize in the white pulp of the spleen during the time when the cells failed to enter

LN [174]. This finding strongly suggests that the entry of lymphocytes to LN and to the white pulp of the spleen is controlled by separate mechanisms. In this respect, Woodruff and Gesner proposed that trypsin specifically inhibits LN homing by cleaving certain constituents of the lymphocyte surface membrane which normally enable the cells to penetrate the walls of postcapillary venules.

Woodruff and Gesner [175] demonstrated that lymphocyte migration was also altered when cells were incubated in vitro with *Vibrio cholerae* neuraminidase; this enzyme cleaves terminal sialic acid from heterosaccharides and glycoproteins. ^{51}Cr labeling studies indicated that treatment of TDL with neuraminidase greatly increased their localization in the liver after intravenous injection. This increase was associated with a three- to fourfold reduction in homing to both spleen and LN. The altered distribution to liver, spleen, and LN persisted for about 24 hr and then gradually returned to the pattern obtained with untreated TDL.[10] Neuraminidase treatment caused a delay of about 24 hr in the mean transit time of lymphocyte recirculation from blood to lymph.

Prior to these studies, Gesner [181] had proposed that lymphocytes express neuraminidase-sensitive "receptors" which control their entry to the lymphoid tissues. The simplest explanation for the above findings, however, is that neuraminidase treatment caused the cells to agglutinate, thus making them susceptible to being trapped temporarily in the liver.[11] Although Woodruff and Gesner conceded this explanation, they believed that the results generally supported Gesner's original postulate. Since treatment with neuraminidase reduced LN homing by no more than two- to fourfold and caused a parallel reduction in homing to the spleen, it is difficult to follow the authors' rationale for concluding that cell surface sugars play a *specific* role in enabling lymphocytes to enter the lymphoid tissues.

It has long been known that certain viral infections are associated with a transient lymphocytopenia (reviewed in Ref. 182). Recent evidence suggests that, in many instances, this lymphocytopenia probably reflects an alteration in lymphocyte migration rather than a decrease in cell production.

Woodruff and Woodruff [182,185-187] studied the severe lymphocytopenia which develops in rats infected with Newcastle disease virus (NDV). The lymphocytopenia lasted for 1 to 2 days, was evident within 12 hr of infection, and was associated with a profound depletion of lymphocytes from the LN paracortex and the PALS of the spleen. There was also a two- to threefold reduction in TDL outputs. Stress did not appear to play a role in these findings, since similar results were obtained in adrenalectomized recipients. Within 3 days of infection, the concentration of lymphocytes in the blood, lymphoid tissues, and thoracic duct lymph returned to normal levels. [^{3}H]TdR labeling studies showed that most of the cells that reappeared at this time were not newly formed. The key question of where the cells had localized before their reappearance was not discussed.

NDV was shown to express neuraminidase activity. Lymphocytes incubated in vitro with NDV at 4°C bound the virus reversibly and agglutinated [185]. Since agglutination was specifically inhibited by *N*-acetylneuraminic acid, binding was considered to be controlled by sialic acid residues on the cell surface; indeed, incubation of lymphocytes with NDV led to the release of free sialic acid from the cells. In further studies, the homing pattern of TDL incubated in vitro with NDV was found very similar to that observed after treatment with *V. cholerae* neuraminidase [186]. On the basis of these findings, the authors concluded that the neuraminidase activity of the virus was responsible for the altered pattern of lymphocyte migration in NDV infection.

This conclusion is difficult to reconcile with results of other studies in which ^{51}Cr-labeled TDL were transferred to rats infected with NDV [187]. When the labeled cells were injected either 24 hr before or 4 hr after inoculation of the virus, homing to LN was decreased by up to 50%, whereas that to spleen was increased. Localization of cells in the liver, lungs, kidney, and thymus was not altered. A decrease in LN homing was also observed when the labeled cells and the virus were given simultaneously; in this situation, however, no alteration in homing to the spleen occurred. This distribution of labeled cells clearly differed from that obtained after neuraminidase (or NDV) treatment in vitro, i.e., where cell localization was reduced in both LN and spleen but was increased in liver. It would seem likely therefore that the altered pattern of lymphocyte migration in NDV infection is not due solely to the neuraminidase activity of the virus.

Whereas severe lymphocytopenia is the hallmark of NDV infection, mice infected with *Bordetella pertussis* develop a marked lymphocytosis. Morse demonstrated that absolute small lymphocyte counts in peripheral blood were elevated within 1 day of infection and reached maximum levels after 3 to 6 days [188]. Lymphocyte counts at this time were three to 12 times above normal levels; [^{3}H]TdR labeling studies showed that these cells were not newly formed [189]. The lymphocytosis was associated with a marked depletion of small lymphocytes from LN, spleen, thymus, and bone marrow [188]; TDL outputs were markedly reduced [190].

When ^{51}Cr-labeled LN cells were incubated in vitro with supernatants from cultures of *B. pertussis,* their capacity to home to LN was reduced about fourfold [191]. This reduction was associated with a marked increase in the content of labeled cells in the blood and with a moderate increase in the spleen; there was little change in the localization of cells in the liver. Similar, though less profound, changes occurred when untreated labeled cells were transferred to mice preinjected with either culture supernatants or with whole *B. pertussis* organisms. There was, however, an anomaly in this situation: in recipients of culture supernatants, but not of whole organisms, homing of cells to the spleen was reduced, not increased; this reduction was associated with an increase in cell localization in the liver. Thus, the culture supernatants appeared to exert a mild trypsin-like activity in vitro, whereas in vivo, the action of this material resembled that of neuraminidase. These findings are not easily interpreted.

Spry [192] recently made the interesting observation that seemingly quite trivial procedures can have a marked effect on lymphocyte migration. He reported that the hourly output of TDL from rats draining lymph for 24 hr was reduced about fourfold when the rats were either anesthetized with ether or simply injected intravenously with tissue culture medium. The author reasoned that stress might have played a part in these findings and supported his view by showing that injection of corticotropin had a similar effect. (The injection here was said to be given in such a way that the rats were "not disturbed.") In other experiments, continuous infusion of rats with prednisolone or corticotropin caused a persistent threefold reduction in TDL outputs and delayed blood to lymph recirculation of isotopically labeled TDL; these changes were not observed in rats infused with saline only. Inhibition of lymphocyte recirculation after corticotropin injection has also been observed in sheep [193].

The mechanism by which glucocorticosteroids (CS) reduce lymphocyte recirculation is unknown. In CS-sensitive species, e.g., mice and rats, injection of CS causes a marked depletion of lymphocytes from the thymus, spleen, and LN [194]. Many of these cells are probably short-lived lymphocytes; the latter are considered to be particularly sensitive to direct lysis by CS [194-197]. While there is evidence that long-lived lymphocytes in these organs are comparatively resistant to CS [198], this resistance does not apply to the long-lived cells present in peripheral blood. Thus, lymphocyte counts in blood may be reduced to 1% of normal levels within 3 to 4 days of CS injection and remain below normal levels for many weeks [199-201]. Are these cells destroyed or is their pattern of migration altered? It is difficult to answer this question, particularly since the CS usually used for in vivo experiments are comparatively insoluble and thus have a prolonged "depot effect" [194].

Three lines of evidence suggest that, in certain situations, CS may alter lymphocyte migration without destroying the cells. First, in the experiments of Spry considered above, in which isotopically labeled TDL were injected intravenously into rats infused with corticotropin, labeled cells appeared in thoracic duct lymph shortly after the infusions were terminated. The author pointed out, however, that this finding could not be explained entirely as a manifestation of altered lymphocyte migration, because the absolute recovery of labeled cells over the next 3 days was much less than in rats infused only with saline. Second, Morse [199] reported that the extreme blood lymphocytopenia induced by injection of CS was converted to a lymphocytosis if *B. pertussis* was administered 1 day after CS injection. Third, lymphocytes with the characteristics of T cells become sequestered in the bone marrow soon after parenteral injection of CS [202,203]; here, it should be stressed that although there is no quantitative information on the degree of T-cell sequestration in the bone marrow after CS injection, such sequestration is probably not sufficient to account for the profound lymphocyte depletion that affects other tissues. Taken together, these data suggest that the impairment of lymphocyte recirculation induced by CS is a reflection not only of lymphocyte destruction but also of an altered pattern of migration.

A clear understanding of the factors that control lymphocyte migration will only emerge through further investigation. Nevertheless, the studies on the effect of treating lymphocytes with trypsin provide compelling evidence that the entry of lymphocytes to LN, in contrast to spleen, is controlled by protein-containing components of the lymphocyte surface membrane. As Woodruff and Gesner suggested, these structures probably determine the specific capacity of lymphocytes to penetrate the walls of postcapillary venules (PCV). Whether these "receptors" for PCV (RPCV) contain glycoprotein, i.e., are neuraminidase sensitive, has not yet been proven. Useful information on the nature of RPCV could probably be obtained by screening various enzymes for their capacity to alter lymphocyte migration after in vitro incubation. This approach might also throw light on the mechanism of action of CS.

Although the capacity of lymphocytes to enter the white pulp of the spleen does not appear to involve RPCV, the fact that the splenic white pulp contains few cells other than lymphocytes suggests that cell entry to this region, as to LN, is governed by a selective process. Interference with this process presumably accounts for the observation that, in *B. pertussis* infection, the splenic white pulp shows severe lymphocyte depletion despite a marked blood lymphocytosis. The nature of the process that determines normal entry of cells to the splenic white pulp, however, is obscure.

Whether infection with organisms, such as *B. pertussis* or NDV, induces an alteration in the migration of both T and B lymphocytes is unknown. Indeed, virtually nothing is known of the factors which determine that T and B cells migrate through different regions of the lymphoid tissues. The fact that their migratory properties are dissimilar is perhaps not surprising in view of the marked differences the cells display at the level of their surface membrane. For example, B cells differ from T cells not only with respect to the surface markers considered earlier but also by their electrophoretic mobility [204-206], concentration of H-2 antigens (particularly Ia antigens) [207], radiosensitivity [208], and sensitivity to CS [194]. Whether these various distinguishing features of T and B cells affect their migratory behavior, however, has not yet been established.[12]

As suggested elsewhere [36], the fact that B cells have a limited capacity to home to LN might imply that they have a poor representation of RPCV. The finding that trypsin treatment of TDL (which contain 15-20% B cells) reduces LN homing by 50-fold [72] strongly suggests that this enzyme inhibits the capacity of both B cells and T cells to enter LN. Direct evidence on this point has come from the observation that pretreatment with trypsin will abolish the limited degree of LN homing shown by highly enriched populations of B lymphocytes [112].

IV. Migration of Recirculating Lymphocytes During Antigenic Stimulation

A. Antigen-induced Recruitment of Recirculating Lymphocytes

Induction of immune responses probably occurs in regions of antigen concentration. For example, while antibody production is low in peripheral LN after intravenous injection of antigen, it is high when antigen is injected locally into the area drained by the nodes [169,209]. The lymphocytes that respond to antigen in a particular site could either be of local origin or have been mobilized from other regions. Studies of Hall and Morris [210] strongly support the second possibility. They observed that heavy irradiation of the popliteal LN of sheep had no effect on antibody production in the node after local injection of antigen. They concluded that since lymphocytes are highly radiosensitive, the immune response must have been mediated by cells that entered the node from the circulation.

The entry of lymphocytes into an area of antigen concentration might be nonspecific or, conversely, might involve only lymphocytes with specificity for the antigen. Experimental evidence considered below indicates that both selective and nonselective recruitment of lymphocytes may occur.

1. Nonselective Recruitment

It is well known that subcutaneous injection of antigen [211,212], skin painting with contact-sensitizing agents [213], and skin allografting [214] lead to profound changes in the draining LN. These changes are evident within 1 to 2 days and consist initially of hypercellularity of the paracortex associated with tight aggregation ("plugging") of lymphocytes in the paracortical sinuses [215, 216]; the latter are probably directly connected with the medullary sinus. "Plugging" is most conspicuous at 2 to 4 days after antigen injection and then regresses. Microangiography has shown that these changes are associated with a conspicuous alteration in the vascularity of the affected LN [217]. Beginning on the second day and reaching a peak at 4 to 5 days, there is a marked increase in both the diameter and in the density of the capillaries. These vessels come to form a dense network throughout the LN, particulary beneath the capsule and in the medullary cords.

Lymphocyte migration through the antigen-stimulated LN has been studied extensively in sheep [218-222]. Shortly after antigen is injected into the area that drains the popliteal LN, there is a brief "shutdown" in the cell output from the efferent lymphatic vessel [219,221,222]. "Shutdown" usually lasts for less than 5 hr; it is variable in extent but may at times be profound, particularly when swine influenza virus is used as the antigen [221]. The cause of this phenomenon is unknown. Hall and Morris [219] suggested that it reflects reduced entry of lymphocytes into the nodes, due either to a transient reduction in blood flow or to a block at the level of the PCV. Direct evidence on this point is lacking. The observation that CS may inhibit lymphocyte recirculation (see Sec. III) raises the possibility that "shutdown" is a consequence of stress. In certain situations, "shutdown" is probably due simply to LN edema [223].

A phenomenon analogous to "shutdown" was reported to affect isolated spleens of rats perfused for 10 hr in vitro: Ford [68] observed that when heterologous erythrocytes were added to the perfusate, the release of cells from the spleen was reduced. The physiologic significance of this finding is difficult to assess.

The phase of "shutdown" in the popliteal LN is followed by a very rapid increase in cell output. By 36 hr after antigen injection, cell traffic through the nodes may be more than sevenfold above normal levels [221]. At this stage, nearly all of the cells in the lymph are typical small lymphocytes; [^{3}H]TdR labeling studies have shown that these cells are not newly formed [218]. The increase in lymphocyte traffic at this time presumably reflects either enhanced blood flow through the nodes or an increased permeability of the walls of the PCV [220]. Blast cells first appear in lymph after 2 to 3 days. Increased cell output persists for a variable time, usually 3 to 5 days.

Several workers have concluded that the hypercellularity of lymphoid tissues during antigenic stimulation reflects nonspecific "trapping" of lymphocytes [224-227]. Zatz and Lance [225] reached this conclusion by studying the homing pattern of ^{51}Cr-labeled LN cells in mice injected with one of several antigens. When antigen was administered intravenously or intraperitoneally, "trapping" (recovery of above normal levels of radioactivity) occurred in the spleen at the expense of the LN. Conversely, after subcutaneous injection of antigen, "trapping" was restricted to the draining LN.

In the spleen, "trapping" was observed within 1 hr of antigen injection but was not demonstrable in LN before 24 hr. "Trapping" usually lasted for 24 to 48 hr.

Zatz and Lance suggested that "trapping" is a reflection of a temporary and predominantly nonspecific sequestration of lymphocytes from the RLP. They cited the phenomena of LN "shutdown" and "plugging" as supporting this view. For LN "trapping," this reasoning is difficult to follow. As mentioned earlier, "shutdown" is evident only within the first few hours of antigen injection, whereas "trapping," at least in mice, is not conspicuous before 24 hr. Thus, "trapping" occurs at a time when, in the sheep popliteal LN, lymphocyte traffic is greatly *increased.* With respect to this point, although paracortical "plugging," which is intense during the period of "trapping," has been considered to reflect impaired migration [216], the opposite view would seem more tenable, i.e., that "plugging" is a manifestation of increased traffic. The possibility arises therefore that "trapping" in LN is a misnomer. Thus, in mice injected with labeled lymphocytes, the increased levels of radioactivity found at a particular time in antigen-stimulated lymphoid tissues might reflect simply an overall increase in the numbers of labeled cells migrating through the tissues at that time. Finally, the contention that "trapping" reflects sequestration of lymphocytes during antigenic stimulation is not supported by recent evidence of Cahill et al. [228]. These workers observed that the *speed* at which ^{51}Cr-labeled lymphocytes migrated from the afferent to efferent lymphatics of the popliteal LN of sheep was not altered during antigenic stimulation. In marked contrast, the *proportion* of the injected lymphocytes which entered and then recirculated through the node increased enormously (e.g., by fivefold or more) within 24 to 36 hr of antigen injection.

Taken together, the above data suggest that shortly after an antigen reaches a particular lymphoid organ, the rate at which the cells of the RLP perfuse that organ is markedly increased. As Hall and Morris [210,218] pointed out, this phenomenon might play a crucial role in determining the rate at which the affected organ can screen the RLP for lymphocytes with specificity for the antigen concerned (see Sec. IV.A.2).

2. *Selective Recruitment*

Several studies have produced evidence that injection of antigen is followed by a transient selective withdrawal of specifically reactive recirculating lymphocytes from the RLP to the lymphoid tissues.

Kreth et al. [229] studied the immune reactivity of PBL from patients infused intravenously for 5 days with streptokinase. During this treatment, the patients' lymphocytes lost their capacity to respond (synthesize DNA) in vitro to streptokinase but responded well to PHA and tuberculin. Reactivity to the injected antigen usually disappeared within 4 hr of commencing treatment and persisted until the infusion was terminated. In most cases, a full return in reactivity to streptokinase was observed when responses were tested 2 weeks later.

Experiments in mice [230,231] and rats [232] demonstrated that the adoptive immune response of TDL to antigens such as heterologous erythrocytes or hapten-protein conjugates was specifically reduced or abolished if the cells were collected at 1 to 2 days after intravenous injection of antigen. This transient incompetence of TDL affected both IgM and IgG antibody production. It appeared to be unrelated to classic tolerance, since the TDL donors themselves gave high antibody responses to the injected antigen. The specific unresponsiveness of TDL in this situation involved both T and B lymphocytes. Thus, with rats immunized 6 weeks previously with dinitrophenylated bovine γ globulin (DNP-BGG), the secondary antibody response to DNP of TDL adoptively transferred with DNP-BGG was specifically reduced when, 1 day before transfer, the cell donors were injected with either unconjugated BGG or DNP conjugated to an unrelated carrier [232]. This finding suggested that suppression of carrier-specific (T) and hapten-specific (B) cells had been induced separately. Similarly, in mice, the unresponsiveness induced in TDL to sheep red blood cells (sRBC) by preinjection of the cell donors with sRBC was not abrogated when the TDL were transferred together with either normal T cells or normal B cells [112]; since the antibody response to sRBC requires collaboration between T and B cells [83], injection of this antigen must therefore have suppressed the function of both cell types.

A phenomenon similar to that described above was reported by O'Toole and Davies [233], who observed that the antibody response of peripheral LN of mice to a local injection of sRBC could be abolished by a prior intraperitoneal injection of this antigen. This effect, which the authors termed "preemption," differed in two respects from the findings considered above. First, it persisted for up to 2 weeks. Second, it was nonspecific: a profound, though less long-lasting, reduction in the regional LN response to sRBC could be induced by intraperitoneal injection of horse erythrocytes.

In several studies, circulating lymphocytes obtained from donors recently injected with histoincompatible lymphoid cells were found to be specifically unresponsive to the antigens expressed by these cells:

1. Experiments in mice [230] and rats [232] demonstrated that the capacity of parental-strain TDL to induce GVH disease in F_1 recipients was specifically reduced when the cell donors were injected with F_1 spleen cells 1 to 2 days previously. More recently, TDL obtained under such conditions were shown to be markedly and specifically impaired in their capacity to

cause rejection of skin allografts carried by "B" mice and to exert cell-mediated lympholysis when cultured with the determinants concerned in vitro [234]; paradoxically, there was only a partial reduction in the capacity of TDL to respond in MLC.

2. Larner [235] reported that the response in MLC of PBL from rats was specifically reduced when the cells were taken from donors given allogeneic lymphoid cells 1 day previously. Cells taken from the spleen at this time, however, gave above normal responses in MLC.

3. Hay et al. [222] injected allogeneic lymphocytes subcutaneously into the drainage area of the popliteal LN of sheep and studied the MLR of cells collected from the efferent lymphatic vessel; the reactivity of these cells to lymphocytes of donor origin was high within the first 2 days of injection, but it later completely disappeared; this disappearance was specific, since the cells responded well to other antigens.

4. Ford and Atkins [236] and Dorsch and Roser [236a] reversed the approach used in the above studies by injecting parental-strain TDL into irradiated F_1 rats and then testing the reactivity of the cells of donor origin which appeared in thoracic duct lymph. Within 12 hr of injection, these cells were found to be specifically depleted of lymphocytes capable of inducing a GVH reaction or skin allograft rejection against host-type determinants. This specific unresponsiveness of the "filtered" donor cells has since been shown to apply in MLC, both in mice [234] and rats [236b].

The unresponsiveness observed in the above studies was usually of short duration. With TDL from mice or rats given antigen intravenously, the cells were specifically unresponsive for 1 to 2 days after antigen injection but had fully regained their reactivity by 3 to 4 days [230,232]. A return of reactivity at this time was also observed in the systems of Ford and Atkins [236] and Hay et al. [222]. By contrast, Larner [235] reported that the unresponsiveness in MLC of PBL from rats injected with allogeneic lymphocytes persisted for at least 30 days after antigen injection. Larner produced evidence that this prolonged period of unresponsiveness was due in part to the presence of blocking factors directed against the test antigens. He observed that if PBL were washed repeatedly before being placed in culture, their reactivity to the injected antigens returned to normal by 10 days; unwashed cells, by contrast, were unresponsive at this stage. Larner considered it unlikely that blocking factors accounted for the unresponsiveness observed at earlier periods. In this respect, he found that although blocking factors were present in the sera of rats injected with alloantigen 1 week previously, they were not produced by PBL taken from rats at 4 days after antigen injection. These data per se do not exclude the possibility that, despite thorough washing of cells, blocking factors were responsible for the unresponsiveness observed between

4 and 10 days after antigen injection; such factors might have been released in culture from alloantibody-producing cells, which, at least in certain situations [237], probably enter the circulation at this time.

In general, the above findings are consistent with the hypothesis that circulating lymphocytes are selectively withdrawn from the RLP as they traverse areas of antigen concentration [230]. Evidence that directly supports this concept of antigen-induced selective recruitment of recirculating lymphocytes (ASRL) has come from the work of Atkins and Ford [238] and Ford et al. [239]. In an ingenious series of experiments, these workers labeled TDL from F_1 and parental-strain rats with different radioisotopes and injected the two cell populations in a known mixture intravenously into irradiated F_1 rats. By radioactive counting procedures which allowed the ratio of the two populations to be monitored in various regions of the recipients, the authors calculated that about 12% of the parental strain TDL failed to recirculate from blood to lymph and became sequestered in the spleen and, to a lesser extent, in the LN; of the cells recruited to the spleen, approximately 60% transformed to blast cells within 24 hr of injection. It was therefore concluded that at least 7% of the donor lymphocytes were reactive to the major histocompatibility determinants of the host.

Evidence consistent with the concept of ASRL was also obtained by Thursh and Emeson [240]. These workers studied the homing properties of labeled LN cells obtained from mice injected 3 weeks before with sRBC and, shortly afterward, with [^{3}H]TdR. On adoptive transfer to normal mice, these "long-lived" labeled cells showed a 10% greater tendency to localize in regional LN draining the site of local injection of sRBC than in nodes injected with a different antigen. A much greater specific localization was observed with cells taken from recently stimulated mice; the cells here were labeled with [^{3}H]TdR in vitro before transfer [241].

Although it has been suggested that ASRL occurs to regions of antigen concentration, it might be argued that, to some extent, the cells are recruited from the circulation to the lymphoid tissues in general. Studies on the localization of ^{51}Cr-labeled heterologous erythrocytes in mice showed that after intravenous injection of sRBC in numbers sufficient to induce ASRL, most of the radioactive counts localized in the liver and spleen; virtually none were found in the mesenteric lymph nodes (MLN) [231]. This finding suggested that if lymphocytes are, indeed, selectively recruited to regions where antigen is concentrated, intravenous injection of sRBC would lead to a depletion of antigen-reactive cells from MLN and thoracic duct lymph but not from spleen. This suggestion was verified by the observation that spleen cells from mice injected 1 day previously with sRBC gave high responses to this antigen on transfer (although, for extraneous reasons to be discussed later, poor responses were obtained within the first week of transfer). Neither TDL nor MLN cells, by contrast, responded to the "selecting" antigen at any time after transfer. These findings are in agreement with the observations of

Hay et al. [222] that, after injection of allogeneic lymphocytes into the afferent lymphatic vessel of the sheep popliteal LN, the unresponsiveness demonstrated in MLC toward the donor antigens applied not only to cells collected from the efferent lymphatic vessel of the infused node but also to cells from the contralateral node. In more recent studies, these workers have shown that the systemic unresponsive state of the host can be prolonged for many months by removing the infused node after 2 to 3 days [242]. Since trace labeling studies indicated that the infused (irradiated) lymphocytes remained in situ in the node, the authors tentatively suggest that at 2 to 3 days postinfusion, the node contains, as a result of ASRL, the host's entire complement of specifically reactive lymphocytes. Whether or not this explanation is correct (other possibilities such as the production of blocking factors or suppressor T cells have yet to be excluded), the data are clearly relevant to the goal of devising a simple method for inducing selective immunosuppression in man.

Large doses of antigen have usually been required to cause ASRL. In mice, to induce a 20-fold reduction in the capacity of TDL to effect specific rejection of skin allografts, it was necessary to preinject the cell donors with massive numbers (6×10^8) of allogeneic lymphocytes [234]. Similarly, ASRL to sRBC in mice was complete only after injection of at least 10^9 cells [231]; with 10^7 sRBC, it was not detectable. Also, the profound degree of ASRL which was observed after passage of parental-strain TDL through irradiated F_1 hybrid rats [236,238] was probably a reflection of the fact that the selecting antigens in this system were provided by the host itself. Relatively small doses of antigen were needed to induce ASRL in the popliteal LN of sheep: complete depletion of MLC-reactive lymphocytes in efferent lymph was observed after injection of 5×10^8 allogeneic lymphocytes into the afferent lymph vessel [222]; this system, nevertheless, must have provided a high local concentration of antigen to the host lymphocytes entering the node. In marked contrast to the above findings, Larner [235] reported a partial suppression of the MLC reactivity of rat PBL after intravenous injection of as few as 3×10^5 allogeneic lymphocytes; why such small doses of antigen were effective in this system is not clear.

The evidence that ASRL is usually only complete after injection of high doses of antigen requires comment. A priori, one might expect even low doses of antigen to induce ASRL. Why, then, was no evidence of ASRL found after injection of mice with 10^7 sRBC (vide supra), i.e., a dose known to be immunogenic? In this respect, it should be pointed out that ASRL was assayed here by collecting TDL from mice injected with varying "selecting" doses of sRBC and transferring the cells in the presence of a constant high dose of antigen (5×10^8 sRBC) into irradiated mice; numbers of antibody-forming cells in spleens of the recipients were then measured 5 to 11 days later. Consequently, it is possible that ASRL was, indeed, induced after injection of 10^7 sRBC but was not evident because the nonselected antigen-reactive cells that remained in the circulation were stimulated with a much higher dose of antigen when tested on transfer. Thus, ASRL after a low selecting dose of antigen might only be demonstrable if a correspondingly small dose of antigen was employed to test the reactivity of the nonselected population that remained in the RLP. This possibility is currently being explored. An additional point of interest would be to determine, in terms of affinity, the specificity of ASRL. It is tempting to speculate that, in accordance with the concept of "immunologic maturation" [243,244], ASRL induced in the presence of antigen at low concentration would affect only lymphocytes carrying receptors of high affinity for the antigen.

Rowley et al. [232] made the interesting observation that ASRL in rats could be prevented by preinjection of antiserum raised against the selecting antigen. It would seem likely that inhibition of ASRL in this situation was a reflection of impaired localization of antigen.

Little is known of the precise movement of cells during the process of selective recruitment. In situations where the immune response is associated with antibody production, B cells probably become sequestered in primary follicles and germinal centers. This notion is likely because these areas are normally traversed by circulating B cells (see Sec. I), are important sites of antibody production [245], and are the predominant region in which cell proliferation occurs in response to T-independent antigens, e.g., pneumococcal polysaccharide [215]. Since the presence of T cells is required for many (T-dependent) antibody responses, does recruitment to sites of antibody production involve both T cells and B cells? T cells characteristically do not enter the B-dependent areas. It is known, nevertheless, that germinal centers, though not primary follicles, do contain appreciable numbers of T cells [246]. This point raises the possibility that the entry of T cells to germinal centers (and/or primary follicles destined to become germinal centers) is restricted to cells recently in contact with antigen. If so, one would expect the T cells present in a particular germinal center to be specifically engaged in the immune response being generated in that area. Although this hypothesis has not yet been proven, it would be in agreement with the view of other workers that T-B cell collaboration probably occurs largely in these areas [246,247].

If antigen-activated T cells do, indeed, migrate to germinal centers during their differentiation to "helper" cells, they probably first undergo blast transformation in the T-dependent areas. In this respect, studies in which thymus cells were exposed to sRBC in irradiated mice showed that, in the spleen, most of the cells which transformed in response to the antigen were located in the PALS [248,249]; these cells were shown in other studies to possess potent helper activity for sRBC [83]. In situations where antigen leads to cell-mediated rather than to humoral responses, the differentiation of T cells to effector cells is probably restricted to the T-dependent areas. For example, in irradiated F_1 mice injected with parental-strain T cells, the marked cell proliferation which precedes the generation of CL is most prominent in the PALS of the spleen and the LN paracortex [250,251]. Similarly, the state of delayed-type hypersensitivity (DTH) which follows skin painting with contact-sensitizing agents is preceded by extensive blast transformation restricted to the paracortex of the draining LN [213].

The mechanism by which lymphocytes are specifically withdrawn from the circulation during antigenic stimulation is a matter for speculation. As suggested elsewhere [252], it is possible that specific contact of lymphocytes with antigen causes subtle changes in the cell surface membrane, changes which lead the cells to alter their normal pattern of migration and home to regions suitable for their differentation into effector cells. In vitro studies have demonstrated that T and B lymphocytes need to be in close contact for several days to obtain optimal antibody responses to T-dependent antigens [253]. If this requirement also applies in vivo, it would follow that a mechanism would be required to immobilize the cells during this stage of the immune response. In this respect, it could be suggested that once antigen-activated lymphocytes have reached areas conducive to antibody production, the changes in their surface membrane become sufficiently extensive to ensure that the cells remain in these areas for several days.

Circumstantial evidence that favors this notion has come from studies on the immune reactivity of spleen cells obtained from mice 1 day after injection of a high dose of sRBC. When these cells were tested in vitro, they gave enhanced responses to sRBC [254], i.e., as would be expected if the injected antigen had induced specific recruitment of lymphocytes to the spleen. Paradoxically, when the cells were adoptively transferred in vivo [252], they failed to respond to sRBC within the first week of transfer, although they responded well to other antigens during this time; this unresponsiveness was shown to affect both T and B cells. Conversely, if the cells were transferred and then left for 5 days before being challenged with antigen, normal or enhanced responses to sRBC were obtained. Although there are several possible explanations for this finding, the fact that the cells responded rapidly in vitro suggests that their temporary incompetence in vivo reflected an alteration in their homing properties. According to this explanation, recently activated lymphocytes introduced into the bloodstream during adoptive transfer would be unable to enter areas conducive to antibody production until their surface membrane changes had reverted to normal. Direct evidence on this point is lacking.

In view of the diversity of the systems considered above, future studies may well show that ASRL is involved in the induction of most, perhaps all, immune responses. For example, although there is no direct evidence that induction of DTH is associated with ASRL, circumstantial evidence makes this association more than likely. As was pointed out by Rowley et al. [232], the observation that development of DTH after intradermal injection of sRBC in

Freund's adjuvant can be prevented by giving a prior intravenous injection of sRBC [255] (an example of "immune deviation" [256]) is most easily explained in terms of ASRL.

B. The Postrecruitment Phase: Entry of Antigen-stimulated Lymphocytes into the Circulation

Two subsets of cells are generated during most immune responses: *effector* cells, whose function is to combat the intruding antigen, either directly or in association with other cell types, and *memory* cells, potentially long-lived cells which determine that subsequent exposure to the antigen will evoke a more vigorous (effective) response than the initial exposure (see Ref. 257).

The terms "effector" cell and "memory" cell are often used loosely. In considering the function and fate of cells generated during the immune response, it is essential to define these terms clearly. In the present context, effector cells will be defined as cells which, without further differentiation, are capable of countering the presence of the antigens which led to their formation. Likewise, memory cells will be regarded as cells which, on reexposure to antigen, require an initial period of differentiation before they can express their function. It is important to point out here that, according to these definitions, the memory state in certain situations could be a reflection of the presence of memory cells, the persistence of effector cells, or both.

Although the relationship between memory cells and effector cells is not clearly understood, in many situations these cells are probably of the same lineage, the functions they display reflecting their stage of differentiation from common precursors (see Ref. 257). Although this hypothesis has not yet been proven, it is consistent with most of the available evidence. Effector cells are probably derived either from nonrecirculating virgin lymphocytes or from recirculating memory lymphocytes, i.e., cells which, according to earlier discussion, are generated through prior contact with either environmental or experimentally injected antigen. This dual origin of effector cells is almost certainly true for the differentiation of B cells (see Sec. II); it is likely to apply also to the T-cell lineage, although this notion has yet to be clearly established. Whether effector cells differentiate to memory cells is uncertain.

1. T Lymphocytes

a. Effector Cells. It has already been mentioned that T cells comprise at least three subpopulations which collectively express a multiplicity of effector functions. Whether each function is unique to one particular type of T cell or whether one T cell can express more than one effector function is uncertain. For example, although the cells which mediate DTH and act as helper cells for antibody production both have the Ly-1$^+$ phenotype, it should not be concluded that these two functions are necessarily a property of the same T cell; future discovery of additional T cell markers might well show that different cells are involved.

It is probable (though unproven) that in all situations in which T effector functions are manifested, the immune response of T cells is essentially similar: that initial contact with antigen leads to ASRL, which causes the local production of effector T cells which migrate soon afterward into the circulation. Several examples of this pathway of T-cell differentiation are considered below.

(1) Transplantation Immunity. Sensitization to transplantation antigens has been the subject of several extensive reviews (e.g., Refs. 1, 258, and 259). It is generally considered that sensitization to conventional skin allografts occurs centrally, i.e., in the LN draining the graft site; thus, sensitization is very limited unless the lymphatic supply from the graft site is intact [260, 261]. As suggested by Burwell [214], it is probable that the characteristic cellular changes which develop in the draining LN represent a response to antigenic material released from the graft (see also the work of Hall [262]). After extensive proliferation of lymphocytes in the draining nodes, large numbers of blast cells enter the efferent lymphatic vessels after about 4 days [262]. Cells capable of causing specific graft rejection on adoptive transfer appear in the blood after 5 days [263]. Rejection of the sensitizing graft probably results from the random entry of small numbers of these cells into the graft site from the bloodstream [264]. Of the rejection process itself, however, little is known.

In situations where the blood vessels of the allograft are anastomosed directly with vessels of the host, sensitization appears to occur peripherally [237,265]. Such grafts rapidly become infiltrated with blast cells; after several days, large numbers of these cells leave the graft via veins and lymphatic vessels.

Miller's observation [266] that NTx mice are unable to reject skin allografts established the importance of T cells in transplantation immunity. Information on the differentiation of effector cells to transplantation antigens has come from studies on the response of parental-strain T cells (thymus or TDL) to the alloantigens present in irradiated F_1 hybrid rats [1,267] and mice [135,250,251,268]. In both species, the donor T cells were shown to proliferate extensively in the spleen and LN of the host [250,267]. Within the first 3 days of T-cell transfer to mice, the thoracic duct lymph of the recipients contained very few cells [135]. By the use of specific alloantisera, these cells were found to consist almost entirely of radioresistant host lymphocytes. Less than 5% of the cells were labeled when the hosts were pulsed repeatedly with [^{3}H]TdR from the time of cannulation. After 3 to 4 days, however, large numbers of lymphocytes emerged, of which 60 to 80% were pyroninophilic blasts and 95% were labeled. By use of appropriate antisera, 95% or more of the cells present in the lymph at this time were shown to be of donor origin and had the characteristic features of T lymphocytes; they were thus christened "T-TDL."

Studies on the immunologic properties of T-TDL [251,268,269] indicated that the cells responded only to the antigens which provoked their formation, i.e., the alloantigens of the host. This finding applied to their capacity to respond in MLC in vitro or in vivo, to reject skin allografts carried by "B" mice, to lyse allogeneic tumor cells in vitro, and to suppress the growth of allogeneic tumor cells in "B" mice; T-TDL, unlike normal T cells, were unable to act as helper cells for the response of "B" mice to the T-dependent antigen, fowl γ globulin (FγG). These data strongly suggested that T-TDL represent an expanded population of effector cells generated from T cells in the original donor cell inoculum which had specificity for the host antigens. The capacity of T-TDL to cause rapid lysis of appropriate target cells complies with the definition of effector function considered above. It is probable that their ability to reject skin allografts also falls within this definition, since graft rejection occurred more rapidly than with normal T cells, and because there is evidence, which will be considered later, that T-TDL have only a very limited capacity for further differentiation when reexposed to antigen soon after activation.

It is evident from the above studies that selective recruitment of host-reactive lymphocytes from the donor cell inoculum occurred at some time before 3 to 4 days, i.e., prior to the appearance of T-TDL in the circulation. It was not possible to prove this point, however, because the donor cells in the lymph before this time were present in only extremely small numbers. This was not surprising since, with TDL as donor cells, a total of only 2×10^6 cells were injected. In rats, Ford and Atkins [236] circumvented this difficulty by injecting the donor TDL in very large numbers (2×10^9). This massive injection enabled the authors to recover sufficient numbers of donor-type lymphocytes from thoracic duct lymph of the host to test their reactivity to the host antigens on transfer. ASRL in this situation (measured by a GVH assay) was evident between 12 and 36 hr of cell injection; similar results have since been obtained in mice [234]. Subsequently, the recirculating donor cells partly regained their reactivity to the host antigens; this return in reactivity corresponded with the appearance of large numbers of blast cells in the lymph.

(2) Helper Cells. With a double adoptive transfer system, Miller and Mitchell [83] demonstrated that thymus cells, activated in the presence of T-dependent antigens in spleens of syngeneic irradiated mice, would stimulate B cells to produce specific antibody to these antigens. More recent studies with this system have shown that specific helper cells can be recovered not only from spleen but also from thoracic duct lymph [270]. For example, with keyhole limpet hemocyanin (KLH) as the activating antigen, the cells obtained from lymph after 4 to 5 days were three- to 12-fold more effective

than those from spleen at promoting antibody production in vitro by DNP-primed B cells; help was specific, in that antibody production occurred in the presence of DNP-KLH, but not with DNP-FγG.

Similar results were also obtained with a different system. Whereas thoracic duct lymph of normal mice injected 1 to 2 days previously with a high dose of sRBC contained virtually no cells capable of responding to this antigen on adoptive transfer, cells collected after 3 days gave normal antibody responses [230]. By 5 days, the response was markedly enhanced. The response to unrelated antigens during this time remained unchanged or gradually decreased. Since the antibody response to sRBC is T dependent, these findings suggest that, after the period of ASRL, specifically reactive helper T lymphocytes reenter the circulation after about 3 days.

Can the helper T cells in the above studies be regarded as effector cells? Feldmann and Basten [271] demonstrated that T cells from spleens of mice primed several months before to sRBC (memory T cells) failed to express helper activity when cultured in vitro in the presence of antiproliferative drugs, e.g., mitomycin C. Such drugs, however, had no effect on the helper activity of "activated" T cells, i.e., T cells obtained from spleens of irradiated mice injected 6 days before with thymus cells and sRBC. It would seem highly likely that this apparent capacity of these cells to express their function without further differentiation was shared by the T cells which entered the circulation in the two studies considered above; if so, such cells could be regarded as effector cells rather than as memory cells.

(3) Delayed-type Hypersensitivity. Several studies collectively provide strong evidence that the state of systemic DTH which follows the local application of certain sensitizing agents results from dissemination of lymphocytes activated in the regional LN (reviewed in Ref. 272). Turk and Stone [273] demonstrated that by the fourth day after sensitization, the draining LN contained cells capable of transferring sensitivity adoptively. At later stages, sensitized cells were detected in peripheral blood [274] and thoracic duct lymph [275,276]. Development of DTH was prevented if the draining LN were excised before 4 days but not at later times [273]. Eltringham and Weissman [277] showed that DTH could be prevented by heavy local irradiation of the nodes; for reasons not clearly apparent, this procedure was effective when administered between 6 and 8 days but not at 3 to 5 days.

The cells that mediate DTH qualify as effector cells, in that treatment with antiproliferative drugs does not appear to suppress their function [278]. Evidence from several sources indicates that these cells are activated T lymphocytes [279-282] which can migrate nonspecifically to sites of inflammation [283]; they manifest nonspecific cytotoxicity in vitro [284].

(4) Immunity to Bacteria, Viruses, and Parasites. Evidence that circulating T cells play a role in bacterial immunity has come largely from work

on rodents infected with *Listeria monocytogenes.* McGregor and his colleagues [285-290] demonstrated that TDL from rats infected with *L. monocytogenes* 1 week previously conferred immunity to this organism on adoptive transfer to noninfected rats. The protective effect of TDL collected at this time appeared to be mediated by recently divided nonrecirculating lymphocytes which showed a propensity to home nonspecifically to sites of inflammation. Most of these cells were probably T cells, since they could not be demonstrated in infected TxBM rats. In mice, other workers have demonstrated that immunity to *L. monocytogenes* is determined by rapidly dividing, short-lived θ-positive lymphocytes [282,291-294]. The mechanism by which these cells destroy or inactivate bacteria is unknown.

Little is known of the identity of cells which participate in immune responses to viruses. T cells appear to be involved in certain situations, e.g., in the response of mice to Sindbis virus [295]. After subcutaneous injection of this virus, the regional LN contained cells which mounted a proliferative response when exposed to the virus in vitro. These cells were first detected at 2 to 4 days after inoculation, reached maximal levels by 6 days, and disappeared after 16 days. Pretreatment of the cells with anti-θ serum before culture greatly reduced their proliferative response; treatment with anti-immunoglobulin antiserum, by contrast, was ineffective. Cells responsive to the virus first appeared in the spleen at 6 days postinoculation and reached peak levels after 10 to 13 days. The response of spleen cells, however, was always much less than that of cells from the regional LN. These data imply that, as with other antigens, lymphocytes were specifically recruited to the LN, proliferated there in response to the virus, and then reentered the circulation. Although it was not demonstrated that these virus-activated T cells expressed effector function, it is now well documented that in many different viral infections, T cells harvested from the spleen exert specific cell-mediated lympholysis against target cells bearing the infecting virus (reviewed in Ref. 295a).

According to Ogilvie and Jones [296], immunity to all helminths studied so far is T dependent. Thus, immunity to these parasites is reduced by such procedures as neonatal thymectomy, treatment with ALS, or thymectomy combined with CTDD. The precise role played by T cells in helminthic infection has not yet been elucidated. From work on rats infected with *Nippostrongylus brasiliensis,* Ogilvie and Jones concluded that "the adult worms are expelled by a complex mechanism which requires the sequential action of antibodies and sensitized lymphocytes"; they speculated that the sensitized cells act by releasing lymphokines which interfere with the metabolism of the worms. Whether immunity to parasites other than helminths is T dependent has not yet been established.

Eosinophilia is often a feature of parasitic infection. While the function of these cells is controversial [297], their production, at least in certain situations, appears to be T dependent. Basten et al. [298,299] observed that in rats infected with the nematode *Trichinella spiralis,* eosinophilia was marked in normal rats but very limited in NTx rats or rats treated with ALS and/or CTDD. The eosinophilia in normal rats was associated with the appearance of large numbers of blast cells in thoracic duct lymph. These cells, unlike normal TDL, induced eosinophilia on adoptive transfer to noninfected rats. This effect was shown to be mediated by the blast cells in the population and was observed even when the cells were enclosed in cell-impermeable diffusion chambers. Although the identity of these cells was not established, it would seem highly probable that they were T cells.

b. Memory Cells. Direct information on memory carried by recirculating T cells is limited. Of necessity, the following discussion is restricted to a consideration of memory to foreign proteins and transplantation antigens.

(1) Nontransplantation Antigens. A variety of approaches have demonstrated that, in such organs as the spleen, memory to T-dependent antigens is expressed by both T cells and B cells [300-304]. Evidence that recirculating T cells carry memory arose from studies on the relative helper activity of T cells obtained from thoracic duct lymph of primed and unprimed mice [301]: T cells from mice primed 2 months previously to FγG were, cell for cell, 10 times more effective at stimulating antibody production by FγG-primed B cells on adoptive transfer than were T cells from normal mice or mice primed with another antigen. From this and other evidence, it was concluded that memory in the T-cell lineage constitutes an increase in the numbers of T cells in the RLP with reactivity to the antigen concerned. This view is supported by the observation that memory to the T-dependent antigen TIGAL (a synthetic polypeptide) is associated with increased numbers of antigen-binding T cells (in spleen) [305]. Whether T-cell memory also reflects qualitative changes in the antigen-reactive cells is unknown, although evidence that the avidity with which T cells bind antigen does not increase after priming [306,307] is against this possibility. It is probable that recirculating T memory cells, like other recirculating lymphocytes, are long-lived cells. Definite evidence on this point, however, is lacking. Thus, although the above studies on memory to FγG are consistent with T memory cells having a long life-span, they do not exclude the possibility that the cells, in fact, were recently generated through exposure to antigen that persisted from the time of immunization.

(2) Transplantation Antigens. Memory to major transplantation antigens is difficult to define (see Ref. 259). It is well accepted that allograft rejection leads to a state of sensitization where a second graft is rejected with an accelerated tempo. Allosensitization by skin grafting or transfer of lymphoid cells, however, has little or no effect on the capacity of recirculating lymphocytes to induce GVH reactions [308] or respond in MLC [259]. This paradoxical observation has stimulated intensive investigation of the genetic control of transplantation immunity.

A variety of evidence suggests that the majority of cells which proliferate in the MLR are not the precursors of effector cells [309-316]. Thus, with certain mouse strain combinations, lymphoid cells may give high responses in the MLR, yet fail to differentiate into CL [310,313]; with other strain combinations, by contrast, CL may be generated in the absence of a strong MLR [313]. In the mouse, the antigenic determinants responsible for allograft rejection and cell-mediated lympholysis (CML) are coded for predominantly by the K and D regions of the *H-2* complex [314,315]. These determinants are closely related to those which stimulate the production of classic *H-2* alloantibody and therefore have been termed "serologically defined" (SD) [310]. Stimuli for the MLR and GVH reactions, by contrast, are controlled largely by the *I* region of the *H-2* complex [314,315]; MLR can also be elicited by (non-H2-linked) *M* locus differences [317]. MLR and GVH determinants have been referred to as "lymphocyte defined" (LD) [310], since, unlike SD determinants, they seem to be expressed predominantly by lymphoid cells. From this evidence, Bach et al. [311] have proposed that lymphocytes responsible for producing allograft rejection and CML (SD-reactive cells) have a different specificity from those involved in the MLR and GVH reactions (LD-reactive cells).

While, broadly speaking, this notion is probably correct, recent evidence suggests that the LD-SD classification will require modification. For example, it is now known that antisera can be raised against *I*-region determinants [318]. Furthermore, certain *I*-region determinants induce strong rejection of skin allografts and also stimulate CML (provided that B blasts are used as targets, *I*-region determinants being expressed strongly on B cells but not on T cells) [319]. For these reasons it may prove more convenient in future to refer to the subsets of H-2 reactive lymphocytes in terms of their Ly phenotype. [It was mentioned in an earlier section that CL and the cells that respond in MLC express different surface Ly antigens (Ly-23$^+$ and Ly-1$^+$, respectively)].

The generation of T-TDL might be considered a suitable model for studying the differentiation and fate of T cells that carry memory for alloantigens. In fact, the information provided by this model has proved difficult to interpret. For this reason, however, it may be of heuristic value to consider the results obtained in some detail. Most of the work with this model has involved the activation of CBA (H-2^k) thymus cells to the alloantigens present in irradiated [CBA × C57BL (H-2^b)] F_1 or [CBA × DBA/2 (H-2^d)] F_1 mice. With these recipients, the injected T cells encounter determinants that differ at the *K, I,* and *D* regions of the *H-2* complex.

When T-TDL labeled with ^{51}Cr were transferred intravenously, their distribution in the lymphoid tissues differed from that of TDL [135,320]. Within 4 hr of injection, both populations were found predominantly in the spleen. Whereas TDL then became redistributed to the lymph nodes, T-TDL localized predominantly in the intestines. The reduced capacity of T-TDL to home to lymph nodes (fourfold less than with TDL), however, did not interfere with their capacity to recirculate.

Thus, when T-TDL were labeled in vivo with [^{3}H]TdR and transferred intravenously to syngeneic recipients, approximately 50% of the injected labeled cells appeared in thoracic duct lymph over a period of 2 days [135]. Similar numbers of labeled cells were collected from the lymph of mice injected with [^{3}H]TdR-labeled normal TDL. Thus, within the first 2 days of transfer, T-TDL resembled normal TDL in being able to recirculate rapidly between blood and lymph soon after transfer.[13] Subsequently, however, most T-TDL soon left the RLP. This was established by injecting mice with T-TDL or TDL labeled either with [^{3}H]TdR or ^{51}Cr and collecting TDL from the recipients at various times thereafter [322]. With [^{3}H]TdR-labeled cells (detected by autoradiography), numbers of labeled cells in TDL from recipients of T-TDL declined much more rapidly than in mice given TDL. By 3 weeks posttransfer, the recovery of labeled cells from recipients of T-TDL was 17-fold less than with TDL. Similar results were obtained with recipients of ^{51}Cr-labeled cells (detected by scintillation counting). Radioactive counts in TDL from recipients of ^{51}Cr-labeled T-TDL declined 22-fold between 1 and 10 days post-transfer. In recipients of labeled TDL, by contrast, the decrease in counts over this period was only threefold.

An objection to the above approach is that some of the transferred cells might have proliferated. If so, with [^{3}H]TdR-labeled cells, this proliferation would have led to dilution of grain counts to below background levels. Labeling with ^{51}Cr is reported to inhibit the capacity of cells to proliferate [323]; whether this inhibition leads to cell death and/or loss of label is not known. To answer this objection, the θ antigen was used as a cell marker, i.e., a marker known to be retained by proliferating cells. It was calculated that in "B" mice given T-TDL 1 month previously, the total numbers of θ-positive cells collected from lymph of the recipients over 12 hr represented 8% of the number of T-TDL (>99% θ-positive) originally injected [322]. This figure compared with a recovery of 59% at this time for recipients of TDL. Although the ratio of these recoveries was similar to that found with radiolabeled cells, the absolute recoveries were much higher. This finding suggested therefore that a proportion of the T-TDL which remained in the RLP for several weeks did, indeed, undergo proliferation during this time. Why this proliferation should have occurred is obscure. It was not unique to T-TDL, however, since proliferation was no less evident in recipients of TDL.

Collectively, these data showed that T-TDL joined the RLP for several days but, unlike normal TDL, most then disappeared. This disappearance could either have reflected cell death or withdrawal of cells from the RLP to other tissue compartments. Since autoradiographs from recipients of [^{3}H]TdR-labeled T-TDL showed a rapid disappearance of labeled cells from all organs examined [320], cell death seemed the most likely possibility. While showing that cells survive on transfer is relatively easy, proving that they die is more difficult. The approach used here was to study the migratory properties of labeled cells recovered from the spleens of mice given T-TDL labeled with ^{51}Cr. This approach was based on the fact that when ^{51}Cr-labeled cells die in the lymphoid tissues, their label becomes associated with a class of cell which, on secondary transfer, becomes localized in the liver, not in the lymphoid tissues; these cells are presumably phagocytes. With this system, it was concluded that of ^{51}Cr-labeled T-TDL which homed to the spleen, most died in situ between 1 and 10 days posttransfer. Cell death in recipients of labeled TDL, by contrast, was minimal during this time.

Although cell death seemed to be the most likely explanation for the rapid disappearance of T-TDL from the RLP, there was also evidence that a small number of cells were excreted via the intestines. Studies with cells labeled with [^3H]TdR or ^{51}Cr all showed that a large proportion of T-TDL (>20%) localized in the intestines on transfer [320]. Of these cells, scintillation counting indicated that approximately 40% were situated in Peyer's patches (compared with >70% for TDL). Autoradiography showed that the cells were concentrated in the T-dependent areas, although they were not restricted to these areas. Labeled cells were also present in the adjacent lamina propria, and some were situated within the surface epithelium. Intraepithelial lymphocytes, or "theliolymphocytes" [324], have been described by several workers [324-326]. Most are probably T cells, since they are rare in nude mice [327] and stain with antisera raised against "mouse-specific lymphocyte antigen (MSLA)," a marker held to be specific for T lymphocytes [328]. Intraepithelial lymphocytes have a rapid turnover: more than 70% were shown to be labeled within 3 days in mice continuously infused with [^3H]TdR [326]. The fate of these cells is controversial. Some workers claim that they migrate into the gut lumen [325]. Others refute this possibility and prefer to consider the epithelial lining of the gut as the mammalian equivalent of the avian bursa [324]. To examine the first possibility, levels of radioactivity were measured in the intestinal contents flushed from recipients of ^{51}Cr-labeled T-TDL [320]. At 1 to 2 days postinjection, the counts detected, though very low (0.3% of those injected), were five- to sixfold higher than in recipients of labeled TDL. This finding suggested that a small proportion of T-TDL did, indeed, migrate into the gut lumen, presumably via the surface epithelium.

It should be emphasized that although most T-TDL soon left the RLP, studies with [^3H]TdR-labeled cells showed that a small number continued to recirculate for at least 3 months. Did these lymphocytes represent memory cells? This possibility was investigated by transferring either T-TDL or TDL to syngeneic "B" mice and testing the immune reactivity of TDL or spleen cells harvested from the recipients 4 to 6 weeks later [329]. Three parameters were used: the MLR, GVH reaction, and allograft rejection.

With respect to the MLR and GVH reactions, TDL from recipients of T-TDL gave significant responses when confronted with the determinants to which the cells had originally been activated; responses against third-party determinants were very low. The response against the activating determinants was lower than that obtained with TDL from "B" mice injected with TDL. When the number of θ-positive cells in the two harvested TDL populations was considered, however, the specific response of TDL from T-TDL-injected mice was comparable to or slightly above that of TDL from TDL-injected mice, both for the MLR and GVH reaction.

Allograft rejection was assessed by studying the capacity of TDL from T-TDL-injected mice to suppress the growth of allogeneic tumor cells in sublethally irradiated mice. (The TDL were mixed with the tumor and injected subcutaneously; the recipients were syngeneic with the TDL.) TDL from TDL-injected mice gave poor protection against the growth of the tumor. By contrast, TDL from mice given T-TDL conferred excellent protection, even at lymphocyte:tumor cell ratios as low as 2:1. This protection was specific and exceeded that of passaged TDL by 30- to 50-fold; it was also T-cell dependent, i.e., was abrogated by treatment with anti-θ serum. Whether protection resulted from the differentiation into cytotoxic lymphocytes was not ascertained. With respect to this point, however, it should be mentioned that, unlike T-TDL per se, TDL from T-TDL-injected mice were not directly cytotoxic for the tumor cells in vitro.

These findings indicated that transfer of T-TDL to "B" mice induced marked qualitative changes in their properties. With regard to allograft rejection, the cells retained their capacity for suppressing the growth of tumor cells in vivo but not for direct lysis of these cells in vitro. In MLC, the kinetics of the response of the passaged T-TDL were similar to those of normal or passaged TDL; i.e., the response developed slowly and peaked after 4 to 6 days. This finding was in striking contrast to the response of T-TDL before passage. In this respect, when T-TDL per se were reexposed to the host antigens in MLC, up to 25% synthesized DNA rapidly and specifically [269]. These responding cells failed to divide, however, and soon reverted from blasts to small lymphocytes. This failure to divide seemed to account for the fact that DNA synthesis in the cultures as a whole reached a maximum on Day 2 but was no longer detectable after Day 3. The "MLR" of T-TDL before passage therefore did not appear to denote proliferation but simply asynchronous entry of a large proportion of the cells into DNA synthesis. This anomalous behavior of the cells may have been related to the fact that T-TDL were unable to induce GVH reactions before passage, even at high doses [251]. While the pathogenesis of GVH disease is not clearly understood, its development appears to depend, at least to some extent, on division of the grafted cells [271,330]. This notion would imply that the inability of T-TDL to induce GVH disease reflected exhaustion of their potential to proliferate. The simplest explanation for the capacity of T-TDL passaged through "B" mice to produce GVH reactions and a "normal" MLR might thus be that adoptive transfer allowed the cells to recover their proliferative potential.

Since cells from T-TDL-injected mice were no more effective at producing GVH reactions or responding in MLC than were cells from mice given TDL, there was no evidence for the production of a state of memory to LD determinants. This finding is consistent with the observation mentioned previously that allosensitization to major histocompatibility (AgB) determinants fails to alter the number of lymphocytes that respond to the sensitizing cells in MLC [259]. Furthermore, there is only minimal alteration in the capacity of TDL to evoke GVH reactions [308]; indeed, the "factor of immunization" for this reaction may be less than unity. This situation is in striking contrast to that with minor histocompatibility determinants, where the factor of immunization may be enormous [308]. The one exception to the apparent lack of memory to LD determinants is the finding of Howard and Wilson [259,331] on the fate of blast cells generated from rat TDL during an MLR against AgB determinants in vitro. When the blasts were transferred to syngeneic "B" rats, TDL harvested from the recipients several weeks later gave high and specific responses against the sensitizing determinants in MLC. In contrast to the present studies with T-TDL, these responses were much higher than those with TDL from "B" rats preinjected with similar numbers of TDL. To account for the discrepancy between these findings and the data obtained with T-TDL is clearly difficult, particularly since the two populations were generated with different systems and in different species.

The finding that cells from T-TDL-injected mice were far superior at suppressing the growth of allogeneic tumor cells than were cells from TDL-injected mice indicated excellent memory for the determinants that control allograft rejection. This finding is consistent with the observation of Billingham et al. [263] that allosensitization, i.e., by skin grafting, greatly increased the capacity of cells from blood or draining LN to cause specific rejection of skin allografts borne by tolerant mice; the sensitized cells appeared at about 6 days after grafting and persisted for 1 year or more. Since, in recipients of T-TDL, the protective cells resided within the RLP and were not directly cytotoxic, these data suggest that, as with nontransplantation antigens, memory to allograft determinants is carried by a population of clonally expanded, long-lived recirculating lymphocytes. This suggestion should not be taken to imply that all cells that control allosensitization reside within the RLP. With most regimes used to induce allosensitization, e.g., skin grafting or injection of allogeneic tumor cells, the sensitizing antigens probably persist for long periods, thus leading to local retention of the responding cells and constant production of effector cells. Such retention might explain the failure of prolonged thoracic duct drainage to abrogate allosensitization induced by skin grafting [1]. Alternatively, sensitization in this situation could be maintained by a class of long-lived, nonrecirculating effector cells that persist in the absence of antigen. Some support for this possibility comes from the report of Häyry and Andersson [332]. These workers observed that when blast cells generated during an MLR in vitro were transferred to TxBM mice, cells capable of mediating direct CML were found in the spleen for several weeks but were not detectable in lymph nodes.

In toto, the data on the fate of T-TDL can be interpreted from two points of view. According to the hypothesis of Bach et al. [311], it can be argued that since T-TDL were raised between strains that differed at the *K, I,* and *D* regions of the *H-2* complex, the activated lymphocytes comprised a mixture of cells reactive either to SD or LD determinants, with LD-reactive cells predominating. On transfer, there was selective survival of the SD-reactive component, most of these cells differentiating into long-lived lymphocytes carrying memory for allograft determinants. The majority of the LD-reactive cells died soon after injection, a few surviving cells accounting for the residual activity of the host against MLR and GVH determinants. Conversely, all of the LD-reactive cells might have died, the reactivity against MLR and GVH determinants being mediated by the (clonally expanded) SD-reactive population.

Alternatively, the data could be interpreted in terms of the view of Wilson et al. [259] that lymphocytes that mediate responses to major H determinants have a common origin, their manifold functions reflecting simply their stage of differentation after contact with antigen. These workers envisage that cells deprived of continuous stimulation with antigen either die or revert to quiescent precursors (cells able to respond in MLR). According to this view, the function of the few descendents of T-TDL which survived after transfer to a neutral environment should have been qualitatively similar to that of normal unstimulated T cells (passaged TDL). The fact that this was not the case makes the data difficult to interpret from this point of view.

The important question of the Ly phenotype of the descendents of T-TDL recovered from "B" mice has yet to be investigated. Clearly one might predict a high enrichment for Ly-23$^+$ cells. In this respect, preliminary studies suggest that, like TDL, T-TDL tested before passage consist predominantly of Ly-1$^+$ and Ly-123$^+$ cells with smaller numbers of Ly-23$^+$ cells [42e].

2. *B Lymphocytes*

a. Effector Cells. The effector cells of the B-cell lineage consist of antibody-forming cells (AFC). Antibody production is a feature of nearly all immune responses, including those due to infection with microorganisms and parasites [333-335].

Evidence was considered in Sec. IV.A that B-cell immune responses, like

T-cell responses, are initiated in regions of antigen concentration. After ASRL to these regions, differentiation of B lymphocytes to AFC proceeds rapidly. AFC are detectable in the spleen within 2 to 3 days of intravenous injection of antigen and at a similar time in the regional LN after subcutaneous injection [169,209,336-338]. Small numbers of AFC appear shortly afterward in the bloodstream [339-342].

When LN are involved in the immune response, AFC also appear in the central lymph [341,343]. Although these cells are rarely present in large numbers (as assayed by the Jerne technique [337]), the lymph at this time frequently contains large numbers of blast cells [343,344-348]. The identity of these cells is uncertain. Studies of Hay et al. [346,347] in sheep suggest that many synthesize antibody but in quantities insufficient to be detectable by conventional techniques. By electron microscopy, they demonstrated that after injection of horseradish peroxidase into the area drained by the popliteal LN, up to two thirds of the blast cells that appeared in the efferent lymph contained intracytoplasmic antibody specific for this antigen. Most of these cells had features of plasmablasts; i.e., they contained scattered short segments of endoplasmic reticulum; typical plasma cells were rare. Whether these findings are applicable to the blast cells generated in response to other antigens and in species other than the sheep has not yet been established.

TDL of unstimulated mice [36] and rats [1] normally contain 2 to 10% large lymphocytes. Morphologically, these cells closely resemble the blast cells generated during antigenic stimulation [349]. Most large lymphocytes seem to be of B-cell origin, since they contain varying amounts of endoplasmic reticulum and intracellular immunoglobulin, particularly IgA [64,350,351]. In mice, less than 10% are θ positive [82]. Large lymphocytes are less common in specific-pathogen-free animals. Their presence therefore probably reflects the natural turnover of B cells that respond to environmental antigens [351]. Since the daily productionof large lymphocytes is high in "B" mice [82] and rats [351], the turnover of these cells (which is very rapid) is probably largely independent of T cells.[14]

The above data suggest that plasmablasts account for most of the large lymphocytes in the central lymph, both in normal and in antigen-stimulated animals. The fate of these "B blasts" has been studied by several approaches. Intravenous injection of [^{3}H]TdR-labeled large lymphocytes from normal rats showed that very few of the cells were able to recirculate [39]. Autoradiography indicated that most of the cells migrated to the lamina propria of the intestines, where they differentiated into typical plasma cells [351]. A more quantitative approach is to label cells in vitro with [^{125}I]UdR and measure radioactivity levels in whole organs from the recipients. Hall and his coworkers, who pioneered this approach, showed that up to 40% of lymph-borne blast cells from antigen-stimulated rats homed to the small intestine [352-355]. Localization in the spleen, LN, and large intestine was much lower. Similar results have since been obtained with lymph-borne cells from normal mice [320]. When these cells were treated with anti-θ serum before labeling, approximately 20% of the injected cells localized in the small intestine (higher than in any other region). Of these cells, nearly all probably settled in the lamina propria of the gut, since more than 90% of the counts were situated in regions outside Peyer's patches. Since radioactivity levels decline very rapidly in recipients of [^{125}I]UdR-labeled B blasts, most of the cells probably die within a few days of injection.

As with T blasts, the factors that control the localization of B blasts in the intestines are unknown. The possibility that intestinal localization might be influenced by antigens that enter from the gut is unlikely, since B blasts have been shown to home to the small intestine of unsuckled neonatal rats delivered by cesarean section [356] and also to fetal gut implanted subcutaneously in adults [328,354,357], i.e., situations where the antigen content of the gut would presumably be very low.

Studies of Guy-Grand et al. [328] suggest that the expression of surface-bound IgA may control the homing of B blasts to the gut. They demonstrated that while IgA-positive blasts homed in large numbers to the lamina propria, blasts that carried either IgG or IgM were unable to localize in the gut and preferentially localized in the spleen and LN. They suggested that the secretory component of IgA, which is synthesized in the gut and binds to IgA, might play a role in attracting the cells to the lamina propria.

The above studies indicate that B blasts have certain properties in common with T blasts. Both cell types, for example, appear to be short-lived and home predominantly to the intestines after intravenous injection. As summarized in Table 1, however, it should be emphasized that T and B blasts show distinct differences in their properties, particularly in their capacity to recirculate and the regions of the intestines in which they localize.

b. Memory Cells. Priming with antigen is known to induce memory in B cells found not only in the secondary lymphoid organs, e.g., the spleen [300,302,303,358,359], but also in TDL [117,301]. Indeed, as mentioned earlier (see Sec. II), it is probable that most long-lived B memory cells reside in the RLP. The sequence of events which leads to the generation of B memory cells is not clearly understood. The work of Strober suggests that when short-lived, nonrecirculating virgin B cells encounter antigen, they are driven to generate long-lived, recirculating B memory cells (see Sec. II). B-cell memory might thus be envisaged simply as a relative expansion and persistence of cells with reactivity to the antigen in question (see also Refs. 243 and 360); this notion would be consistent with evidence that immunization leads to an increase in numbers of specific antigen-binding B cells [307]. According to this explanation, the specificity of B memory cells would not be expected to differ qualitatively from that of unprimed cells.

TABLE 1
Properties of Small and Blast T and B Lymphocytes

Cells	Capacity to Recirculate	Speed of Recirculation	Localization After Intravenous Injection				Average Life-span
			Spleen	Lymph nodes	Small Intestine (distribution)	Large Intestine	
Small T lymphocytes	++++	Fast	++++	+++	++ (Peyer's patches)	+	Many months
T blasts	++++	Fast	+++	+	+++ (Peyer's patches, adjacent lamina propria and surface epithelium)	++	Several days
Small B lymphocytes	++(rats) +(mice)	?Slow ?Fast but infrequent	++++	+	+ (Peyer's patches)	+	>1 Month (but less than T cells)
B blasts	+	Fast	++	+	+++ (lamina propria)	+	Several days

Three lines of evidence might be considered to be inconsistent with this view.

1. Studies on the adoptive antibody response of mice to FγG indicated that small numbers (10^5) of primed T cells would stimulate primed B cells [301]; primed T cells in such numbers failed to stimulate unprimed B cells, however, even when the latter were transferred in large numbers.

2. Evidence from several sources suggests that, in certain forms of tolerance, unresponsiveness may be a reflection of a suppressive action exerted by T cells (reviewed in Ref. 361). Recent studies have shown that while such "suppressor" T cells (obtained from mice that exhibit high-zone tolerance to FγG) fail to induce unprimed B cells to produce antibody, they will, at least in small numbers, stimulate optimal antibody production by primed B cells [362].

3. Populations of primed B cells have, on the average, a higher avidity of antigen binding [307] and produce higher-affinity antibody [243] than do unprimed B cells.

While these data clearly suggest that qualitative differences exist between primed and unprimed B-cell populations, they do not necessarily imply that B memory cells differ qualitatively from their precursors. Indeed, the above-mentioned differences might be explained by the concept of immunologic maturation, namely, that memory cells are selectively generated from the few unprimed precursor cells which express receptors of high affinity for the antigen in question (see Sec. IV.A). The observed differences in the sensitivity of primed and unprimed B-cell populations to the helper activity of T cells might thus be a reflection of parallel differences in the affinity of the responding cells in the two populations. Consideration of this possibility clearly begs the question of the fundamental nature of T-B cell collaboration.

Although TDL are known to express B-cell memory within a few weeks of priming [117,301], the time at which these cells first enter the circulation is unknown. This phenomenon may well occur more slowly than with T cells: Cunningham and Sercarz [302] observed that, in mice primed with sRBC, B-cell memory in the spleen was very limited within a week of priming but then increased gradually over the next 2 months.

As with T cells, little direct evidence is available on the life-span of recirculating B memory cells. TDL from mice show typical secondary adoptive antibody responses for several months after priming [142,301]. This finding, however, does not necessarily imply that memory cells generated during the primary response survive in interphase until antigen challenge; persistence of antigen might maintain the cells in a state of slow turnover. This problem could be avoided by studying the duration of memory in recipients of primed

TDL, i.e., a population where carry-over of antigen would be negligible. By use of this approach in rats, Ellis and Gowans [363] demonstrated that when TDL from rats primed with tetanus toxoid were transferred without antigen to irradiated intermediate hosts, TDL collected from these hosts 4 weeks later gave secondary adoptive responses to the antigen.

Acknowledgments

I wish to thank Drs. J. F. A. P. Miller and W. L. Ford for their valuable comments on this review. I am also indebted to the following members of the Basel Institute for Immunology for their helpful advice and criticism: Drs. H. von Boehmer, R. N. P. Cahill, L. Hudson, L. Lafleur, I. Lefkovits, B. Kindred, M. Nabholz, and G. Roelants. I am most grateful to Miss P. Hamilton for typing the manuscript.

Notes

1. Although only about 1% of spleen cells from nude or TxBM since stain with anti-θ antisera raised in mice, 20% or more show weak staining with antisera raised in rabbits against mouse brain (some brain cells being θ-positive) [42a]. A variety of evidence suggests that these "θ^{+weak}" cells may represent or be derived from prethymic stem cells [42b]. Such findings imply that the stem cells which enter the thymus are not strictly pluripotential but are precomitted to T cell differentiation.

2. LN homing may be delayed in situations where a large proportion of the injected cells localize initially in the lungs, e.g., with the injection LN cells into rats [73].

3. Studies on mice treated with the bone-seeking isotope ^{89}Sr indicate that B-cell differentiation can still proceed despite ablation of the marrow [106]. This finding cannot be said to disprove that in *normal* adult mice, the marrow is the chief source of B cells.

4. Studies of Droege and Zucker [126] suggest that there is a third subpopulation which exerts a suppressive effect on other T cells.

5. Recent studies of Pearson et al. [154a] challenge this hypothesis. These workers reported finding large numbers of small lymphocytes in thoracic duct lymph of fetal lambs cannulated in utero, i.e., in an environment essentially free of exogenous antigen. The majority of the TDL were probably T cells since thymectomy reduced their number by 75%. Of particular interest was the finding that the cells were able to recirculate after intravenous injection. The authors therefore concluded from these findings that the formation of the RLP does not depend critically upon the presence of antigen. This conclusion would be inescapable if it had been shown that the recirculating cells studied had a long lifespan. As the

data stand, however, it could be argued that most of the cells in the central lymph were short-lived. If this were the case, how could such a finding be reconciled with the evidence from (adult) mice that short-lived T cells fail to recirculate? While it would be premature to discuss this point in detail, it may be relevant that, in mice, cell migration from the thymus *at birth* occurs not to the spleen but predominently to LN and Peyer's patches [19,138a]; likewise, very similar migratory patterns were exhibited by the fetal sheep TDL of Pearson et al. The possibility arises, therefore, that the failure of recent thymic emigrants to recirculate in the adult is due simply to their being trapped by the spleen, thereby being prevented from reaching LN and subsequently the central lymph.

6. More recently, it has been found that the cells that control the secondary response to ferritin have a higher density of surface Ig than do those that give a primary response [156].

7. It should be mentioned that in certain strains of rats, appreciable numbers of fully immunocompetent lymphocytes enter the marrow from the circulation [163].

8. Recent evidence suggests that B_V cells increase considerably in size when they reach the spleen [156]. Significantly, this phenomenon is not observed with germfree animals [164]. Therefore, it is probably a nonspecific event, perhaps reflecting stimulation by products (lymphokines?) released by other cells that respond to specific antigen.

9. More recent studies have shown that trypsin-treated cells also regain their LN-seeking capacity when cultured in vitro; this recovery is temperature dependent and requires protein synthesis [173].

10. A similar effect on lymphocyte homing has also been reported for cells treated in vitro with sodium periodate [176], concanavalin A [177-180], or phytohemagglutinin [179]; like neuraminidase, these agents all attach to carbohydrate-containing moieties on the cell surface.

11. In this respect, it may be mentioned that liver cells express receptors which nonspecifically bind glycoproteins stripped of terminal sialic acid residues [183,184].

12. Scanning electron microscopy has revealed the interesting finding that both T and B cells display numerous surface microvilli while in circulation but have have a smooth surface when in their respective microenvironments in the lymphoid tissues [208a]. The significance of this finding is unknown.

13. Similar results have been observed with cytotoxic blast cells generated during an MLR in vitro. Rouse and Wagner [321] observed that although most of the cells localized in the liver after intravenous injection, appreciable numbers recirculated.

14. This assumption may not necessarily be correct, because large lymphocytes, though common in NTx and TxBM mice, are rare in nude mice [36].

References

1. J. L. Gowans and D. D. McGregor, *Progr. Allergy* **9**, 1 (1965).
2. J. F. A. P. Miller, A. Basten, J. Sprent, and C. Cheers, Cell. Immunol. **2**, 469 (1971).
3. M. C. Raff, Transplant. Rev. **6**, 52 (1971).
4. M. F. Greaves, J. J. T. Owen, and M. C. Raff, *T and B Lymphocytes,* American Elsevier, New York, 1973.
5. A. Basten, J. F. A. P. Miller, J. Sprent, and J. Pye, J. Exp. Med. **135**, 610 (1972).

5a. H. Cantor and E. A. Boyse, J. Exp. Med. **141**, 1376 (1975).

5b. I. F. C. McKenzie and G. D. Snell, J. Immunol. **114**, 848 (1975).

6. J. F. A. P. Miller and A. J. S. Davies, Annu. Rev. Med. **15**, 23 (1964).
7. J. F. A. P. Miller and D. Osoba, Physiol. Rev. **47**, 437 (1967).
8. R. Benner, F. Meima, G. M. van der Meulen, and W. B. van der Muiswinkel, Immunology **26**, 247 (1974).
9. J. E. Kindred, Amer. J. Anat. **71**, 207 (1942).
10. G. Sante-Marie and C. P. Leblond, Proc. Soc. Exp. Biol. Med. **98**, 909 (1958).
11. E. Andreasen in *The Kinetics of Cellular Proliferation* (F. Stohlman, Jr., ed.), Grune and Stratton, New York, 1959, p. 19.
12. D. Metcalf in *Ciba Symposium on the Thymus: Experimental and Clinical Studies* (G. E. W. Wolstenholme and R. Porter, eds.), Churchill, London, 1966, p. 242.
13. W. D. Mickalke, M. W. Hess, H. Riedwyl, R. D. Stoner, and H. Cottier, Blood **33**,541 (1969).
14. B. J. Bryant, Eur. J. Immunol. **2**, 38 (1972).
15. G. Sainte-Marie and F. Peng, Rev. Can. Biol. **30**, 51 (1971).
16. G. J. V. Nossal, Ann. N. Y. Acad. Sci. **120**, 171 (1964).
17. T. J. Linna, Blood **31**, 727 (1968).
18. R. J. Iorio, A. D. Chanana, E. P. Cronkite, and D. D. Joel, Cell Tissue Kinet. **3**, 161 (1970).
19. D. D. Joel, M. W. Hess, and H. Cottier, J. Exp. Med. **135**, 907 (1972).
20. I. L. Weissman, J. Exp. Med. **126**, 291 (1967).
21. M. Kotani, K. Seiki, A. Yamashita, and I. Horii, Blood **27**, 511 (1966).
22. M. Kotani, M. Kawakita, M. Fukanogi, A. Yamashita, K. Seiki, and I. Horii, Okajimas Fol. Anat. Jap. **43**, 61 (1967).
23. G. Sainte-Marie, in *Contemporary Topics in Immunobiology* (A. J. S. Davies and R. L. Carter, eds.), Vol. 2, Plenum Press, New York, 1973, p. 111.
24. I. Toro and I. Olah, J. Ultrastruct. Res. **17**, 439 (1967).
25. G. Sainte-Marie and C. P. Leblond, Blood **23**, 275 (1964).
26. U. Ernström, L. Gyllensten, and B. Larsson, Nature (London) **207**, 540 (1965).
27. R. M. Williams, A. D. Chanana, E. P. Cronkite, and B. H. Waksman, J. Immunol. **106**, 1143 (1971).

28. A. J. S. Davies, E. Leuchars, V. Wallis, and M. J. Doenhoff, Proc. Roy. Soc. London Ser. B **176**, 369 (1971).
29. A. J. S. Davies and R. L. Carter, in *Contemporary Topics in Immunobiology* (M. G. Hanna, Jr., ed.), Vol. 1, Plenum Press, New York, 1972, p. 1.
30. M. A. S. Moore and J. J. T. Owen, J. Exp. Med. **126**, 715 (1967).
31. J. J. T. Owen and M. A. Ritter, J. Exp. Med. **129**, 431 (1969).
32. M. A. S. Moore and J. J. T. Owen, Lancet **ii**, 658 (1967).
33. J. F. A. P. Miller, Brit. Med. Bull. **21**, 111 (1965).
34. K. Komuro and E. A. Boyse, Lancet **i**, 740 (1973).
34a. *Biological Activity of Thymic Hormones* (D. W. van Bekkum, ed.), Kooyker Scientific Publications, Rotterdam.
34b. O. Stutman, in *Biological Activity of Thymic Hormones* (D.W. van Bekkum, ed.) Kooyker Scientific Publications, Rotterdam, p. 87.
35. J. F. A. P. Miller, G. F. Mitchell, and N. S. Weiss, Nature (London) **214**, 992 (1967).
36. J. Sprent, Cell. Immunol. **7**, 10 (1973).
37. H. D. Agnew, Proc. Soc. Exp. Biol. Med. **125**, 132 (1967).
38. I. Goldschneider and D. D. McGregor, J. Exp. Med. **127**, 155 (1968).
39. J. C. Howard, J. Exp. Med. **135**, 185 (1972).
40. W. O. Reinhardt and J. M. Yoffey, Amer. J. Physiol. **187**, 493 (1956).
41. G. J. Cole and B. Morris, Aust. J. Exp. Biol. Med. Sci. **49**, 33 (1971).
42. J. F. A. P. Miller and J. Sprent, Nature [New Biol.] **230**, 267 (1971).
42a. G. E. Roelants, F. Loor, H. von Boehmer, J. Sprent, L.-B. Hägg, K. Mayor, and A. Rydén, Eur. J. Immunol. **5**, 127 (1975).
42b. G. E. Roelants, K. Mayor, L.-B. Hägg, and F. Loor, Eur. J. Immunol. **6**, 75 (1976).
42c. M. A. Vadas, J. F. A. P. Miller, I. F. C. McKenzie, S. E. Chism, F.-W. Shen, E. A. Boyse, J. R. Gamble, and A. M. Whitelaw, J. Exp. Med. **144**, 10 (1976).
42d. M. Feldmann, P. C. L. Beverley, M. Dunkley, and S. Kontiaien, Nature (London) **258**, 614 (1975).
42e. P. C. L. Beverley and J. Sprent, unpublished data.
43. J. D. Mann and G. M. Higgins, Blood **5**, 177 (1950).
44. J. L. Gowans, Brit. J. Exp. Pathol. **38**, 67 (1957).
45. D. D. McGregor, Fed. Proc. **25**, 1713 (1966).
46. T. K. Dineen and D. B. Adams, Immunology **19**, 11 (1970).
47. H. Schnappauf and U. Schnappauf, *Blut* **16**, 209 (1968).
48. H. E. Sarles, A. R. Remmers, Jr., J. C. Fish, C. O. Canales, F. D. Thomas, K. R. T. Tyson, G. A. Beathard, and S. E. Ritzmann, Arch. Intern. Med. **125**, 443 (1970).
49. W. S. Tunner, P. P. Carbone, and G. L. Irvin, Surg. Gynecol. Obstet. **121**, 334 (1965).
50. J. L. Gowans, J. Physiol. (London) **146**, 54 (1959).
51. N. B. Everett, W. O. Reinhardt, and J. M. Yoffey, Blood **15**, 82 (1960).
52. R. W. Caffrey, W. O. Rieke, and N. B. Everett, Acta Haematol. **28**, 145 (1962).

53. H. Frost, R. N. P. Cahill, and Z. Trnka, Eur. J. Immunol., **5**, 839 (1975).
54. S. Perry, G. L. Irvin, and J. Whang, in *The Lymphocyte in Immunology and Haemopoiesis* (J. M. Yoffey, ed.), Edward Arnold, London, 1967, p. 99.
55. R. M. Binns and J. G. Hall, Brit. J. Exp. Pathol. **47**, 275 (1966).
56. M. C. Raff, Immunology **19**, 637 (1970).
57. J. L. Gowans and E. J. Knight, Proc. Roy. Soc. London Ser. B **159**, 257 (1964).
58. W. L. Ford and S. J. Simmonds, Cell. Tissue Kinet. **5**, 175 (1972).
59. D. M. V. Parrott, M. A. B. de Sousa, and J. East, J. Exp. Med. **123**, 191 (1966).
60. M. A. B. de Sousa, D. M. V. Parrott, and E. M. Pantelouris, Clin. Exp. Immunol. **4**, 637 (1969).
61. D. M. V. Parrott, J. Clin. Pathol. Suppl. **20**, 456 (1967).
62. H. Cottier, E. P. Cronkite, C. R. Jansen, K. R. Rai, S. Singer, and C. R. Sipe, Blood **24**, 241 (1964).
63. W. L. Ford, Brit. J. Exp. Pathol. **49**, 502 (1968).
64. V. T. Marchesi and J. L. Gowans, Proc. Roy. Soc. London Ser. B **159**, 283 (1964).
65. G. L. Schoefl, J. Exp. Med. **136**, 568 (1972).
66. L. Weiss, *The Cells and Tissues of the Immune Response,* Prentice-Hall, Inc., Englewood Cliffs, N. J., 1972, p. 49.
67. J. Mitchell, Immunology **22**, 231 (1972).
68. W. L. Ford, Cell. Tissue Kinet. **2**, 171 (1969).
69. W. L. Ford, Brit. J. Exp. Pathol. **50**, 257 (1969).
70. J. Mitchell, Immunology **24**, 93 (1973).
71. M. M. Zatz and E. M. Lance, Cell Immunol. **1**, 3 (1970).
72. J. Woodruff and B. M. Gesner, Science **161**, 176 (1968).
73. B. F. Heslop and B. E. Hardy, Transplantation **11**, 128 (1971).
74. J. M. Yoffey and F. C. Courtice, *Lymphatics, Lymph and Lymphoid Tissue,* Arnold, London, 1956.
75. J. Otteson, Acta Physiol. Scand. **32**, 75 (1954).
76. K. E. Buckton, P. Jacobs, W. M. Court-Brown, and R. Doll, Lancet **ii**, 676 (1962).
77. A. Norman, M. S. Sasaki, R. E. Ottoman, and A. G. Fingerhut, Science **147**, 745 (1965).
78. N. B. Everett, R. W. Caffrey, and W. O. Rieke, Ann. N. Y. Acad. Sci. **113**, 887 (1964).
79. N. B. Everett and R. W. Tyler, Int. Rev. Cytol. **22**, 205 (1967).
80. J. R. Little, G. Brecher, T. R. Bradley, and S. Rose, Blood **19**, 236 (1962).
81. S. H. Robinson, G. Brecher, I. S. Lourie, and J. E. Haley, Blood **26**, 281 (1965).
82. J. Sprent and A. Basten, Cell. Immunol. **7**, 40 (1973).
83. J. F. A. P. Miller and G. F. Mitchell, Transplant. Rev. **1**, 3 (1969).
84. C. Ruchti, H. Cottier, E. P. Cronkite, C. R. Jansen, and K. R. Rai, Cell. Tissue Kinet. **3**, 301 (1970).

85. E. P. Cronkite and A. D. Chanana, in *Formation and Destruction of Blood Cells* (T. J. Greenwalt and G. A. Jamieson, eds.), Lippincott, Philadelphia, 1970, p. 284.
86. D. Metcalf and M. A. S. Moore, *Haemopoietic Cells,* North-Holland, Amsterdam, 1971.
87. P. W. Kincade, K. S. Self, and M. D. Cooper, Cell. Immunol. **8**, 93 (1973).
88. R. A. Peterson, M. D. Cooper, and R. A. Good, Amer. J. Med. **38**, 579 (1965).
89. D. Y. E. Perey, M. D. Cooper, and R. A. Good, Science **161**, 265 (1968).
90. F. Melchers, H. von Boehmer, and R. Phillips, Transplant. Rev. **25**, 26 (1975).
91. M. C. Raff, M. Megson, J. J. T. Owen, and M. D. Cooper, Nature (London), **259**, 224 (1976).
92. J. J. T. Owen, M. D. Cooper, and M. C. Raff, Nature (London) **249**, 361 (1974).
93. G. J. V. Nossal and B. L. Pike, Immunology **25**, 33 (1973).
94. J. M. Yoffey and F. C. Courtice, *Lymphatics, Lymph and the Lymphomyeloid Complex,* Academic Press, London and New York, 1970.
95. D. G. Osmond and G. J. V. Nossal, Cell. Immunol. **13**, 132 (1974).
96. D. G. Osmond and G. J. V. Nossal, Cell. Immunol. **13**, 117 (1974).
97. J.-E. Ryser and P. Vassalli, J. Immunol. **113**, 719 (1974).
98. L. Lafleur, B. J. Underdown, R. G. Miller, and R. A. Phillips, Ser. Haematol. **5**, 50 (1972).
99. L. Lafleur, R. G. Miller, and R. A. Phillips, J. Exp. Med. **137**, 954 (1973).
100. C. Röpke and H. P. Hougen, in *Proceedings of the First International Workshop on Nude Mice* (J. Rygaard and C. O. Poulsen, eds.), Gustav Fischer Verlag, Stuttgart, 1974, p. 51.
101. C. Röpke, H. P. Hougen, and N. B. Everett, Cell. Immunol. **15**, 82 (1975).
102. H. P. Hougen and C. Ropke, Clin. Exp. Immunol. **22**, 528 (1975).
103. F. Brahim and D. G. Osmond, Anat. Rec. **168**, 139 (1970).
104. F. Brahim and D. G. Osmond, Anat. Rec. **175**, 737 (1973).
105. T. J. Linna and S. Liden, Int. Arch. Allergy Appl. Immunol. **35**, 35 (1969).
106. R. A. Phillips and R. G. Miller, Nature [New Biol.] **251**, 446 (1974).
107. A. Basten, J. Sprent, and J. F. A. P. Miller, Nature [New Biol.] **235**, 178 (1972).
108. S. Strober, Nature [New Biol.] **237**, 247 (1972).
109. D. M. V. Parrott and M. A. B. de Sousa, Clin. Exp. Immunol. **8**, 663 (1971).
110. J. C. Howard, S. V. Hunt, and J. L. Gowans, J. Exp. Med. **135**, 200 (1972).
111. H. G. Durkin, G. A. Theis, and G. J. Thorbecke, Nature [New Biol.] **235**, 118 (1972).
112. J. Sprent, unpublished data (1974-1976).
113. W. L. Ford, Progr. Allergy **19**, 1 (1975).
113a. P. Nieuwenhuis and W. L. Ford, Cell. Immunol. **23**, 254 (1976).

114. N. B. Everett and R. W. Tyler, in *Formation and Destruction of Blood Cells* (T. J. Greenwalt and G. A. Jamieson, eds.), Lippincott, Philadelphia, 1970, p. 264.
115. C. Bianco, R. Patrick, and V. Nussenzweig, J. Exp. Med. **132**, 702 (1970).
116. W. O. Rieke and M. R. Schwartz, in *The Lymphocyte in Immunology and Haemopoiesis,* (J. M. Yoffey, ed.), Arnold, London, 1967, p. 224.
117. S. Strober, J. Exp. Med. **136**, 851 (1972).
118. J.-C. Cerottini and K. T. Brunner, Immunology **13**, 395 (1967).
119. M. Schlesinger and U. K. Golakai, Science **155**, 1114 (1967).
120. E. M. Lance, S. Cooper, and E. A. Boyse, Cell. Immunol. **1**, 536 (1970).
121. M. C. Raff and J. J. T. Owen, in *Proceedings of the 3rd International Conference on Lymphatic Tissue and Germinal Centers* (K. Lindahl-Kiessling, G. Alm, and M. G. Hanna, Jr., eds.), Plenum Press, New York, 1971, p. 11.
122. M. Schlesinger, Progr. Allergy **16**, 214 (1972).
123. M. C. Raff, Nature [New Biol.] **229**, 182 (1971).
124. H. Blomgren and B. Andersson, Exp. Cell Res. **57**, 185 (1969).
125. H. Blomgren and B. Andersson, Cell. Immunol. **1**, 545 (1971).
126. W. Droege and R. Zucker, Transplant. Rev. **25**, 3 (1975).
127. K. Shortman and H. Jackson, Cell. Immunol. **12**, 230 (1974).
128. I. L. Weissman, J. Exp. Med. **137**, 504 (1973).
129. K. Zeiller, G. Pascher, G. Wagner, H. G. Liebich, E. Holzberg, and K. Hannig, Immunology **26**, 995 (1974).
130. C. G. Fathman, M. Small, L. A. Herzenberg, and I. L. Weissman, Cell. Immunol. **15**, 109 (1975).
131. B. Andersson and H. Blomgren, Cell. Immunol. **1**, 363 (1970).
132. H. Blomgren and E. Svedmyr, Cell. Immunol. **2**, 285 (1971).
133. H. Blomgren and B. Andersson, Clin. Exp. Immunol. **10**, 297 (1972).
134. M. Schlesinger, S. Gottesfeld, and Z. Korzash, Cell. Immunol. **6**, 49 (1973).
135. J. Sprent and J. F. A. P. Miller, Cell. Immunol. **3**, 385 (1972).
136. I. Goldschneider and D. D. McGregor, Lab. Invest. **18**, 397 (1968).
137. M. A. B. de Sousa, in *Contemporary Topics in Immunobiology* (A. J. S. Davies and R. L. Carter, eds.), Vol. 2, Plenum Press, New York, 1973, p. 119.
137a. I. L. Weissman and G. F. Mitchell, Personal communication (1976).
138. E. V. Elliott, Nature [New Biol.] **242**, 150 (1973).
138a. I. L. Weissman, T. Masuda, C. Olive, and S. H. Friedberg, Isr. J. Med. Sci. **11**, 1267 (1975).
139. R. Wilson, M. Bealmear, and R. Sobonya, Proc. Soc. Exp. Biol. Med. **118**, 97 (1965).
140. J. Kruml, J. Ludvik, and I. Trebichavsky, Folia Microbiol. (Prague) **14**, 441 (1969).
141. G. J. Thorbecke, H. A. Gordon, B. Wostman, M. Wagner, and J. A. Reyniers, J. Infect. Diseases **101**, 237 (1957).
142. J. Sprent and J. F. A. P. Miller, Unpublished observations (1974).

143. S. D. Waksal, L. Weprin, and R. L. St. Pierre, J. Reticuloendothel. Soc. **13**, 343 (1973).
144. M. C. Raff and H. Cantor, in *Progress in Immunology* (B. Amos, ed), Academic Press, New York, 1971, p. 83.
145. J.-F. Bach, M. Dardenne, and A. J. S. Davies, Nature [New Biol.] **231**, 110 (1971).
146. J.-F. Bach and M. Dardenne, Cell. Immunol. **6**, 394 (1973).
147. L. Olsson and M. H. Claesson, Nature [New Biol.] **244**, 50 (1973).
148. H. Cantor and R. Asofsky, J. Exp. Med. **131**, 235 (1970).
149. H. Cantor and R. Asofsky, J. Exp. Med. **135**, 764 (1972).
150. R. E. Tigelaar and R. Asofsky, J. Exp. Med. **137**, 239 (1973).
151. R. E. Tigelaar and R. Asofsky, J. Immunol. **110**, 567 (1973).
152. L. Cohen and M. L. Howe, Proc. Nat. Acad. Sci. USA **70**, 2707 (1973).
153. H. Wagner, Science **181**, 1170 (1973).
154. H. Wagner, J. Exp. Med. **138**, 1379 (1973).
154a. L. D. Pearson, M. W. Simpson-Morgan, and B. Morris, J. Exp. Med. **143**, 167 (1976).
155. S. Stober and J. Dilley, J. Exp. Med. **138**, 1331 (1973).
156. S. Strober, Transplant. Rev. **24**, 84 (1975).
157. S. Strober and J. Dilley, J. Exp. Med. **137**, 1275 (1973).
158. R. Schlegel, H. von Boehmer, and K. Shortman, Cell. Immunol. **16**, 203 (1975).
159. J. W. Schrader, Cell. Immunol. **10**, 380 (1974).
160. G. J. V. Nossal and B. L. Pike, J. Exp. Med. **141**, 904 (1975).
161. N. R. Klinman and J. L. Press, Transplant. Rev. **24**, 41 (1975).
162. L. Hudson, personal communication, (1974).
163. J. C. Howard and D. W. Scott, Cell. Immunol. **3**, 421 (1972).
164. K. Shortman, J. M. Fidler, R. A. Schlegel, G. J. V. Nossal, M. Howard, J. Lipp, and H. von Boehmer, Contemp. Topics Immunobiol., in press (1976).
165. D. D. McGregor and J. L. Gowans, J. Exp. Med. **117**, 303 (1963).
166. M. E. Phillips, F. Quagliata, and G. J. Thorbecke, Immunology **22**, 565 (1972).
167. E. B. Jacobson and G. J. Thorbecke, J. Exp. Med. **130**, 287 (1969).
168. J. J. Miller, J. Immunol. **92**, 673 (1964).
169. J. J. Miller and S. Koskimies, Cell. Immunol. **3**, 231 (1972).
170. J. B. Smith, A. J. Cunningham, K. J. Lafferty, and B. Morris, Aust. J. Exp. Biol. Med. Sci. **48**, 57 (1970).
171. F. M. Burnet, *The Clonal Selection Theory of Acquired Immunity*, Cambridge University Press, London, 1959.
172. W. S. Bullough, *The Evolution of Differentiation*, Academic Press, London, 1967.
173. J. J. Woodruff and J. F. Woodruff, Cell. Immunol. **10**, 78 (1974).
174. B. M. Gesner, J. J. Woodruff, and R. T. McCluskey, Amer. J. Pathol. **57**, 215 (1969).
175. J. J. Woodruff and B. M. Gesner, J. Exp. Med. **129**, 551 (1969).
176. M. Zatz, A. L. Goldstein, O. O. Blumenfield, and A. White, Nature [New Biol.] **240**, 252 (1972).

177. R. W. Gillette, G. O. McKenzie, and M. H. Swanson, J. Immunol. **111**, 1902 (1973).
178. R. N. Taub, Cell. Immunol. **12**, 263 (1974).
179. M. Schlesinger and E. Israel, Cell. Immunol. **14**, 66 (1974).
180. B. A. Rodriguez, R. R. Rich, and R. D. Rossen, J. Immunol. **115**, 771 (1975).
181. B. M. Gesner, Ann. N. Y. Acad. Sci. **129**, 758 (1966).
182. J. F. Woodruff and J. J. Woodruff, Cell. Immunol. **1**, 333 (1970).
183. W. E. Pricer, Jr. and G. Ashwell, J. Biol. Chem. **246**, 4825 (1971).
184. L. Van Lenten and G. Ashwell, J. Biol. Chem. **247**, 4633 (1972).
185. J. F. Woodruff and J. J. Woodruff, Cell. Immunol. **5**, 296 (1972).
186. J. J. Woodruff and J. F. Woodruff, Cell. Immunol. **10**, 78 (1974).
187. J. J. Woodruff and J. F. Woodruff, Cell. Immunol. **5**, 307 (1972).
188. S. I. Morse, J. Exp. Med. **121**, 49 (1965).
189. S. I. Morse and S. K. Riester, J. Exp. Med. **125**, 401 (1967).
190. S. I. Morse and S. K. Riester, J. Exp. Med. **125**, 619 (1967).
191. R. N. Taub, W. Rosett, A. Adler, and S. I. Morse, J. Exp. Med. **136**, 1581 (1972).
192. C. J. F. Spry, Cell. Immunol. **4**, 86 (1972).
193. H. Schnappauf and V. Schnappauf, Nouvelle Rev. Franc. Hematol. **8**, 555 (1968).
194. H. N. Claman, N. Engl. J. Med. **287**, 388 (1972).
195. J. N. Esteban, Anat. Rec. **162**, 349 (1968).
196. R. J. North, Cell. Immunol. **3**, 501 (1972).
197. A. A. van den Broek, in *Microenvironmental Aspects of Immunity* (B. D. Janković and K. Isaković, eds.), Plenum Press, New York and London, 1973, p. 337.
198. J. J. Miller and L. J. Cole, J. Exp. Med. **126**, 109 (1967).
199. S. I. Morse, J. Exp. Med. **123**, 283 (1966).
200. E. V. Elliot and N. R. St. C. Sinclair, Immunology **15**, 643 (1968).
201. J. Thompson and R. van Furth, J. Exp. Med. **131**, 429 (1970).
202. J. J. Cohen, J. Immunol. **108**, 841 (1972).
203. J. V. Moorehead and H. N. Claman, Cell. Immunol. **5**, 74 (1972).
204. G. Bert, J. A. Forrester, and A. J. S. Davies, Nature [New Biol.] **234**, 86 (1971).
205. K. Zeiller, E. Holzberg, G. Pascher, and K. Hannig, Hoppe-Seyler's Z. Physiol. Chem. **353**, 105 (1972).
206. H. von Boehmer, K. Shortman, and G. J. V. Nossal, Cell. Physiol. **83**, 231 (1974).
207. Transplant. Rev. Vol. 30 (1976).
208. R. A. Anderson, J. Sprent, and J. F. A. P. Miller, Eur. J. Immunol. **4**, 199 (1974).
208a. W. van Ewijk, N. H. C. Brons, and J. Rozing, Cell. Immunol. **19**, 245 (1975).
209. A. J. Cunningham, Aust. J. Exp. Biol. Med. Sci. **46**, 141 (1968).
210. J. G. Hall and B. Morris, Lancet **i**, 1077 (1964).

211. D. M. V. Parrott and M. A. B. de Sousa, Nature (London) **212**, 1316 (1966).
212. A. J. S. Davies, R. L. Carter, E. Leuchars, V. Wallis, and P. C. Koller, Immunology **16**, 57 (1969).
213. J. Oort and J. L. Turk, Brit. J. Exp. Pathol. **46**, 147 (1965).
214. R. G. Burwell, Ann. N. Y. Acad. Sci. **99**, 821 (1962).
215. M. A. B. de Sousa and D. M. V. Parrott, J. Exp. Med. **130**, 671 (1969).
216. R. H. Kelly, R. A. Wolstencroft, D. C. Dumonde, and B. M. Balfour, Clin. Exp. Immunol. **10**, 49 (1972).
217. P. G. Herman, I. Yamamoto, and H. Z. Mellins, J. Exp. Med. **136**, 697 (1972).
218. J. G. Hall and B. Morris, J. Exp. Med. **121**, 901 (1965).
219. J. G. Hall and B. Morris, Brit. J. Exp. Pathol. **46**, 450 (1965).
220. J. G. Hall, Quart. J. Exp. Physiol. **52**, 76 (1967).
221. J. B. Smith and B. Morris, Aust. J. Exp. Biol. Med. Sci. **48**, 33 (1970).
222. J. B. Hay, R. N. P. Cahill, and Z. Trnka, Cell. Immunol. **10**, 145 (1974).
223. P. K. Pattengale, W. M. Stahl, and G. J. Thorbecke, Amer. J. Pathol. **67**, 527 (1972).
224. D. W. Dresser, R. N. Taub, and A. R. Krantz, Immunology **18**, 663 (1970).
225. M. M. Zatz and E. M. Lance, J. Exp. Med. **134**, 224 (1971).
226. E. E. Emeson and D. R. Thursh, J. Exp. Med. **137**, 1293 (1973).
227. G. L. Asherson and R. M. R. Barnes, Immunology **24**, 885 (1973).
228. R. N. P. Cahill, H. Frost, and Z. Trnka, J. Exp. Med. **143**, 870 (1976).
229. H. W. Kreth, G. Thiessen, and H. Deicher, Clin. Exp. Immunol. **7**, 109 (1970).
230. J. Sprent, J. F. A. P. Miller, and G. F. Mitchell, Cell. Immunol. **2**, 171 (1971).
231. J. Sprent and J. F. A. P. Miller, J. Exp. Med. **139**, 1 (1974).
232. D. A. Rowley, J. L. Gowans, R. C. Atkins, W. L. Ford, and M. E. Smith, J. Exp. Med. **136**, 499 (1972).
233. C. M. O'Toole and A. J. S. Davies, Nature (London) **230**, 187 (1971).
234. J. Sprent and J. F. A. P. Miller, J. Exp. Med. **143**, 585 (1976).
235. B. J. Larner, Transplantation **16**, 134 (1973).
236. W. L. Ford and R. C. Atkins, Nature [New Biol.] **234**, 178 (1972).
236a. S. Dorsch and B. Roser, Aust. J. Exp. Biol. Med. Sci. **52**, 45 (1974).
236b. E. Heber-Katz and D. B. Wilson, J. Exp. Med. **142**, 928 (1975).
237. N. C. Pedersen and B. Morris, J. Exp. Med. **131**, 936 (1970).
238. R. C. Atkins and W. L. Ford, J. Exp. Med. **141**, 664 (1975).
239. W. L. Ford, S. J. Simmonds, and R. C. Atkins, J. Exp. Med. **141**, 681 (1975).
240. D. R. Thursh and E. E. Emeson, J. Exp. Med. **135**, 754 (1972).
241. D. R. Thursh and E. E. Emeson, J. Exp. Med. **138**, 659 (1973).
242. R. N. P. Cahill, unpublished data (1974).
243. G. W. Siskind and B. Benacerraf, Advan. Immunol. **10**, 1 (1969).
244. J. M. Davie and W. E. Paul, J. Exp. Med. **137**, 201 (1973).

245. H. Cottier, N. Odartchenko, R. Schindler, and C. C. Congdon (eds.), *Germinal Centers in Immune Responses,* Springer-Verlag, Berlin, Heidelberg, New York, 1967, p. 1.
246. G. A. Gutman and I. L. Weissman, Immunology **23**, 465 (1972).
247. J. Mitchell, J. Pye, M. C. Holmes, and G. J. V. Nossal, Aust. J. Exp. Biol. Med. Sci. **50**, 637 (1972).
248. G. J. V. Nossal, A. J. Cunningham, G. F. Mitchell, and J. F. A. P. Miller, J. Exp. Med. **128**, 839 (1969).
249. J. F. A. P. Miller and G. F. Mitchell in *Ciba Foundation Symposium: The Thymus* (G. E. W. Wolstenholme and J. Knight, eds.), Churchill, London, 1970, p. 238.
250. J. Sprent and J. F. A. P. Miller, Cell. Immunol. **3**, 361 (1972).
251. J. Sprent and J. F. A. P. Miller, Cell. Immunol. **3**, 213 (1972).
252. J. Sprent and J. F. A. P. Miller, J. Exp. Med. **138**, 143.
253. M. Feldman and A. Basten, Eur. J. Immunol. 2, 213 (1972).
254. J. Sprent and I. Lefkovits, J. Exp. Med. **143**, 1289 (1976).
255. M. A. Axelrad and D. A. Rowley, Science **160**, 1465 (1968).
256. G. L. Asherson, Immunology **10**, 179 (1966).
257. J. F. A. P. Miller, in *Contemporary Topics in Immunobiology* (A. J. S. Davies and R. L. Carter, eds.), Vol. 2, Plenum Press, New York and London, 1973, p. 151.
258. D. B. Wilson and R. E. Billingham, Advan. Immunol. **7**, 189 (1967).
259. D. B. Wilson, J. C. Howard, and P. C. Nowell, Transplant. Rev. **12**, 3 (1972).
260. C. F. Barker and R. E. Billingham, J. Exp. Med. **133**, 620 (1971).
261. N. L. Tilney and J. L. Gowans, J. Exp. Med. **133**, 951 (1971).
262. J. G. Hall, J. Exp. Med. **125**, 737 (1967).
263. R. E. Billingham, W. K. Silvers, and D. B. Wilson, J. Exp. Med. **118**, 397 (1963).
264. E. M. Lance and S. Cooper, Cell. Immunol. **5**, 66 (1972).
265. R. Gruber and Z. J. Lucas in *Microenvironmental Aspects of Immunity* (B. D. Janković and K. Isaković, eds.), Plenum Press, New York and London, 1973, p. 545.
266. J. F. A. P. Miller, Lancet **ii**, 748 (1961).
267. J. L. Gowans, Ann. N. Y. Acad. Sci. **99**, 432 (1962).
268. J. Sprent and J. F. A. P. Miller, Nature [New Biol.] **234**, 195 (1971).
269. C. Cheers, J. Sprent and J. F. A. P. Miller, Cell. Immunol. **10**, 57 (1974).
270. M. Feldmann and J. Sprent, unpublished data (1972).
271. M. Feldmann and A. Basten, Eur. J. Immunol. **2**, 213 (1972).
272. J. L. Turk, *Delayed Hypersensitivity,* North-Holland, Amsterdam, 1967, p. 1.
273. J. L. Turk and S. H. Stone in *Cell-bound Antibodies* (B. Amos and H. Koprowski, eds.), Wistar Institute Press, Philadelphia, 1963, p. 51.
274. H. Haxthausen, Acta Dermato-Venereol. **31**, 659 (1951).
275. T. Wesslen, Acta Tuberc. Scand. **26**, 38 (1952).
276. E. Skog, Acta Dermato-Venereol. **35**, 93 (1955).
277. J. R. Eltringham and I. L. Weissman, *J. Immunol.* **106**, 1185 (1971).

278. B. R. Bloom, L. D. Hamilton, and M. W. Chase, Nature (London) **201**, 689 (1964).
279. M. G. Cooper, Scand. J. Immunol. **1**, 237 (1972).
280. M. G. Cooper and G. L. Ada, Scand. J. Immunol. **1**, 247 (1972).
281. G. L. Asherson, G. G. Allwood, and B. Mayhew, Immunology **25**, 485 (1973).
282. S. Youdin, O. Stutman, and R. A. Good, Cell. Immunol. **8**, 395 (1973).
283. G. L. Asherson and R. M. R. Barnes, Immunology **24**, 885 (1973).
284. G. L. Asherson and J. Ferluger, Immunology **25**, 471 (1973).
285. F. T. Koster and D. D. McGregor, Science **167**, 1137 (1970).
286. D. D. McGregor, F. T. Koster, and G. B. Mackaness, Nature (London) **228**, 855 (1970).
287. D. D. McGregor, F. T. Koster, and G. B. Mackaness, J. Exp. Med. **133**, 389 (1971).
288. F. T. Koster, D. D. McGregor, and G. B. Mackaness, J. Exp. Med. **133**, 400 (1970).
289. F. T. Koster and D. D. McGregor, J. Exp. Med. **133**, 864 (1971).
290. D. D. McGregor, H. H. Hahn, G. B. Mackaness, Cell. Immunol. **6**, 186 (1973).
291. R. V. Blanden and R. E. Langman, Scand. J. Immunol. **1**, 379 (1972).
292. F. C. Lane and E. R. Unanue, J. Exp. Med. **135**, 1104 (1972).
293. R. J. North, Cell. Immunol. **7**, 166 (1973).
294. R. J. North, J. Exp. Med. **138**, 342 (1973).
295. D. E. Griffin and R. T. Johnson, Cell. Immunol. **9**, 426 (1973).
295a. P. C. Doherty, R. V. Blanden, and R. M. Zinkernagel, Transplant. Rev. **29**, 89 (1976).
296. B. M. Ogilvie and V. E. Jones, Progr. Allergy **17**, 93 (1973).
297. M. Samter and D. Czarny, in *Immunological Diseases* (M. Samter, ed.), Little, Brown and Company, Boston, 1971, p. 375.
298. A. Basten, M. H. Boyer, and P. B. Beeson, J. Exp. Med. **131**, 1271 (1970).
299. A. Basten and P. B. Beeson, J. Exp. Med. **131**, 1288 (1970).
300. M. C. Raff, Nature (London) **226**, 1257 (1970).
301. J. F. A. P. Miller and J. Sprent, J. Exp. Med. **134**, 66 (1971).
302. A. J. Cunningham and E. Sercarz, Eur. J. Immunol. **1**, 413 (1971).
303. G. F. Mitchell, E. L. Chan, M. S. Noble, I. L. Weissman, R. I. Mishell, and L. A. Herzenberg, J. Exp. Med. **135**, 165 (1972).
304. D. H. Katz and B. Benacerraf, Advan. Immunol. **15**, 2 (1972).
305. G. Roelants, L. Forni, and B. Pernis, J. Exp. Med. **137**, 1060 (1973).
306. E. Möller, W. W. Bullock, and O. Mäkelä, Eur. J. Immunol. **3**, 172 (1973).
307. G. Roelants and A. Rydén, Nature (London) **247**, 104 (1974).
308. W. L. Ford, W. Burr, and M. Simonsen, Transplantation **10**, 258 (1970).
309. V. P. Eijsvoogel, J. J. Van Rood, E. D. de Toit, and P. T. A. Shellekens, Eur. J. Immunol. **2**, 413 (1972).
310. F. H. Bach, M. B. Widmer, M. L. Bach, and J. Klein, J. Exp. Med. **136**, 1430 (1972).

311. F. H. Bach, M. Segall, K. S. Zier, P. M. Sondel, B. J. Alter, and M. L. Bach, Science **180**, 403 (1973).
312. *The Genetic Determinants and Mechanism of Cell-mediated Immune Responses* (F. H. Bach, ed.) Transplant. Proc. **5**(4), 1315 (1973).
313. M. Nabholz, J. Vives, H. M. Young, T. Meo, V. Miggiano, A. Rijnbeck, and D. C. Schreffler, Eur. J. Immunol. **4**, 378 (1974).
314. M. B. Widmer, B. J. Alter, F. H. Bach, M. L. Bach, and D. W. Bailey, Nature [New Biol.] **243**, 239 (1973).
315. T. Meo, J. Vives, A. Rijnbeck, V. Miggiano, M. Nabholz, and D. C. Shreffler, Transplant. Proc. **5**(4), 1339 (1973).
316. J. Sprent, H. von Boehmer, and M. Nabholz, J. Exp. Med. **142**, 321 (1975).
317. H. Festenstein, Transplant. Rev. **15**, 62 (1973).
318. D. C. Shreffler and C. S. David, Advan. Immunol. **20**, 125 (1975).
319. M. Nabholz, H. Young, A. Rijnbeck, R. Boccardo, C. S. David, T. Meo, V. Miggiano, and D. C. Shreffler, Eur. J. Immunol. **5**, 594 (1975).
320. J. Sprent, Cell. Immunol. **21**, 278 (1976).
321. B. T. Rouse and H. Wagner, Transplantation **16**, 131 (1973).
322. J. Sprent and J. F. A. P. Miller, Cell. Immunol. **21**, 303 (1976).
323. M. J. Doenhoff and A. J. S. Davies, J. Exp. Med. **143**, 660 (1976).
324. K. E. Fichtelius, E. J. Yunis, and R. A. Good, Proc. Soc. Exp. Biol. Med. **128**, 185 (1968).
325. M. Kotani, A. Yamashita, F. Rai, K. Seiki, and I. Horii, Blood **29**, 616 (1967).
326. E. M. Lemmel and K. E. Fichtelius, Int. Arch. Allergy Appl. Immunol. **41**, 716 (1971).
327. D. M. V. Parrott and M. A. B. de Sousa, *Proceedings of the First International Workshop on Nude Mice* (J. Rygaard and C. O. Poulsen, eds.) Gustav Fischer Verlag, Stuttgart, 1974, p. 61.
328. D. Guy-Grand, C. Griscelli, and P. Vassalli, Eur. J. Immunol. **4**, 435 (1974).
329. J. Sprent and J. F. A. P. Miller, Cell. Immunol. **21**, 314 (1976).
330. J. Sprent, R. E. Anderson, and J. F. A. P. Miller, Eur. J. Immunol. **4**, 204 (1974).
331. J. C. Howard and D. B. Wilson, J. Exp. Med. **140**, 660 (1974).
332. P. Hayry and L. C. Andersson, Cell. Immunol. **17**, 165 (1975).
333. E. F. Wheelock and S. T. Toy, Advan. Immunol. **16**, 123 (1973).
334. S. Mudd (ed.), *Infectious Agents and Host Reactions,* Saunders, London, 1970, p. 1.
335. E. J. L. Soulsby (ed.), *Immunity to Animal Parasites,* Academic Press, New York, 1972, p. 1.
336. G. J. V. Nossal, Int. Rev. Exp. Pathol. **1**, 1 (1962).
337. N. K. Jerne, A. A. Nordin, and C. Henry in *Cell-Bound Antibodies* (B. B. Amos and H. Koprowski, eds.), Wistar Institute Press, Philadelphia, 1963, p. 109.
338. I. L. Weissman, M. Peacock, and J. R. Eltringham, J. Immunol. **110**, 1300 (1973).

339. L. Hulliger and E. Sorkin, Nature (London) **198**, 299 (1973).
340. M. Landy, R. P. Sanderson, M. T. Bernstein, and A. L. Jackson, Nature (London) **204**, 1320 (1964).
341. K. Hummeler, T. N. Harris, N. Tomassini, M. Hechtel, and M. B. Farber, J. Exp. Med. **124**, 255 (1966).
342. B. S. Rabin and N. R. Rose, Cell. Immunol. **7**, 389 (1973).
343. J. G. Hall and B. Morris, Quart. J. Exp. Physiol. **48**, 235 (1963).
344. A. J. Cunningham, J. B. Smith, and E. H. Mercer, J. Exp. Med. **124**, 701 (1966).
345. O. Nilsson, Acta Pathol. Microbiol. Scand. Sec. B **79**, 534 (1971).
346. J. B. Hay, M. J. Murphy, B. Morris, and M. C. Bessis, Amer. J. Pathol. **66**, 1 (1972).
347. M. J. Murphy, J. B. Hay, B. Morris, and M. C. Bessis, Amer. J. Pathol. **66**, 25 (1972).
348. E. J. Delorme, J. Hodgett, J. G. Hall, and P. Alexander, Proc. Roy. Soc. London Ser. B **174**, 229 (1969).
349. C. Griscelli, P. Vassalli, and R. T. McClusky, J. Exp. Med. **130**, 1427 (1969).
350. A. Basten, N. L. Warner, and T. Mandel, J. Exp. Med. **135**, 627 (1972).
351. A. F. Williams and J. L. Gowans, J. Exp. Med. **141**, 335 (1975).
352. J. G. Hall and M. E. Smith, Nature (London) **226**, 262 (1970).
353. J. G. Hall, D. M. Parry, and M. E. Smith, Cell. Tissue Kinet. **5**, 269, (1972).
354. A. R. Moore and J. G. Hall, Nature (London) **239**, 161 (1972).
355. A. R. Moore and J. G. Hall, Cell. Immunol. **8**, 112 (1973).
356. T. E. Halstead and J. G. Hall, Transplantation **14**, 339 (1972).
357. D. M. V. Parrott and A. Ferguson, Immunology **26**, 571 (1974).
358. E. L. Chan, R. I. Mishell, and G. F. Mitchell, Science **170**, 1215 (1970).
359. A. Schimpl and E. Wecker, Nature (London) **226**, 1258 (1970).
360. F. Celada, Progr. Allergy **15**, 223 (1971).
361. W. Droege, Current Titles Immunol. Transplant. Allergy **1**, 95, 131 (1973).
362. A. Basten, J. F. A. P. Miller, J. Sprent, and C. Cheers, J. Exp. Med. **140**, 199 (1974).
363. S. T. Ellis and J. L. Gowans, Proc. Roy. Soc. London Ser. B **183**, 125 (1973).

SECTION II

Origins of Lymphocytes and the Lymphatic System

CHAPTER 3

Ontogenetic Emergence of Immunocytes

P. W. Kincade*
M. A. S. Moore*

Cancer Research Unit
The Walter and Eliza Hall Institute
of Medical Research
Royal Melbourne Hospital
Victoria, Australia

The ontogeny of immunologic function and analysis of cellular differentiation that accompanies immunologic reactions has been reviewed extensively both in this volume and elsewhere [1,2]. Consequently, the main theme of this chapter is to review the sequence of differentiation from the most primitive stem cell through the emergence of cells that can perform the various types of reactions classed as immunologic.

The lymphoid system may be divided vertically into the T- and

*Present address: Laboratories of Developmental Hematopoiesis, Sloan-Kettering Institute for Cancer Research, New York, New York.

B-lymphocyte pathways of development and horizontally into the primary and secondary lymphoid tissues. While these divisions are valid for T-cell development in both mammals and birds, it remains uncertain whether in mammals there is a clear distinction between primary and secondary tissues involved in the maturation of B cells, such as exists in the avian bursal system. It is, however, possible to consider, as primary, the antigen-independent differentiation step from uncommitted stem cell to progenitor cells committed to B and T pathways of differentiation and, as secondary, antigen-dependent further proliferation and differentiation of T and B lymphocytes.

I. Emergence of T Lymphocytes

A. Development of the Thymus

The genesis of this primary lymphoepithelial organ involves a chronologic series of tissue interactions initiated early in ontogeny at the site of the III and IV pharyngeal pouches. In the dorsal part of the pharyngeal pouch, interaction between branchial ectoderm and endoderm leads to the development of an epithelial thymic anlage [3]. Shortly thereafter, beginning on the seventh to eighth days of incubation in a chick embryo and on the 11th day of gestation in the mouse, a second population of cells appears within the thymic epithelium, characterized by intense cytoplasmic basophilia [4]. The migratory characteristic of these basophilic cells is suggested by their irregular nuclear and cytoplasmic outlines and by the presence of tails of cytoplasm which sometimes traverse the epithelial basement membrane. Basophilic cells appear in the mesenchyme that surrounds the thymus prior to their appearance within the epithelium, and their subsequent appearance in the thymus precedes vascularization. Consequently, if the intraepithelial basophilic cells are, indeed, immigrant stem cells, they have traversed the epithelial basement membrane and migrated between the closely packed epithelial cells.

Direct evidence for the circulatory origin of cells that colonize the thymic epithelium and subsequently develop into T lymphocytes has come from several studies. In experiments that utilized sex chromosomes as markers, the mitotic composition of the developing thymic lymphocyte cell population was assessed in pairs of chick embryos of opposite sex united by a vascular anastomosis of chorioallantoic or yolk sac blood vessels produced either artificially by parabiosis or occurring naturally in dizygotic twin embryos. When vascular anastomosis was established prior to the onset of thymic lymphopoiesis, high levels of thymic chimerism were subsequently found, which suggested that lymphoid stem cells were entering the avian thymus at 7 to 9 days of incubation at the time of first appearance of basophilic cells within the thymus [4]. Since chromosome marker techniques can only measure the dividing cell compartment, it was not possible to exclude a separate and possibly nonimmigrant origin for minor subpopulations of T lymphocytes, such as the population of thymocytes that are TL negative, cortisone resistant, and have a low density of θ alloantigen, a population which may have an alternative pathway of differentiation from the majority of thymic lymphocytes [5]. Recently, it has become possible to show that all T lymphocytes ultimately originate from stem cells that enter the thymic rudiment early in development. By use of interspecies differences in the structure of interphase nuclei in chick-quail combinations, Le Douarin and Jotereau [6] have shown that presumptive quail thymic endoderm grafted into 3-day chick embryos developed into a lymphoid thymus in which all lymphocytes (and connective tissue mesenchyme) were of chick origin and the epithelium was of quail origin. Grafts of 4-day thymic rudiments composed of quail mesenchyme and endoderm likewise developed normally; all lymphocytes were chick derived, and epithelium and connective tissue mesenchyme were of quail origin. These results indicate that neither thymic epithelium nor mesenchymal components can develop into T lymphocytes, even to a minor degree.

The isolation of thymic rudiments during the phase of stem cell entry and their subsequent grafting or culture in systems that prevent further stem cell inflow have shown that the extent of lymphopoiesis sustained by the rudiment correlates with the number of basophilic cells within the epithelium [4,7,8]. The rudiments excised prior to the localization of such cells fail to develop lymphocyte populations [7]. By 9 days in the chick and 12 days in the mouse embryo, the rudiments contain sufficient basophilic stem cells (100-200) to sustain normal lymphoid development for 7 to 10 days. A conservative estimate of the potential of these cells suggests that each may generate a minimum of 10^4 lymphocytes. A prerequisite for the proliferation and differentiation of immigrant stem cells is an inductive interaction between perithymic mesenchyme and thymic epithelium, since 12-day thymic epithelium, which contained stem cells but separated from adjacent mesenchyme by trypsinization, failed to undergo lymphoid differentiation in culture [9]. Lymphopoiesis could be restored by addition of thymic mesenchyme, and this effect could be mediated across a Millipore filter membrane [9,10]. In this context, the failure of development of the thymus in the nude (*nu/nu*) mouse [11] may be due to a defect in this epithelial-mesenchymal inductive interaction so necessary for further lymphoid development of the thymus. The thymic rudiment of the nude mouse embryo develops normally to a stage equivalent to that of a normal 13- to 14-day embryo, becoming colonized by basophilic cells which undergo a limited degree of lymphoid differentiation during this period [12]. By 15 days of gestation, the nude thymus epithelium becomes vacuolated, and lymphopoiesis is not sustained.

The stem cells which migrate into the thymus originate in myelopoietic tissue, and, developmentally, the only organs with thymus-repopulating capacity that function during the first wave of stem cell migration to the thymus are the yolk sac and the fetal liver in mammals and the yolk sac and spleen in birds. Analysis of the development of chimerism in hematopoietic tissues of parabiosed chick embryos and studies of the development of hematopoiesis in in vitro organ cultures of whole mouse embryos with or without their attached yolk sacs have shown that the initiation of intraembryonic hematopoiesis is dependent on a migration stream of hematopoietic stem cells which develop *ab initio* within the yolk sac blood islands and colonize developing hematopoietic microenvironments of the liver (in mammals), spleen (in birds), and the epithelial environment of the thymus [4,8,13,14]. In lower vertebrates, the yolk sac does not appear to be the sole site of origin of hematopoietic stem cells, since some evidence suggests that these cells may develop in mesenchyme associated with the neural folds [15].

The functional characterization of the stem cells that migrate into the thymus remains unclear. Ultimately, these cells are derived from multipotential stem cells which are capable of differentiating into all lines of myeloid and lymphoid differentiation and may be detected by the in vivo spleen colony assay (CFU-s) [8,16]. CFU-s are present in the yolk sac and in the circulation during the period of stem cell migration into the thymus and may be detected within the thymus rudiment of the mouse during the 12th day of gestation [8,14]. It does, however, remain possible that there is an intermediate differentiation step between the multipotential stem cell and the cell that colonizes the thymus epithelium. This differentiation step may involve the restriction of differentiation potential, so that the colonizing cell is, in fact, a lymphoid rather than a multipotential stem cell. Preliminary studies of marrow-derived cells capable of T-cell differentiation in adult mouse radiation chimeras have indicated the existence of a possible pre-T cell which possesses a model buoyant density different from that of the multipotential stem cell [17]. If such a cell population could be demonstrated in early embryonic hematopoietic tissue, it would provide support for the necessity of a differentiation stage between the multipotential stem cell and the thymus-populating cell.

Since both the embryonic and adult thymus lack cells capable of repopulating the thymus of adult irradiated animals, it is evident that immigrant stem cells rapidly undergo a differentiation step within the thymus which precedes the appearance of T-cell differentiation antigens. This early thymic lymphoid population predominates in the first 2 to 3 days of thymic development and appears to be cortisone resistant and remarkably radio resistant [18].

Although cell surface alloantigens are not detected by cytotoxicity assays in this population, it is possible that more sensitive methods of detection, e.g., absorption tests, may demonstrate small amounts of θ or TL antigen, even at this early stage.

By the 16th day of gestation, 70% of thymic lymphocytes display θ alloantigen, and by 18 days, 90% are θ positive [19]. TL and θ alloantigens do not appear simultaneously on T lymphocytes, and between 16 and 18 days of gestation, considerably more thymocytes are θ positive than TL positive.

At no stage during the development of the avian or mammalian thymus are substantial numbers of immunoglobulin (Ig) -containing cells detectable by autoradiography or immunofluorescence with anti-immunoglobulin sera [20]. In amphibians, however, Du Pasquier et al. [21] have reported Ig synthesis by thymocytes at 6 to 8 days postfertilization and prior to the appearance of Ig-synthesizing cells in the spleen. Up to 80% of thymus cells were Ig positive in amphibian larvae, but after metamorphosis, the numbers of positive cells decreased markedly, possibly due to diminished expression of Ig on the cell surface.

The further development of the thymus is marked by the appearance of corticomedullary organization and functional heterogeneity within the lymphocyte population. A minor population of thymic lymphocytes (15%) are TL negative, with a low density of θ alloantigen and a high concentration of H2 antigen. The majority (85%) of thymocytes are TL positive, with a high density of θ alloantigen and low concentration of H-2 antigen. The latter population is cortisone sensitive and appears to be immunologically inactive, whereas the former population is cortisone resistant and shares many of the functional characteristics of peripheral T cells [5,22].

Although it has been presumed that the minor cortisone-resistant population was derived from the immunologically inactive cortisone-sensitive cells, recent studies that utilized cell separation techniques and autoradiography suggested that the two populations are essentially unrelated and represent separate lines of differentiation within the thymus [5]. The TL-positive high-θ population may be mature but blocked lymphocytes destined to undergo death within the thymus possibly due to their self-reactivity, whereas the TL-negative population is the source of the virgin reactive T cells of the peripheral lymphoid tissue. In this context, Jerne [23] has suggested that the somatic generation of immune recognition may involve the generation within the thymus of two populations of lymphocytes, one of which reacts against the histocompatibility antigens that the individual happens to possess and is therefore subject to self-tolerance and another that is responsible for alloaggression and diversification by spontaneous random somatic mutation.

The functional maturation of T lymphocytes within the thymus has been monitored by assessment of responsiveness to plant lectins. Phytohemagglutinin (PHA) reactivity of mouse thymocytes has been reported as early as 15 to 16 days of gestation [24], reaching its greatest magnitude by 18 days and declining thereafter [25]. In the first few days after birth, thymocytes appear to be refractory to PHA, even after cortisone treatment (which increases the reactivity of the adult thymus). Reactivity to concanavalin A has been reported as early as 17 to 18 days of gestation but remained low at subsequent stages of thymic development [24]. Responsiveness to pokeweed mitogen was maximum 3 days after birth [25].

More specific measures of immunologic function have shown that cells capable of producing a graft-versus-host reaction (GVHR) and of a mixed lymphocyte reaction (MLR) appear in the thymus earlier than in peripheral lymphoid tissue [26,27]. Neonatal thymocytes are capable of eliciting a GVHR and are as effective as adult thymocytes in this regard; however, even as many as 10^8 thymocytes from fetuses 1 to 2 days before birth failed to elicit a detectable GVHR [26,27]. Reactivity of thymocytes to allogeneic cells, as detected by mixed lymphocyte culture (MLC) responsiveness, first appears at 18 days of gestation, reaches a maximum 3 days after birth, and falls to adult levels by 2 to 3 weeks [24,27]. Proliferative responses to allogeneic cells have been reported in neonatal rat thymocyte cultures, and the ontogenic emergence of allogeneic reactivity preceded the development of xenogeneic reactivity, as revealed in mixed rat-mouse thymocyte cultures [28]. Self-reactivity has been reported as early as 18 days of gestation in syngeneic mouse thymocyte cultures [24]; reactivity reached a maximum 3 days after birth and declined thereafter to undetectable levels [29].

The emergence of T cells with helper function follows closely the development of T cells capable of allogeneic reactivity. Neonatal thymocytes are as effective as adult thymocytes in collaborating with B cells, although late-term fetal thymocytes were considerably less effective [30].

Due to differing sensitivities of the various assays of immunocompetence, it cannot be concluded that functional T cells emerge as a single population at a particular stage of development or whether several distinct populations are emerging at different stages of development. The apparent modulation of the different reactivities of thymus cells during the late fetal and neonatal periods may be attributed to the rate of development of immunocompetent T cells within the thymus, the rate of migration of such cells to the peripheral lymphoid tissue, dilution of reactive cells with nonreactive populations, and emergence of subpopulations of suppressor T cells required to control self-reactivity.

B. Development of T Cells in Peripheral Lymphoid Tissue

Evidence for the peripheralization of T cells from the thymus to the thymus-dependent areas of spleen and lymph node has come from many experimental systems that employed chromosome marker, grafting, and adult parabiosis techniques [8,31]. Local tritiated thymidine labeling of the neonatal thymus in situ has also clearly shown that a minor population of T cells migrates from the thymus to the peripheral lymphoid tissue in the immediate postnatal period [32], and since a residual population of θ-positive cells is present, even after neonatal thymectomy, it may be presumed that peripheralization of T cells is initiated prior to birth in the mouse fetus.

θ-Positive T cells are detectable in the peripheral lymphoid tissue of 1-day-old mice; however, some discrepency exists as to the incidence of such cells in the circulation, mesenteric and peripheral lymph nodes, and Peyer's patches, as determined by cytotoxicity [33] or indirect immunofluorescence [34]. The latter technique revealed a considerably higher incidence of T cells in the tissues studied, with 60% θ-positive cells in the mesenteric and peripheral lymph nodes on Day 1, which rose to 80 to 90% by 3 days after birth. Spear et al. [35] report detection of θ-positive cells in the mouse spleen as early as 15 days of gestation, and at birth the percentage of θ-positive cells was three fourths of adult values. This percentage was considerably higher than the 1/30th of adult values reported by Stobo and Paul [36] in the neonatal BALB/c spleen. This early peripheral θ-positive population in fetal and neonatal mice appears to be functionally immature; these cells are incapable of responding normally to T-cell mitogens, such as concanavalin A or PHA, and do not appear to be antigen binding.

The gradual increase in resistance of the neonatal mouse to allogeneic lymphocytes between 2 and 4 days after birth suggests that immunocompetent cells, as measured by their ability to resist a graft-versus-host (GVH) attack, arise soon after birth, and GVH and MLC reactivities of spleen cells are generally detectable shortly after birth [25,27]. Considerable strain variation in onset of GVH reactivity of the spleen has been reported; for example, neonatal C57 spleen cells are capable of eliciting an in vivo GVHR, whereas CBA spleen cells are not reactive until 2 days after birth [37].

With the more sensitive in vitro assay for GVH reactivity, in which paired F_1 cell suspensions, GVH reactivity was detected in spleen cell suspensions on the first day after birth, and by 4 days, the spleen was fully competent [38].

II. Emergence of B Lymphocytes

A. Development of B Lymphocytes in Birds

Much of what is known about early events in plasma cell differentiation has accrued from studies that employed chickens. Attention was directed to this species after the recognition by Glick et al. [39] of the importance of the bursa of Fabricius in the functional maturation of antibody responsiveness. Subsequent studies of the role of the chicken bursa and thymus led to the concept of separate origins for cells that mediate humoral and cell-mediated immune responses [40-42]. It is therefore appropriate to begin this discussion of the development of B cells with an outline of lymphopoiesis in the chicken bursa.

1. Gross Development of the Bursa

This lymphoepithelial organ first appears at 4 to 5 days of incubation as an evagination of the dorsal wall of the cloaca. By the 11th day, the luminal surface of the bursa is plicated, and on the 12th day, localized thickenings of epithelium occur within these plicae. Bursal lymphopoiesis begins by the 14th day within these epithelial buds, which then detach from the luminal epithelium and develop as circumscribed lymphoid follicles surrounded by a basement membrane [43]. These follicles rapidly expand in size, primarily due to lymphocyte accumulation, and after hatching, distinct cortical and medullary regions separated by a basement membrane are present. The cortex is comprised of densely packed lymphocytes in rapid division, and the periphery of the medulla likewise contains many dividing cells, but the central medulla is more diffusely populated with lymphocytes and a network of epithelial cells. Breaks within the basement membrane suggest migration of cells between these two compartments [44], and the order of their development, thymidine labeling studies [45], and recovery after irradiation [46] suggest that the direction of this migration is from medulla to cortex. The bursa attains maximum size at 5 to 12 weeks, begins involution at sexual maturity, and completely involutes by 6 to 12 months of age.

2. Ancestry of Bursal Lymphocytes

The question of the derivation of bursal lymphocytes was a parallel controversy to that of the origin of thymic lymphocytes. In a series of sex chromosome marker studies, Metcalf and Moore [8] and Moore and Owen [43,47] obtained evidence for a blood born immigrant stem cell. Dividing bursal cells of parabiotic or twin dizygotic chick embryos were examined for chromosomes of the opposite sex. When sampling was done prior to lymphoid differentiation between 11 and 13 days of incubation, little or no chimerism was evident. In the critical period of lymphoid transition between 14 and 15 days, chimerism was highly variable. As soon as lymphopoiesis was initiated in bursal follicles, chimerism was obtained and was sometimes as high as 50% in both partners. Thus, the vascular union of the two embryos allowed an exchange of bursal lymphocyte progenitors. Further, grafts of bursas from 10- to 14-day embryos placed on the chorioallantoic membrane of 10- to 12-day embryos were able to accept host stem cells and developed in parallel with the host bursa. A very high degree of chimerism was observed, even when the host bursa was prevented from development by testosterone treatment. The origin of these stem cells was studied by using the chromosome marker system to determine chimerism in irradiated embryos injected with hematopoietic cells of opposite sex [48]. Embryonic blood, bone marrow, spleen, yolk sac, and thymus were tested for their bursa-repopulating capacity. Spleen, yolk sac, and peripheral blood cells all were capable of reconstituting the irradiated bursa in the critical 13- to 14-day period, whereas thymus cells were ineffective. Bone marrow became a consistent donor of repopulating cells only later. The timing of bursal seeding by immigrant stem cells was further investigated by injecting tritiated thymidine-labeled embryo marrow and spleen cells to chick embryos. Maximum bursal localization of injected cells was attained when cells were administered on Day 14. This stage of development corresponds to the time when the bursa contains many large undifferentiated cells with prominent nucleoli and basophilic cytoplasm, indistinguishable from cells present in the developing thymus. The immigrant nature of these cells was established by injecting tritiated thymidine-labeled hematopoietic cells from various organs into embryos at various stages of development. A few hours after injection of 14-day embryos, labeled cells were found in the bursal blood vessels and adjacent mesenchyme which were morphologically identical to the basophilic cells of normal 14-day embryos. By 24 hr after injection, a significant proportion of labeled cells were within follicles. By 48 hr, increasing numbers of labeled cells were present in follicles, and some were morphologically identified as lymphocytes.

3. *Immunoglobulin Synthesis by Bursal Cells*

A striking feature of bursal lymphopoiesis is the synthesis of Ig. This phenomenon was first demonstrated by Thorbecke et al. [49] and subsequently confirmed with a variety of techniques [50-53]. Ig is first detectable within bursal cells of 14-day embryos by use of μ- or light chain-specific antibody. Cells that contain γ chains have not been observed until the time of hatching, and α chains are detectable in bursal follicles within a few days of hatching [54]. Cells that contain demonstrable Ig are restricted to the medulla, except for occasional plasma cells in the cortex and lamina propria.

Several characteristics distinguish Ig synthesis by bursal cells from that of plasma cells. The intensity of immunofluorescent staining of bursal cells, as compared to that of mature plasma cells, suggests that very modest quantities of intracellular Ig are present [51]. Physiochemical studies have revealed little Ig secretion of bursal cells and the presence of a unique μ chain with deficient carbohydrate [52,55]. Individual plasma cells, with rare exceptions, contain only a single major class, subclass, and allotype of immunoglobulin [56,57]. Bursal cells, however, may lack Ig class exclusion [51]. In studies of bursal sections, IgG-containing cells were only found superimposed in areas rich in IgM-containing cells, whereas collections of cells that stained for IgM alone were often seen. Furthermore, individual cells of bursal cell suspensions often stained for more than one class of Ig, whereas spleen cells only rarely did so.

The Ig synthesized by bursal cells is rapidly incorporated into the cell membrane. Immunofluorescence of viable bursal cell suspensions has revealed IgM-bearing cells as early as 15 days of incubation [54,58]. By the time of hatching, a majority of bursal cells have detectable surface Ig [58-61]. Surface Ig on bursal cells seemed to have less tendency to aggregate to polar caps with labeled anti-Ig than did that of peripheral blood lymphocytes, but a variety of staining conditions has not been employed [59]. Sallstrom and Alm [62] recently noted that bursal cells are less able to coalesce surface-bound molecules of concanavalin A than are peripheral blood cells.

4. *Bursal Development and Exogenous Antigens*

The events described above that occur during the embryonic development of the bursa, including the onset of IgM and IgG synthesis, appear to be unrelated to exogenous antigens [49,51]. Their timing is remarkably reproducible with different strains of chicken embryos, including those from specific pathogen-free flocks. Deliberate immunization or life in a germfree environment has little discernible influence on bursal development. Most attempts to demonstrate antibody-producing cells in the bursa after systemic or intrabursal immunization have been unsuccessful [63-65]. Recently, the appearance of cells in the bursa a few days after hatching that produce specific antibodies to organisms of the gut microflora has been demonstrated [66]. Since the bursal cortex forms after hatching, and it occasionally contains plasma cells, some of the cell proliferation in that site could be due to stimulation by substances from the gut lumen.

The data discussed thus far indicate that immigrant stem cells of yolk sac origin migrate into specialized buds of gut epithelium around the 13th day of incubation. The size of this colonizing population of cells has been estimated to be between 100 and 1,000 [8]. Probably within hours of this event, IgM synthesis is initiated, and these molecules are rapidly placed in the cell membrane. Numbers of these primitive lymphocytes steadily increase, and two other major classes of Ig sequentially make their appearance. Exogenous antigens apparently play no role in these events.

5. *Relationship Between Bursal Lymphopoiesis and Emergence of B Lymphocytes in Peripheral Lymphoid Tissues*

a. Effect of Bursectomy. Bursectomy has been extensively employed to define the role of that organ in B-cell development. A summary of the effects of bursectomy will be presented to show that the primary role of the bursa is to seed B lymphocytes or their progenitors to peripheral lymphoid tissues and to allow some speculations about the timing of this process and the differentiation potential of the disseminated cells.

Surgical bursectomy, when performed at its earliest practical stage (approximately 17 days of incubation), results in a profound immune deficiency. Such animals are often agammaglobulinemic, lack plasma cells and germinal centers, and fail to produce antibody [67]. A deficiency of circulating cells with easily detectable surface immunoglobulin also exists [68]. If surgical bursectomy is carried out at progressively later stages of development, the resultant deficiency of circulating Ig-bearing cells is progressively less severe.

The various classes of serum Ig are differentially sensitive to bursectomy. If the operation is performed at hatching, reduced levels of both IgG and IgA result, with coexistently elevated IgM levels [68-70]. Some individual birds bursectomized just prior to hatching selectively lack IgA-containing plasma cells and serum IgA. IgG synthesis is the next most sensitive to bursectomy, and chickens bursectomized slightly earlier may have little or no serum IgG or IgA and greatly elevated IgM. This overproduction of IgM has been explained as a lack of feedback regulation, which normally is a function of low-molecular-weight antibodies [69].

The responsiveness of bursectomized animals to deliberate immunization or environmental antigens is also differentially affected by bursectomy. Removal of the bursa at late stages of embryonic life or during the first 2 weeks of life results in deficient or absent primary immune responses, whereas secondary responses are generally normal [71,72]. Titers of natural agglutinins to foreign erythrocytes reflect an animal's responsiveness to environmental antigens. Profound agglutinen deficiencies result from bursectomy, and the duration of these deficiencies decreases the later the bursectomy is performed [68,73].

The varying degrees of immune deficiency produced by surgical bursectomy can be obtained by other techniques or combinations of techniques. One of the most widely used of these methods is testosterone treatment. The observation that the bursa involutes at sexual maturity led Glick and Sadler [74] to investigate the possibility that this process was under gonadal control. Bursal development was found to be virtually absent in testosterone-treated embryos. The exact mode of action of testosterone is unknown, but it has been demonstrated that stem cells capable of populating the bursa are unaffected in treated embryos [43]. In addition to failure of lymphoid follicular development, testosterone treatment causes morphologic alterations in the bursal epithelium. Cells of the lining epithelium in treated bursas are considerably elongated and hypertrophied, and cystic spaces that contain mucoid secretion are present. Some testosterone treatment regimens lead to agammaglobulinemia, lack of plasma cells, and lack of germinal centers, i.e., complete bursectomy [75]. Others lead to partial deficiences indistinguishable from those of chickens surgically bursectomized in late embryonic life [76].

It is difficult by either hormonal or surgical means to eliminate the bursa early enough to consistently prevent all vestiges of bursa-dependent structures from developing. For this reason, irradiation or immunosuppressive drugs have been used alone or in combination with surgical bursectomy to achieve "total" bursectomy [77-81].

Yet another way of preventing the development of bursa-dependent cells is by antibody-mediated suppression. Since Ig is associated with bursal lymphocytes from their earliest appearance, administration of foreign antibodies to Ig is sufficient to arrest their development. When given on the 13th day of incubation, antibodies specific for IgM suppress development of IgM-, IgG-, and IgA-producing cells [82,83]. This suppression is dose dependent and is transient unless followed by bursectomy at hatching. The combination of antibody treatment and bursectomy at hatching completely prevents development of bursa-dependent cells, and agammaglobulinemia is the result. Differential effects of anti-IgM treatment result if the antibody is not given until after bursectomy at hatching. Under these conditions, selective retardation of IgM synthesis has been observed. The precise mechanism of antibody-mediated suppression is unknown, but Fab fragments of anti-Ig are sufficient to produce immune deficiency [83]. Therefore, complement-mediated lysis of Ig-bearing cells is an unlikely mechanism. It is conceivable that antibody-dependent cell-mediated cytotoxicity is involved [84].

A few generalizations about the long-term effects of bursectomy are possible. Absolute numbers of circulating lymphocytes are normal in bursectomized birds [85,86]. Deficiencies in circulating Ig levels in adult chickens which result from bursectomy are permanent, and completely agammaglobulinemic birds have survived as long as 9 months of age without any recovery of Ig-synthesizing capability. Also, selective deficiencies of IgA or IgG and IgA are not repaired with time. Reduced numbers of circulating Ig-bearing cells which exist in young bursectomized chickens likewise persist. On the other hand, once the ability to produce Ig of a given class is attained, the bursa can be removed without a resultant acquired immune deficiency [68,87].

An important point to be made about the various bursectomy procedures described is that removal of the bursa and ablation of bursa-dependent cells can be achieved without a lasting effect on the development of thymus-derived cells. Chickens that completely lack bursa-dependent cells are normal in their ability to reject skin homografts or display delayed hypersensitivity responses [42].

b. Reconstitution of Bursectomized Chickens. The above discussion describes the variety of techniques which can be employed to obviate the function of the bursa of Fabricius. In principle, such B-less animals should provide an assay system for the proliferative and differentiation potential of cells of various stages of development in the plasma cell line. However, the lack of syngeneic chicken flocks has severely limited the application of reconstitution experiments in this model.

Cooper et al. [88] first restored the ability to form germinal centers, plasma cells, and Ig to bursectomized irradiated recipients with autologous bursal cells, but specific antibody responsiveness was not restored. Other experiments with autologous bursal cells or implants for newly hatched chicks have failed to achieve full reconstitution [89,90].

Other reconstitution attempts have employed semihistocompatible cell transfers. Gilmour et al. [91] demonstrated that bursal cells from 4-week-old donors could transfer responsiveness to *Brucella* organisms but not sheep erythrocytes to irradiated recipients. Cain and David partially reconstituted the response to sheep erythrocytes of neonatally bursectomized chickens with large numbers of bursal cells from 5-week-old donors [92]. Bone marrow from normal, but not bursectomized, 6- to 8-week-old chickens likewise restores immune competence to newborn bursectomized chickens [90].

c. Other Approaches. Toivanen et al. [80,93] studied the reconstituting capacity of various cell suspensions in cyclophosphamide-treated 4-day-old chickens. In this system, embryonic yolk sac, liver, bone marrow, and spleen cells had no effect, whereas embryonic (17 days of incubation, 4 days posthatching) bursal cells were capable of repopulating the treated bursas and restoring some immune competence in a portion of the animals. Bursal cells from young chickens (3½-10 weeks of age) most consistently restored immune competence but failed to restore normal bursal morphology. Later transplants from bone marrow (10 weeks of age) and spleen (14 weeks of age) consistently produced recovery of immune competence.

Weber [81] transferred chromosomally marked 4-week-old bursal cells to 4-week-old chicks rendered agammaglobulinemic by combined testosterone and cyclophosphamide treatment. He found that x-irradiation of the recipients and intravenous, rather than intraperitoneal, transfer of donor cells were essential for successful reconstitution. Donor cells proliferated in response to antigen primarily in the spleen and to a lesser extent in the bone marrow. Specific antibodies to *Brucella* and sheep erythrocytes were produced by the restored animals, and plasma cells, but not germinal centers, were present. Donor cells in these animals were also responsive to lipopolysaccharide [94]. The chimerism produced in these experiments was not permanent, and by 10 weeks after cell transfer, the animals had returned to an agammaglobulinemic state.

The reconstitution experiments demonstrate that the lesion of bursectomized chickens can be repaired with bursal or bursa-derived lymphoid cells. Thus, the primary role of the bursa is lymphopoiesis. Other, possibly humoral, functions which are often postulated have not been substantiated [95-97].

More difficult to discern is the nature of the cells which leave the bursa. The defective primary immune responses and persistent deficiencies of B cells in bursectomized chickens are subject to two interpretations. The development of B lymphocytes in peripheral lymphoid tissues may only be related to the traffic of mature cells from the bursa, and these effects could result from a limited population of these extra bursal cells. Alternately, the cells which escape the bursa in embryonic or neonatal life may differ in proliferative potential [98] and in other properties from those which emerge later. Young bursal cells may differ from older bursal cells in their ability to repopulate cyclophosphamide-treated bursas [80,93], the nature of the Ig they produce [51], the mobility of their membrane components [62], and their ability to achieve permanent chimerism in agammaglobulinemic chickens [81]. However, with the possible exception of Ig class expression, there is no evidence that cells with immature characteristics normally leave the bursa.

An experimental approach to the above question might be possible if truly syngeneic flocks were available. Ideally, grafts of B lymphocytes should be exchangeable without the necessity of irradiation or immunosuppressive drug treatment. Then, limiting-dilution transfers of adult lymphocytes could be made to agammaglobulinemic recipients in an effort to reproduce the symptoms of embryonic bursectomy.

Some idea of the normal development of bursa-dependent cells in peripheral lymphoid tissues can be obtained from the appearance of Ig-containing cells in the tissues of chickens that bear vertically transmitted viruses and that have been reared in a conventional environment [51]. The order of appearance of Ig-containing cells in such tissues recapitulates their appearance in the bursa. Very rare IgM-containing cells have been seen before the time of hatching; the earliest was found at 17 days of incubation. A rapid increase in numbers of these cells occurred on the third day after hatching. Peripherally located IgG-containing cells were not found until the fourth day after hatching, and their rapid expansion occurred on approximately the eighth day of life. Development of Ig-containing cells in tissues other than the bursa is defective in chickens reared in a germfree environment.

Precise determination of the time of appearance Ig-bearing cells in peripheral lymphoid tissues of the chicken has not been made, but the bursal origin of these cells appears to be certain [59,60].

A limited number of studies have employed local labeling of bursal cells to study their fate in vivo. Aside from demonstrating that bursal cells migrate to nonthymus-dependent areas of peripheral lymphoid tissue, including germinal centers, these studies shed little light on the kinetics and direction of early migration streams of cells that originate in the bursa [99,100].

B. Development of B Lymphocytes in Mammals

A mammalian analog of the bursa of Fabricius has not been critically defined. Therefore, studies on early events in mammalian B-lymphocyte differentiation are not strictly comparable to those conducted with chickens. While controversy over the bursal equivalent continues, recent identification of markers for cells of the plasma cell series have made it possible to determine when cells of this lineage make their appearance in ontogeny. When fully exploited, these techniques should reveal the migration patterns of young B lymphocytes and perhaps will implicate the site of their origin.

1. Immunoglobulin-bearing Cells

Of the markers for B lymphocytes of mice and humans, surface Ig is the most useful. As previously discussed, the earliest Ig produced by bursal cells is destined to be incorporated into the cell membrane rather than to be secreted. There is now ample evidence that, in mice and in humans, readily detectable surface Ig, demonstrated by anti-Ig blast transformation in vitro, immunofluorescence, or autoradiography, is as distinctive for nonthymus-derived lymphocytes as it is for bursa-derived cells in the chicken [101,102].

IgM-bearing cells have been detected in the human fetus as early as 9.5 weeks of gestation [103]. Shortly thereafter, IgG- and IgA-bearing cells make their appearance, and by 14.5 weeks the proportion of peripheral blood cells that bears these immunoglobulins is comparable to that of adults. At the earliest stages of gestation, only the liver was suitable for examination, but later, Ig-bearing cells were demonstrated in the spleen, thymus, and peripheral blood.

Recently, it has been shown that IgD is present on the majority of IgM-bearing cells in newborn and adult human peripheral blood [104,105]. This finding suggests that the δ chain might precede the μ chain in appearance on the surface of developing B lymphocytes. The failure of previous attempts to demonstrate IgD synthesis by human fetal tissues may reflect the bias of the methods used for Ig intended for secretion rather than for formation of membrane-bound Ig [106].

Similar techniques have been used to reveal Ig-bearing cells in tissues of fetal mice. By the 16th day of gestation, Ig-bearing cells are present in the spleen, liver, and peripheral blood and are regularly demonstrable in the bone marrow after the 18th day (Fig. 1). Their development in lymph nodes and Peyer's patches occurs mainly after birth, and adult proportions are attained in the spleen by 3 weeks of age [20,35].

It should be emphasized that the methods currently available for demonstrating Ig-bearing cells require cell suspensions to be made which contain reasonable numbers of viable nucleated cells. This requirement places constraints on the interpretation of the presence of Ig-bearing cells in very young embryos. Young bursal follicles, for example, are very difficult to disrupt, and the resultant cell suspensions often contain many damaged cells and clusters of undissociated cells [54]. Therefore, failure to demonstrate Ig-bearing cells in a particular young organ does not preclude their presence in low proportions relative to structural elements.

Soloman has devised a procedure for equating developmental stages of various species [2]. By use of his constants for calculating age equivalence $K(t - t')$, remarkably close agreement is seen between the earliest detection of Ig-bearing cells in mice and humans and the initiation of bursal Ig synthesis in the chicken (Table 1). B cells have been demonstrated in the human fetus within 4 days of the predicted onset of Ig synthesis. It is likely, then, that this first appearance of Ig-bearing cells occurs as a normal event in differentiation, independent of influence by exogenous antigens. Furthermore, newborn germfree mice have a normal distribution and number of Ig-bearing cells [107].

2. *Immunoglobulin-containing Cells*

In the chicken, two categories of cells contain Ig in sufficient quantities to be detectable by immunofluorescence. One is a weakly staining lymphoblastic cell that contains one or multiple classes of nonsecretory Ig and is found in the medulla of bursal follicles. The other cell type usually contains more substantial quantities of Ig of a single class, secretes Ig, and is distributed contiguously with cells of the plasma cell series. The former cell type shows no obvious dependence on exogenous antigens, whereas the latter develops normally only through antigenic exposure.

Cells superficially analogous to bursal Ig-containing cells have been seen in the gut-associated tissues of mammals [108], but little information is available as to their development. Technical difficulties have thus far prevented determining whether they precede the emergence of Ig-bearing cells [109].

Ig-containing cells of the plasmacytic type have been detected in

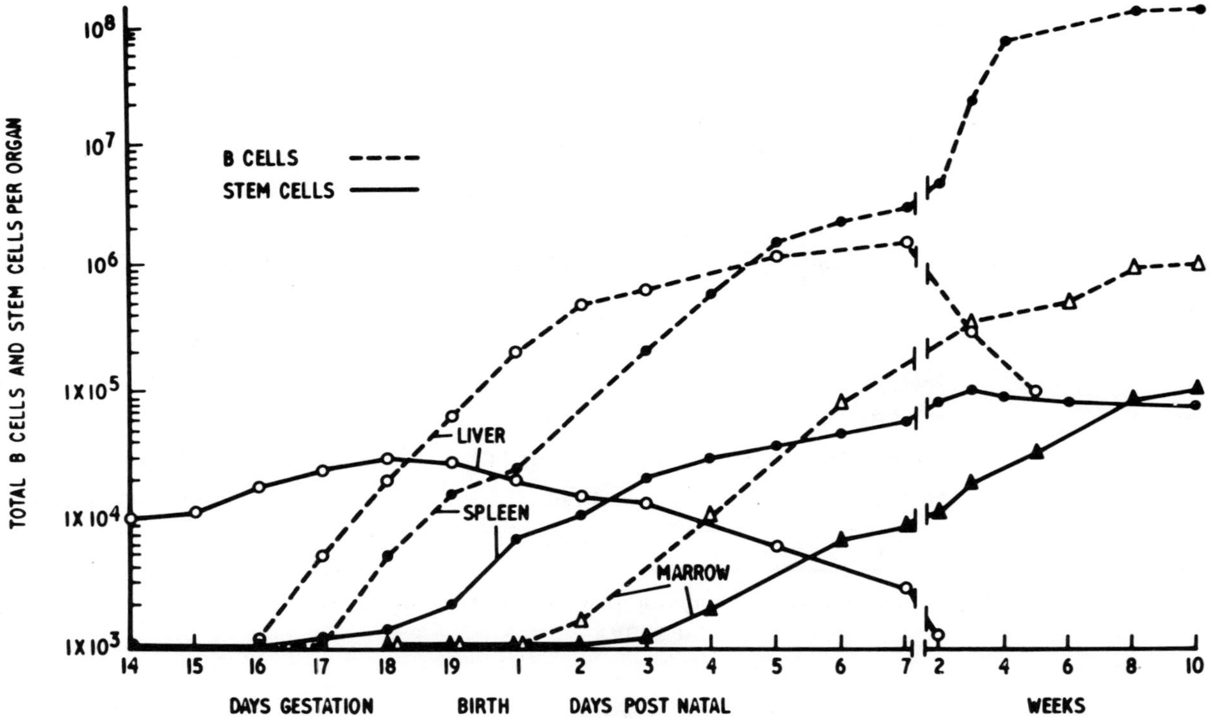

FIG. 1. Emergence of B lymphocytes (---) and stem cells (–) (CFU-s adjusted for seeding efficiency) in hematopoietic tissues of fetal and neonatal mice. Note that the liver not only provides stem cells for B-lymphocyte differentiation but also is an early and consistent location for B lymphocytes. Data are from Metcalf and Moore [8] and Nossal and Pike [20].

TABLE 1
Events in Embryogenesis Associated with Lymphocyte Development in Three Species

	Chicken	Man	Mouse
Initiation of circulation	39 Hr	21 Days	9 Days
Onset of intraembryonic myelopoiesis	11 Days (spleen)	42 Days (liver)	10 Days (liver)
Thymus rudiment appears	6 Days	40 Days	10-11 Days
Large lymphocytes present in thymus	7 Days	70 Days	12-13 Days
Bursal rudiment appears	8 Days		
Colonization of bursa by stem cells	12-14 Days		
Earliest B cells detectable	14 Days (0.102)	66.5 Days (0.157)	16 Days (0.097)

developing human fetuses after the emergence of Ig-bearing cells [103]. The presence of these cells may also be indicated by assays of in vitro Ig-synthesizing capability of various tissues, such as the spleen, or by the presence of Ig of fetal origin in the circulation. Because of different sensitivities of these methods, and due to the varying influences of antigenic stimuli, there is no uniformity apparent in the emergence of these cells.

3. *The Stem Cell for Mammalian B-lymphocyte Differentiation*

There is no reason to suspect that the as yet undefined bursal analog is not populated with blood-borne immigrant stem cells which originally developed in the yolk sac. It is therefore useful to consider the nature of the cells which initially settle in the bursal equivalent and from which the plasma cell line descends.

In the mouse, multipotential stem cells of liver origin or daughter lymphoid stem cells probably enter the bursal equivalent on the 14th to 16th days of gestation. The multipotential nature of the stem cells is indicated by the ability of cloned cells in spleen colonies to completely reconstitute both thymus-derived and nonthymus-derived responsiveness of irradiated animals to a variety of antigens [110-112]. At the gestational age when Ig-bearing cells are first detectable in mice and humans, only the liver contains large numbers of yolk sac-derived hematopoietic stem cells [8,14]; therefore, it is the probable donor. It is not known whether this initial entry of stem cells is followed by continual recruitment or whether this early immigrant population possesses sufficient proliferation potential for the life of the animal. Furthermore, there is no information available as to whether the differentiation of stem cells to B lymphocytes occurs at a high rate throughout life or if the population of B cells present in the neonate is normally self-sustaining.

By inference from studies of the bursa and both chicken and mammalian thymus development, the immigrant stem cell which normally enters the bursal equivalent would be large and have a basophilic cytoplasm. This does not mean, however, that other morphologic types of stem cells (e.g., transitional cells, lymphocytes) do not have the potential to differentiate within the bursal equivalent to B lymphocytes.

B-lymphocyte differentiation can be demonstrated in the adult lethally irradiated mouse provided with a source of syngeneic stem cells [20,110,112-114]. The stem cells may be obtained from either fetal liver or from spleen colonies (CFU-s). It is known that stem cells from these two sources differ greatly, not only in physical properties but also in proliferative potential [115-117]. Regardless of which type of stem cell is administered to the irradiated adult, approximately 1 week is required before B lymphocytes can be detected. As previously discussed, this process occurs within the embryonic chicken bursa within 1 day. Reconstitution of the plasma cell line of an immune deficient human has been accomplished with fetal liver cells, and approximately 3 weeks were required for B-cell emergence [118].

4. *Theories for the Mammalian Bursal Equivalent*

The available information on B-lymphocyte development in mammals suggests many similarities with the situation described for the chicken. In that species, production of virgin B cells is absolutely dependent on a single organ, the bursa of Fabricius, and is not influenced in any obvious way by the thymus. Without question, the analogous differentiation pathway in mammals is thymus independent. Agreement as to the actual bursal equivalent, however, has not been reached. At various times, such candidate tissues as the thymus, tonsils, appendix, Peyer's patches, germinal centers, bone marrow, and skin have entered the debate which has continued for more than 10 years. It is not the purpose of this chapter to extensively review the literature on this issue but rather to recount the key points of the most favored theories. Before doing so, it is necessary to consider the minimum requirements for any candidate bursal analog. It must accept immigrant multipotential stem cells and commit them irrevocably to B-lymphocyte differentiation, be present and function before Ig-bearing cells are detectable elsewhere, and perform without intervention by exogenous antigens. In addition to these absolute requirements, it should also be the first location of easily detectable Ig synthesis, should be important for Ig class diversification, should involve a large cell to small cell maturation sequence, and may have a follicular structure.

a. Gut-associated Lymphoepithelial Tissues (GALT). Interest in the importance of the appendix and Peyer's patches in the development of humoral immunity began with the observation that lymphopoiesis in the appendix occurred in neonatally thymectomized rabbits [119]. Subsequent studies in the rabbit have shown that appendectomy [120], appendectomy plus x-irradiation [121], or appendectomy plus Peyer's patch removal plus x-irradiation [122,123] depresses the primary immune response but does not impair the function of thymus-derived cells. Peyer's patches are not sites of active antibody formation after local or parenteral immunization, but germinal centers can be induced by direct injection of the patches [124]. The structural relationships of the GALT have recently been redescribed with respect to the partitioning of thymus- and nonthymus-derived areas and their development [108,125,126]. At some time during embryogenesis, Peyer's patches develop beneath a dome of epithelium, which later becomes pinocytotic and is distinguishable by its lack of goblet cells [127]. After birth, a cortical area develops that partially surrounds the central medulla but is not separated from it by a basement membrane. Interspersed between these areas, thymus-derived cells accumulate. The ratio of thymus-dependent to non-thymus-dependent areas varies widely from appendix to Peyer's patch and from species to species; the thymus-dependent area predominates in newborn mice [33,128]. Cell proliferation is especially pronounced in the cortex, as in the bursal cortex, and this mitotic activity seems to be related to exposure to gut microflora [129-132]. Although Ig-containing cells of the plasma cell type are sparse, Ig-containing cells can be demonstrated in the central medulla (corona), and multiple heavy-chain classes appear to be superimposed [108]. The resemblance of these cells to bursal follicles is striking when the plane of section is longitudinal and far enough from the gut lumen to exclude the thymus-dependent areas. In one species, the pig, rudimentary Peyer's patches are detectable morphologically [109] before Ig-bearing cells emerge [133]. Precise timing of the first appearance of Ig-containing cells in these tissues has been difficult to determine for technical reasons. Peyer's patches are poorly developed and lack corticomedullary distinctions in young mice which have undergone anti-Ig treatment [134].

Several types of information are sorely needed to substantiate the GALT as a bursal analog. The precise chronologic sequence of first appearance and development of these tissues in several species must be determined in relation to onset of Ig synthesis and appearance of Ig-bearing cells. It must then be shown that this process is dependent on imigrant stem cells. Finally, the influence of exogenous antigen on early GALT development must be elucidated. An interesting collection of lymphoid tissue associated with the bronchus bears several similarities to GALT and deserves further study [135,136].

b. Bone Marrow. Mitchell and Miller [137] first demonstrated the presence of precursors for antibody-forming cells within adult bone marrow. The relative absence of thymus-derived cells in this location, together with the infrequency of B cells in the thymus, made possible the demonstration of functional collaboration between B and T cells in the immune response [138]. Studies of cell kinetics have indicated a rapid turnover of cells in the marrow morphologically identifiable as lymphocytes [139,140], and evidence has been obtained that these cells disseminate to other tissues [141]. It has been tempting to deduce from these findings that B lymphocytes are produced in the bone marrow, and the term "bone marrow derived" has become synonymous with mammalian B cells in popular usage. This is an unfortunate and confusing classification, since there is as yet no direct evidence that Ig-bearing B lymphocytes originate de novo in the marrow.

The data available to date do not allow acceptance of the bone marrow as the strict equivalent of the avian bursa. Substantial development of the bone marrow, including its content of Ig-bearing cells and colonization by stem cells, occurs after B lymphocytes have emerged elsewhere. The liver and not the bone marrow is the probable initial donor of multipotent stem cells for the bursal equivalent, although these cells could conceivably be recruited from the marrow if needed in adult life. Approximately 25% of the nucleated cells in bone marrow of mice or humans are classifiable as lymphocytes, but only 8 to 10% are Ig bearing by immunofluorescence [142], and no structural organization of these lymphocytes, e.g., follicular aggregates, have been found in normal adult bone marrow [143]. No direct relationship has been established between the Ig-negative and Ig-positive lymphocytes, but the thymidine labeling kinetics of the two populations are compatible with a maturation sequence from small Ig-negative cells to small Ig-positive lymphocytes [144].

Bone marrow B cells in mice may have properties distinctive from those of B lymphocytes in other tissues. They have been reported to be relatively resistant to anti-Ig killing [145], do not collaborate with irradiated T cells [146], resist inactivation by radioactive antigen [147], and may have a distinct distribution of Ig classes [148]. Some of these properties may be attributable to the nonuniformity of Ig density on bone marrow B lymphocytes [149].

It is quite possible that the bone marrow plays an important role in B-lymphocyte function and/or maturation in the adult. Considerably more information is needed about the marrow B-cell population, especially as regards the possible relationship of Ig-negative to Ig-positive lymphocytes, the migration of Ig-positive bone marrow cells, and the extent to which antigen affects the marrow.

c. Hematopoietic Tissue. The difficulty encountered in demonstrating a precocious nonthymus-derived lymphoid tissue in young mammals and the failure thus far of efforts to detect a focus of B-lymphocyte emergence in embryos or irradiated stem cell-reconstituted adults have led some to believe that multiple sites may be involved in B-lymphocyte differentiation [20,114]. According to this view, B lymphopoiesis could occur in any hematopoietic tissue, and since there is a shift of this activity from liver to spleen to bone marrow in development, all of these sites could at some time be involved. The liver would appear to satisfy some requirements for a bursal equivalent. Like the bursa, it originates from interaction between gut epithelium and mesenchyme, is populated by hematopoietic stem cells, and is an early location for detectable B cells in human and mouse embryos. There is little data to either substantiate or refute this multiple origin concept, and, by definition, it may resist direct critical evaluation. It is likely, rather, that the validity of the theory will be measured by the failure of the others we have discussed.

5. Development of Immunoglobulin Class Diversity in Mammals

One of the most intriguing aspects of B-lymphocyte maturation is the sequential expression of the various heavy-chain classes. Each class first makes its appearance in prescribed order as a B-lymphocyte surface receptor, and the sequence is recapitulated later by antibody-forming cells. Previously we have discussed the evidence for μ as the earliest heavy chain expressed in chickens, followed by γ and α. There is now evidence that the situation in mice and humans is similar. Development of B cells in mice can be severely depressed by treatment with anti-μ antibodies [134,150]. It is also possible to selectively influence the γ- and α-producing capability of young mice by a regimen of anti-γ antibody treatment [151]. IgM is the earliest of these classes found on B cells in humans [103]. The evidence in the chicken suggested an irrevocable intrabursal switch in the commitment of cells to the synthesis of these Ig classes, but information on this point has been difficult to obtain in other species. Even the number of classes present on individual B lymphocytes in peripheral lymphoid tissues of mammals is unresolved. By immunofluorescence, single heavy-chain major classes, subclasses, and allotypes are borne by cells [152-154]. Other, perhaps more sensitive, techniques provide evidence of considerable overlap [155-157]. B cells which produce IgG after adoptive transfer [158] or during a primary immune response in vitro [159] are sensitive to anti-μ treatment, but it is not certain that these assays are equally sensitive to all categories of cells. Recently, both IgM and IgG responses in an adoptive secondary in chickens was suppressed with anti IgM [98]. Some evidence has been obtained for the segregation of IgM- and IgG-committed lymphocytes from the bone marrow by cell separation [160] or limiting-dilution [161] techniques. It appears certain that some peripheral B lymphocytes destined to become IgG antibody-producing cells bear IgM receptors [162], but the frequency of this population of çells is not known. A change in the Ig class within a B-cell clone can occur without change in the specificity [163]. An exception to the condition that immunofluorescence reveals single Ig classes per individual B lymphocyte is found in the recent descriptions of IgD distribution on human B cells [105,164]. Most IgM-bearing cells also stain for IgD and vice versa. These coexistent molecules share the same type of light chain and can be separately moved or removed from the cell surface with anti-Ig. No doubt these findings will encourage determinations of the emergence of IgD-bearing cells in utero and spur efforts to identify related Ig classes in other species.

a. Diversification of Antibody Specificity. Current dogma holds that individual antibody-forming cells secrete Ig molecules of homogeneous specificity, and it is assumed that these cells arose from precursor B cells that bore surface Ig receptors of the same specificity. This position is controversial in the sense that while an immune response to a given antigen can be prevented by removing B cells with receptors for it, formal proof is not available that some immunocompetent B cells do not have receptors which differ somewhat from the Ig their progeny will secrete. Without entering this debate, it is safe to assume that at some time during B-cell development, the extensive repertoire of antibody specificities which are either encoded in the genome of stem cells or generated through somatic mutation is distributed evenly over the population of virgin immunocompetent cells, with each cell expressing one or a few of these specificities.

The role played by the bursa in the commitment of B lymphocytes to particular Ig classes suggests that it might also be the location where Ig specificity is determined [165]. Impaired recovery of bursectomized chickens from tolerance [166,167] could be due to the fact that new clones of B cells for a given specificity can only originate there. That is, cells committed to antibody synthesis of a given specificity do not later change to new specificities after leaving the bursa. Also in support of this concept is the recent finding that stable patterns of unresponsiveness to defined haptens result from bursectomy [46].

Antigen-binding techniques should be applicable in determining the emergence of specificities. Thus far, only a small group of antigens has been employed, but antigen-binding cells are present in embryonic mice and chickens as early as are Ig-bearing cells [35,168,169]. It is uncertain whether the equivalent studies of human fetal cells relate to B lymphocytes or thymus-derived cells [170,171].

III. Functional Maturation of Immune Responsiveness

We have avoided discussion of development of immune competence to various antigens since this phenomenon no doubt involves maturation of macrophages, B cells, and T cells and other complications, such as feedback from maternal antibodies [172]. The previous discussion has focused on the emergence and dissemination of recognizable members of the plasma cell and thymus-derived lines of cells. More subtle differentiation steps than mere acquisition of surface antigens and proliferation may only be recognizable by tests of functional capability. Initially, these tests must be artificial in the sense that their relationship to normal in vivo differentiation processes is unknown. Application of a sufficient number of tests to the study of developing cells can lead to a definition of subpopulations whose interrelationship may be eventually revealed. In recent studies of the development of immunocompetence in the mouse, attempts have been made to "tailor make" assays to detect the function of a single population of cells. For example, to assay for the presence of functional B cells from young tissues, T and adherent (A) cell requirements can be fulfilled with lipopolysaccharide and reducing agents, respectively [173-175], and B cells can be made limiting in adoptive transfers by adding an excess of irradiated spleen cells and thymus cells [176].

Detection of young B cells can be favored by multiple immunizations [177], high dosages of antigen [177-179], and delays in various steps of the assay [176-180,181]. T cell-independent antigens provide a further refinement of such assays.

The potential usefulness of these approaches can be illustrated by some recent studies of the developing mouse. More extensive reports of this rapidly expanding area can be found elsewhere in this volume.

Press and Klinman [182] have recently employed a focus-forming assay to study developing B lymphocytes with competence for dinitrophenol (DNP). Limiting dilutions of cells were used to produce foci in the spleens of carrier-primed irradiated recipients. These foci were then individually tested in an in vitro assay to DNP. As early as 16 days of gestation in the mouse, precursors for antibody-producing cells were demonstrated in fetal liver. Antigen requirements and frequency of precursors were similar to those of adults after birth, but the amount of antibody produced by the progeny of fetal cells was less than that produced by adult B cells. This study suggests a very early potential for immune competence in fetal B cells, but, in any assay of this kind, it could be argued that some maturation of the cells under study took place during the test (e.g., in the spleens of the irradiated recipients).

Although antibody-forming potential exists early, it normally is difficult to demonstrate in the intact animal until a few days after birth. Some strains are more precocious than others in responding to antigens like sheep red blood cells, and the magnitude of the responses increases logarithmically with age [183]. Increasing responsiveness with age has been attributed to various factors, but recent reports suggest that T cells capable of interacting with B cells are the most limiting factor in neonatal responsiveness [175,184,185] and indicate that the earliest thymus-derived cells to populate the spleen are incapable of helper function. Acquisition of responsiveness to various antigens has been shown to occur at different times in some species [186], but since this is not reflected in studies of antigen binding, the full meaning of these observations is unclear.

Lafleur and coworkers [176,187,188] have defined a subpopulation of B lymphocytes, by a delayed adoptive transfer assay, which has the following characteristics. It is a rapidly sedimenting Ig-bearing cell with restricted antibody-forming potential. It exists in the bone marrow and spleen but is absent from the lymph nodes. From a related study, it appears likely that this cell is cortisone resistant but requires a cortisone-sensitive environment for conversion to the smaller, presumably more mature, B lymphocyte [180]. At present, it is not known if B cells with the above characteristics are obligate precursors for mature cells or, alternatively, if they represent a specialized reservoir of cells. Another population of B lymphocytes which is resident in the bone marrow has been defined by its inability to cooperate with irradiated T cells [146].

Addendum

In the interim since this review was prepared, progress in understanding the development of lymphocytes has been steady. In this short space, we wish to direct the reader's attention to some of the more exciting areas which either did not receive adequate attention in the initial writing or in which advances have since been significant.

The basic outline of early development of and within the thymus has been confirmed and extended by the elegant recent studies of Le Douarin and Jotereau with quail-chick embryo chimeras [189]. Their depiction of cycles of attraction by thymic epithelium for circulating stem cells, intrathymic lymphoid development, and peripheralization suggests that an understanding of the molecular mechanisms which govern these recognition and induction events is not far away.

At least one factor which is responsible for T-cell differentiation has now been chemically characterized. Goldstein and colleagues have taken advantage of the associated effects of a thymic hormone, thymopoietin, on the neuromuscular junction to purify and characterize it [190-192]. This factor specifically induces the appearance of T-cell markers and at least some functional capability on thymus-seeking progenitors. A similar factor with specificity for B-cell differentiation has not been discovered, but the fact that several nonspecific factors mimic thymopoietin's effects has been employed to determine the probable sequence through which B cells acquire various surface receptors [193,194].

Some progress in understanding the attainment of functional capability by T cells has come from the recognition that various T-cell functions are associated with subsets of cells that bear different alloantigens [195,196] or receptors [197].

The nature of the mammalian bursal equivalent is still unresolved. However, one B-lymphocyte maturation event, acquisition of surface Ig, occurs in isolated cultures of fetal liver, spleen, or bone marrow [198-200]. There are now indications that intracytoplasmic Ig may be present at a much earlier stage [201,202]. The bone marrow is still of considerable interest as a site of B-lymphocyte differentiation, but it is certainly not obligate for this process [203,204]. It is hoped that ways will be found to discriminate between primary induction events which commit stem cells to B lymphoid differentiation and subsequent maturation to functional capability.

Several characteristic features have been noted for given states of B-cell differentiation. These features include characteristic high turnover rate and ease of modulation of membrane Ig on immature cells [201,205,206] and sensitivity to various mitogens [207,208]. Size, density, and electrophoretic mobility changes, in addition to adherence properties, accompany transitions from immature to mature to memory stages [201,209-211] and possibly also changes in cell surface Ig density [210-212]. Acquisition of the murine equivalent of human IgD seems to represent a late stage of development [213].

References

1. J. Sterzl and I. Riha (eds.), *Developmental Aspects of Antibody Formation and Structure,* Czechoslovak Academy of Science and Academic Press, 1971, Vol. I and II.
2. J. B. Soloman, *Foetal and Neonatal Immunology,* North-Holland Publishing Co., Amsterdam, 1971.
3. W. S. Hammond, J. Morphol. **95**, 501 (1954).
4. M. A. S. Moore and J. J. T. Owen, J. Exp. Med. (1967).
5. K. Shortman and H. Jackson, Cell. Immunol. **12**, 230 (1974).
6. N. M. Le Douarin and F. V. Jotereau, Nature [New Biol.] **246**, 25 (1973).
7. J. J. T. Owen and M. A. Ritter, J. Exp. Med. **129**, 431 (1969).
8. D. Metcalf and M. A. S. Moore, *Haemopoietic cells,* North-Holland Publishing Co., Amsterdam, 1971.
9. R. Auerbach, Develop. Biol. **3**, 336 (1961).
10. R. Auerbach, Develop. Biol. Suppl. **1**, 254 (1967).
11. E. M. Pantelouris, Nature (London) **213**, 370 (1968).
12. M. A. S. Moore and A. Szenberg, Unpublished observations, 1973.
13. M. A. S. Moore and J. J. T. Owen, Lancet **1**, 658 (1967).
14. M. A. S. Moore and D. Metcalf, Brit. J. Haematol. **18**, 279 (1970).
15. P. Slonimsky, Arch. Biol. (Liege) **42**, 415 (1931).
16. A. M. Wu, J. E. Till, L. Siminovitch, and E. A. McCulloch, J. Exp. Med. **127**, 455 (1968).
17. M. O. El-arini and D. Osoba, J. Exp. Med. **137**, 821 (1973).
18. Y. Sidky, Anat. Rec. **161**, 187 (1968).
19. J. J. T. Owen and M. C. Raff, J. Exp. Med. **132**, 1216 (1970).
20. G. J. V. Nossal and B. L. Pike, Immunology **25**, 33 (1973).
21. L. Du Pasquier, N. Weiss, and F. Loor, Eur. J. Immunol. **2**, 366 (1972).
22. J. C. Cerottini and K. T. Brunner, Immunology **13**, 395 (1967).
23. N. K. Jerne, Eur. J. Immunol. **1**, 1 (1971).
24. D. E. Mosier, Fed. Proc. **32**(3), 1011A (1973).
25. M. L. Howe and B. Manziello, J. Immunol. **109**, 534 (1972).
26. M. W. Cohen, G. J. Thorbecke, G. M. Hochwald, and E. B. Jacobsen, Proc. Soc. Exp. Biol. Med. **114**, 242 (1963).
27. A. L. Goldstein, A. Guha, M. L. Howe, and J. White, J. Immunol. **106**, 773 (1971).
28. S. C. Knight and G. J. Thorbecke, Cell. Immunol. **2**, 91 (1971).
29. M. L. Howe, A. L. Goldstein, and J. R. Battisto, Proc. Nat. Acad. Sci. USA **67**, 613 (1970).
30. M. H. MacGillivray, B. Mayhew, and N. R. Rose, Proc. Soc. Exp. Biol. Med. **133**, 688 (1970).

31. D. Metcalf, *The Thymus,* Springer-Verlag, Berlin and New York, 1966.
32. I. L. Weissman, J. Exp. Med. **126**, 291 (1967).
33. M. C. Raff and J. J. T. Owen, Eur. J. Immunol. **1**, 27 (1971).
34. A. D. Chanana, J. Schaedeli, M. W. Hess, and H. Cottier, J. Immunol. **110**, 283 (1973).
35. P. G. Spear, A. Wang, U. Rutishauser, and G. M. Edelman, J. Exp. Med. **138**, 557 (1973).
36. J. D. Stobo and W. E. Paul, J. Immunol. **110**, 362 (1973).
37. B. Argyris, Transplantation **3**, 618 (1965).
38. R. Auerbach and A. Globerson, Exp. Cell Res. **42**, 31 (1966).
39. B. Glick, T. S. Chang, and R. G. Jaap, Poultry Sci. **35** (1956).
40. N. L. Warner, A. Szenberg, and F. M. Burnet, Aust. J. Exp. Biol. Med. Sci. **40**, 373 (1962).
41. B. D. Jankovic and M. Isvaneski, Int. Arch. Allergy Appl. Immunol. **23**, 188 (1963).
42. M. D. Cooper, R. D. A. Peterson, M. A. South, and R. A. Good, J. Exp. Med. **123**, 75 (1966).
43. M. A. S. Moore and J. J. T. Owen, Develop. Biol. **14**, 40 (1966).
44. E. Lar, I. Olsah, and I. Toro, Acta Biol. Acad. Sci. Hung. **20**, 93 (1969).
45. E. Rubin, M. D. Cooper, and F. W. Kraus, Bacteriol. Proc. **67** (1971).
46. M. D. Cooper, Personal communication.
47. M. A. S. Moore and J. J. T. Owen, Nature (London) **208**, 956 (1965).
48. M. A. S. Moore and J. J. T. Owen, Nature (London) **215**, 1081 (1967).
49. G. J. Thorbecke, N. L. Warner, G. M. Hochwald, and S. H. Ohanian, Immunology **15**, 123 (1968).
50. C. E. Grossi, V. Genta, M. Ferrarini, and D. Zacceco, Rev. Franc. Etudes Clin. Biol. **8**, 497 (1968).
51. P. W. Kincade and M. D. Cooper, J. Immunol. **106**, 371 (1971).
52. Y. S. Choi and R. A. Good, J. Exp. Med. **136**, 8 (1972).
53. J. Bienenstock, J. Gauldie, and D. Y. E. Perey, J. Immunol. **111**, 1112 (1973).
54. P. W. Kincade and M. D. Cooper, Unpublished observations.
55. Y. S. Choi and R. A. Good, J. Exp. Med. **135**, 1133 (1972).
56. J. J. Cebra, J. E. Colberg, and S. Dray, J. Exp. Med. **123**, 547 (1966).
57. B. Pernis, Cold Spring Harbor Symp. Quant. Biol. **32**, 333 (1967).
58. L. Hudson and I. M. Roitt, Eur. J. Immunol. **3**, 63, 67 (1973).
59. P. W. Kincade, A. R. Lawton, and M. D. Cooper, J. Immunol. **106**, 1421 (1971).
60. E. P. Rabellino and H. M. Grey, Immunology **106**, 1418 (1971).
61. W. P. McArthur, J. Chapman, and G. J. Thorbecke, J. Exp. Med. **134**, 1036 (1971).
62. J. F. Sallstrom and G. V. Alm, Exp. Cell Res. **75**, 63 (1972).
63. B. D. Jankovic and K. Mitrovic, Folia Biol. (Prague) **13**, 406 (1967).
64. P. B. Dent and R. A. Good, Nature (London) **207**, 491 (1965).
65. Y. S. Choi and R. A. Good, J. Immunol. **110**, 1485 (1973).
66. P. J. Van Alten and H. J. Meuwissen, Science **176**, 45 (1972).

67. P. J. Van Alten, W. A. Cain, R. A. Good, and M. D. Cooper, Nature (London) **217**, 358 (1968).
68. P. W. Kincade, K. S. Self, and M. D. Cooper, Cell. Immunol. **8**, 93 (1973).
69. M. D. Cooper, W. A. Cain, P. J. Van Alten, and R. A. Good, Int. Arch. Allergy Appl. Immunol. **35**, 242 (1969).
70. D. Y. E. Perey and J. Bienenstock, J. Immunol. **111**, 633 (1973).
71. B. D. Jankovic and K. Isakovic, Nature (London) **211**, 202 (1966).
72. M. E. Rose and E. Orlans, Nature (London) **217**, 231 (1968).
73. B. D. Jankovic and K. Isakovic, Folia Biol. (Prague) **13**, 401 (1967).
74. B. Glick and C. R. Sadler, Poultry Sci. **40**, 185 (1961).
75. N. L. Warner, J. W. Uhr, G. J. Thorbecke, and Z. Ovary, J. Immunol. **103**, 1317 (1969).
76. K. G. Lerner, B. Glick, and F. C. McDuffie, J. Immunol. **107**, 493 (1971).
77. S. P. Lerman and W. P. Weidanz, J. Immunol. **105**, 614 (1970).
78. B. Glick, Transplantation **11**, 433 (1971).
79. T. J. Linna, D. Frommel, and R. A. Good, Int. Arch. Allergy Appl. Immunol. **42**, 20 (1972).
80. P. Toivanen, A. Toivanen, and R. A. Good, J. Immunol. **109**, 1058 (1972).
81. W. T. Weber, Cell. Immunol. **4**, 51 (1972).
82. P. W. Kincade, A. R. Lawton, D. E. Bockman, and M. D. Cooper, Proc. Nat. Acad. Sci. USA **67**, 1918 (1970).
83. G. A. Leslie and L. N. Martin, J. Immunol. **110**, 959 (1973).
84. P. Ralph, I. Nakoinz, and M. Cohn, Nature [New Biol.] **245**, 157 (1973).
85. B. Glick and K. Sato, Amer. J. Physiol. **27**, 1371 (1964).
86. K. Isakovic and B. D. Jankovic, Int. Arch. Allergy Appl. Immunol. **24**, 296 (1964).
87. P. W. Kincade and M. D. Cooper, Science **179**, 398 (1973).
88. M. D. Cooper, M. L. Swartz, and R. A. Good, Science **151**, 471 (1966).
89. J. H. Thompson and M. D. Cooper, Transplantation **11**, 71 (1971).
90. J. Ivanyi, L. B. Murgatroyd, and P. M. Lydyard, Immunology **23**, 107 (1972).
91. D. G. Gilmour, G. A. Theis, and G. J. Thorbecke, J. Exp. Med. **132**, 134 (1970).
92. W. A. Cain and L. A. David, J. Immunol. **109**, 598 (1971).
93. P. Toivanen, A. Toivanen, T. J. Linna, and R. A. Good, J. Immunol. **109**, 1071 (1972).
94. W. T. Weber, J. Immunol. **111**, 1277 (1973).
95. B. Glick, Poultry Sci. **39**, 1097 (1960).
96. R. L. St. Pierre and G. A. Ackerman, Science **147**, 1307 (1965).
97. P. B. Dent, D. Y. E. Perey, M. D. Cooper, and R. A. Good, J. Immunol. **101**, 799 (1968).
98. J. Ivanyi, Eur. J. Immunol. **3**, 789 (1973).
99. R. Woods and J. Linna, Acta Pathol. Microbiol. Scand. **64**, 470 (1965).

100. H. G. Durkin, G. A. Theis, and G. J. Thorbecke, Nature [New Biol.] **235**, 118 (1971).
101. M. C. Raff, Immunology **19**, 637 (1970).
102. E. R. Unanue, H. M. Grey, E. Rabellino, P. Campbell, and J. Schmidtke, J. Exp. Med. **133**, 1188 (1971).
103. A. R. Lawton, K. S. Self, S. A. Royal, and M. D. Cooper, Clin. Immunol. Immunopathol. **1**, 84 (1972).
104. D. S. Rowe, K. Hug, W. P. Faulk, J. N. McCormick, and H. Gerber, Nature [New Biol.] **242**, 155 (1973).
105. D. S. Rowe, K. Hug, L. Forni, and B. Pernis, J. Exp. Med. **138**, 965 (1973).
106. R. Van Furth, H. R. E. Schuit, and W. Hijmans, Immunology **11**, 19 (1966).
107. A. R. Lawton, Personal communication.
108. M. D. Cooper and A. R. Lawton, in *Contemporary Topics in Immunobiology* (M. G. Hanna, ed.), Plenum Press, New York, 1972, Vol. 1, p. 49.
109. H. A. Chapman, J. S. Johnson, and M. D. Cooper, J. Immunol. **112**, 555 (1974).
110. J. Trentin, N. Wolf, V. Cheng, W. Fahlberg, D. Weiss, and R. Bonlag, J. Immunol. **98**, 1326 (1967).
111. A. M. Wu, J. E. Till, L. Siminovitch, and E. A. McCulloch, J. Exp. Med. **127**, 455 (1968).
112. L. L. L. Yung, T. C. Wyn-Evans, and E. Diener, Eur. J. Immunol. **3**, 224 (1973).
113. M. L. Tyan and L. A. Herzenberg, J. Immunol. **101**, 446 (1968).
114. O. Stutman, Advan. Exp. Med. Biol. **29**, 19 (1973).
115. M. A. S. Moore, T. A. McNeil, and J. S. Haskill, J. Cell. Physiol. **75**, 181 (1970).
116. J. S. Haskill and M. A. S. Moore, Nature (London) **226**, 853 (1970).
117. H. S. Micklem, D. A. Ogden, and A. C. Payne, in *Haemopoietic Stem Cells, A Ciba Foundation Symposium,* North-Holland Publishing Co., Amsterdam, 1973, Vol. 13.
118. R. G. Keightley, A. R. Lawton, L. Y. F. Wu, and M. D. Cooper, Exp. Hematol. in press (1976).
119. O. K. Archer, D. E. R. Sutherland, and R. A. Good, Nature (London) **200**, 337 (1963).
120. M. D. Cooper, D. Y. Perey, A. E. Gabrielsen, D. E. R. Sutherland, M. F. McKneally, and R. A. Good, Int. Arch. Allergy Appl. Immunol. **33**, 65 (1968).
121. S. Konda and T. N. Harris, J. Immunol. **97**, 805 (1966).
122. M. D. Cooper, D. Y. Perey, M. F. McKneally, A. E. Gabrielsen, D. E. R. Sutherland, and R. A. Good, Lancet **1**, 1388 (1966).
123. D. Y. E. Perey, D. Frommel, R. Hong, and R. A. Good, Lab. Invest. **22**, 212 (1970).
124. J. Bienenstock and J. Dolezel, J. Immunol. **106**, 938 (1971).
125. B. H. Waksman, H. Ozer, and H. E. Blythman, Lab. Invest. **28**, 614 (1973).

126. M. D. Cooper, P. W. Kincade, D. E. Bockman, and A. R. Lawton, in *Proceedings of the International Symposium on the Immunoglobulin A System,* Birmingham, Alabama, October 1973.
127. D. E. Bockman and M. D. Cooper, Amer. J. Anat. **136**, 455 (1973).
128. B. H. Waksman, J. Immunol. **111**, 878 (1973).
129. H. J. Menwissen, G. T. Kaplan, D. Y. Perey, and R. A. Good, Proc. Soc. Exp. Biol. Med. **130**, 300 (1969).
130. D. Y. E. Perey and R. A. Good, Lab. Invest. **18**, 15 (1968).
131. A. Stramignoni, F. Mollo, S. Rua, and G. Palestro, J. Pathol. Bacteriol. **99**, 265 (1969).
132. M. Pollard and N. Sharon, Infect. Immunity **2**, 96 (1970).
133. R. M. Binns, A. Feinstein, B. W. Gurner, and R. R. A. Coombs, Nature [New Biol.] **239**, 114 (1972).
134. A. R. Lawton, R. Asofsky, M. B. Hylton, and M. D. Cooper, J. Exp. Med. **135**, 277 (1972).
135. J. Bienenstock, N. Johnston, and D. Y. E. Perey, Lab. Invest. **28**, 686 (1973).
136. J. Bienenstock, N. Johnston, and D. Y. E. Perey, Lab. Invest. **28**, 693 (1973).
137. G. F. Mitchell and J. F. A. P. Miller, J. Exp. Med. **128**, 821 (1968).
138. H. N. Claman and E. A. Chaperon, Transplant. Rev. **1**, 92 (1969).
139. D. G. Osmond and N. B. Everett, Blood **23**, 1 (1964).
140. C. Craddock, Acta Haematol. **33**, 19 (1965).
141. F. Brahim and D. G. Osmond, Anat. Rec. **168**, 139 (1970).
142. E. Rabellino, S. Colon, H. M. Grey, and E. R. Unanue, J. Exp. Med. **133**, 156 (1971).
143. J. M. Yoffey, G. Hudson, and D. G. Osmond, J. Anat. **99**, 841 (1965).
144. D. G. Osmond and G. J. V. Nossal, Cell. Immunol. **13**, 132 (1974).
145. J. J. Mond and G. J. Thorbecke, J. Immunol. **110**, 605 (1973).
146. T. Ito, T. Kino, and G. Cudkowicz, J. Immunol. **110**, 596 (1973).
147. A. Basten, J. F. A. P. Miller, N. L. Warner, and J. Pye, Nature [New Biol.] **231**, 104 (1971).
148. N. I. Abdon and N. L. Abden, Clin. Exp. Immunol. **13**, 45 (1973).
149. D. G. Osmond and G. J. V. Nossal, Cell. Immunol. in press (1976).
150. D. J. Manning and J. W. Jutila, J. Exp. Med. **135**, 1316 (1972).
151. A. R. Lawton, R. M. Asofsky, J. M. Davie, and M. B. Hylton, Fed. Proc. **32**, 4469 (1973).
152. B. Pernis, L. Forni, and L. Amante, J. Exp. Med. **132**, 1001 (1970).
153. J. M. Davie, W. E. Paul, R. G. Mage, and M. B. Goldman, Proc. Nat. Acad. Sci. USA **68**, 430 (1971).
154. S. S. Fröland and J. B. Natvig, J. Exp. Med. **136**, 409 (1972).
155. S. Sell, Transplant. Rev. **5**, 19 (1970).
156. M. F. Greaves, Transplant. Rev. **5**, 45 (1970).
157. G. J. V. Nossal, N. L. Warner, and H. Lewis, J. Exp. Med. **135**, 405 (1972).
158. H. G. Herrod and N. L. Warner, J. Immunol. **108**, 1712 (1972).

159. C. W. Pierce, S. M. Solliday, and R. Asofsky, J. Exp. Med. **135**, 675 (1972).
160. H. C. Miller and G. Cudkowicz, Science **171**, 913 (1971).
161. G. Cudkowicz, G. M. Shearer, and R. L. Pierce, J. Exp. Med. **130**, 481 (1969).
162. B. Pernis, Ann. N. Y. Acad. Sci. **190**, 420 (1971).
163. A. C. Wang, S. K. Wilson, J. E. Hopper, H. H. Fudenberg, and A. Nisonoff, Proc. Nat. Acad. Sci. USA **66**, 337 (1970).
164. W. Knapp, R. L. H. Bohhuis, J. Radl, and W. Hijmans, J. Immunol. **111**, 1295 (1973).
165. M. D. Cooper, A. R. Lawton, and P. W. Kincade, Clin. Exp. Immunol. **11**, 143 (1972).
166. R. D. A. Peterson, G. V. Alm, and S. Michalek, J. Immunol. **106**, 1609 (1971).
167. J. Ivanyi and A. Salerno, Immunology **22**, 247 (1972).
168. J. M. Dwyer and N. L. Warner, Nature [New Biol.] **229**, 210 (1971).
169. R. Back and G. V. Alm, Eur. J. Immunol. **3**, 58 (1973).
170. J. M. Dwyer and I. R. Mackay, Lancet I, 1199 (1970).
171. J. Decker, J. Clarke, L. MacPherson, R. Weinstein, and E. E. Sercarz, Advan. Exp. Med. Biol. **29**, 269 (1972).
172. J. B. Solomon, G. S. Riddell, and D. F. Whyte, Immunology **22**, 219 (1972).
173. O. Sjoberg, J. Andersson, and G. Moller, Eur. J. Immunol. **2**, 326 (1972).
174. C. Chen and J. G. Hirsch, J. Exp. Med. **136**, 604 (1972).
175. P. G. Spear and G. M. Edelman, J. Exp. Med. **139**, 249 (1974).
176. L. Lafleur, R. G. Miller, and R. A. Phillips, J. Exp. Med. **135**, 1363 (1972).
177. R. Auerbach, Curr. Topics Develop. Biol. **7**, 257 (1972).
178. J. Sterzl, Cold Spring Harbor Symp. Quant. Biol. **32**, 493 (1967).
179. E. S. Rector and B. G. Carter, J. Immunol. **110**, 1591 (1973).
180. M. Bennett, J. Cell. Physiol. **76**, 197 (1970).
181. M. O. Chison and E. S. Golub, Transplantation **14**, 368 (1972).
182. J. L. Press and N. R. Klinman, J. Immunol. **111**, 829 (1973).
183. J. H. L. Playfair, Immunology **15**, 35 (1968).
184. M. O. Chison and E. S. Golub, J. Immunol. **108**, 1379 (1972).
185. B. G. Carter and E. S. Rector, J. Immunol. **109**, 1345 (1972).
186. A. M. Silverstein and R. A. Prendergast, in *Developmental Aspects of Antibody Formation and Structure* (J. Sterzl and F. Riha, eds.), Czechslovak Academy of Science, 1970, Vol. 1, p. 69.
187. L. Lafleur, B. J. Underdown, R. G. Miller, and R. A. Phillips, Ser. Hematol. **2**, 50 (1972).
188. L. Lafleur, R. G. Miller, and R. A. Phillips, J. Exp. Med. **137**, 954 (1973).
189. N. M. Le Douarin and F. V. Jotereau, J. Exp. Med. **142**, 17 (1975).
190. G. Goldstein, Ann. N.Y. Acad. Sci. **249**, 177 (1975).
191. R. S. Basch and G. Goldstein, Proc. Nat. Acad. Sci. USA **71**, 1474 (1974).

192. K. Komuro, G. Goldstein, and E. A. Boyse, J. Immunol. **115**, 195 (1975).
193. U. Hammerling, A. F. Chin, J. Abbott, and M. P. Scheid, J. Immunol. **115**, 1425 (1975).
194. J. Abbott, M. K. Hoffman, A. F. Chin, and U. Hammerling, in *Proceedings of the 2nd International Congress on Differentiation* (N. Muller-Berat, ed.), North-Holland Publishing Co., Amsterdam, in press, 1975.
195. H. Cantor and E. A. Boyse, J. Exp. Med. **141**, 1376 (1975).
196. H. Shiku, P. Kisielow, M. A. Bean, T. Takahashi, E. A. Boyse, H. F. Oettgen, and L. J. Old, J. Exp. Med. **141**, 227 (1975).
197. R. D. Stout and L. A. Herzenberg, J. Exp. Med. **142**, 1041 (1975).
198. J. J. T. Owen, M. D. Cooper, and M. C. Raff, Nature (London) **249**, 361 (1974).
199. J. J. T. Owen, M. C. Raff, and M. D. Cooper, Eur. J. Immunol. **5**, 468 (1975).
200. J. J. T. Owen, M. C. Raff, and M. D. Cooper, submitted for publication (1976).
201. F. Melchers, H. Von Boehmer, and R. A. Phillips, Transplant. Rev. **25**, 26 (1975).
202. M. C. Raff, M. Megson, J. J. T. Owen, and M. D. Cooper, Nature **259**, 224 (1976).
203. R. A. Phillips and R. G. Miller, Nature (London) **251**, 444 (1974).
204. P. W. Kincade, M. A. S. Moore, R. A. Schlegel, and J. Pye, J. Immunol. **115**, 1217 (1975).
205. M. C. Raff, J. J. T. Owen, M. D. Cooper, A. R. Lawton, M. Megson, and W. E. Gathings, J. Exp. Med. **142**, 1052 (1975).
206. C. L. Sidman and E. R. Unanue, Nature (London) **257**, 149 (1975).
207. E. Gronowicz, A. Coutinho, and G. Möller, Scand. J. Immunol. **3**, 413 (1974).
208. P. Ralph, I. Nakoinz, and W. C. Raschke, Biochem. Biophys. Res. Commun. **61**, 1268 (1974).
209. R. G. Miller, R. M. Gorczynski, L. Lafleur, H. R. MacDonald, and R. A. Phillips, Transplant. Rev. **25**, 97 (1975).
210. S. Strober, Transplant. Rev. **24**, 84 (1975).
211. R. A. Schlegel and K. Shortman, J. Immunol. **115**, 94 (1975).
212. D. G. Osmond and G. J. V. Nossal, Cell. Immunol. **13**, 132 (1974).
213. E. S. Vitetta, U. Melcher, M. McWilliams, M. E. Lamm, J. M. Phillips-Quagliata, and J. W. Uhr, J. Exp. Med. **141**, 206 (1975).

CHAPTER 4

Phylogenetic Emergence of Lymphoid Tissues and Cells

Nicholas Cohen

Division of Immunology
Department of Microbiology
University of Rochester School
of Medicine and Dentistry
Rochester, New York

I. Introduction

It is an irrefutable fact that *all* representatives of *all* vertebrate classes satisfy anthropocentric criteria of immunologic reactivity. All vertebrates have serum immunoglobulins, possess cells that can synthesize and secrete specific antibodies, can immunologically recognize and destroy transplants of allogeneic tissues, and can display some form of immunologic memory to at least some antigens. Such phylogenetic universality is only one of the many "truths" to be gleaned from perusing the ever increasing number of research papers and reviews that have established comparative immunology as a subspecialty of immunology [1-8].

In my opinion, nearly all our phylogenetic insights into the nature of immunity have stemmed from research directed toward satisfying two distinct goals. One goal has been to define and compare quantifiable end products of immune responses of phylogenetically distant species [1,4-8]. The most obvious end product is antibody [4,6]. The critical studies of several immunochemists in the 1960s indicated that shark immunoglobulins are restricted to pentameric and monomeric forms of IgM [9,10]. We now appreciate that while all vertebrate species have immunoglobulins which resemble mammalian macroglobulin, molecules similar to the mammalian IgG class first appear at the phylogenetic level of anuran amphibians [4,6,9-17]. Such phylogenetic progressions are of obvious interest to those investigating the genetics [18] and the ontogenetic patterns [19] of immunoglobulin synthesis and the nature of the membrane receptors of thymus-derived (T cells) and bone marrow-derived (B cells) lymphocytes [20]. A second and certainly more cumbersome end product of an immune response is "simply" the number of days it takes for a representative of a given species to reject an allograft [1,8]. Ramifications of the extensive studies that have led to the hypothesis that acute rejection reactivity appears to have evolved from interactions that elicit only chronic rejection reactions [1,8,21] may be of eventual interest to those who are striving to fathom the genetics and evolution of the *H-2* and the *HL-A* gene complexes, the nature of these gene products, the structure of the cell membrane, and the evolution of cell-to-cell cooperation [22].

The second research goal has been to understand the evolution of the lymphoid machinery that generates the immunologic end products of antibody and graft destruction. The application of this approach to an avian model has led to the classic studies which made T and B cells "household" words in educational and research facilities in Washington, D.C. and elsewhere. It is also this approach that has spawned the voluminous literature that I shall attempt to collate and review in this chapter.

To me, the most meaningful way of organizing this review has been to use a taxonomic approach in which our current knowledge of the lymphoid complex of living representatives of each class and order of ectothermic (cold-blooded) vertebrates will be presented in separate sequentially arranged sections (Fig. 1). Discussions of lymphoid tissues and lymphocytes of avian and mammalian species will be left to my author colleagues who have contributed to this volume and to my reader colleagues who already have an understanding and appreciation of the immune systems of endotherms. The reader must also be reminded that any generalizations I will make about the evolution of lymphocytes and lymphoid organs have been formulated from studies with living animals. Therefore, they are based solely on the assumption that these vertebrates retained at least some immunologic and morphologic characteristics of their ancestral forms that disappeared millions of years ago.

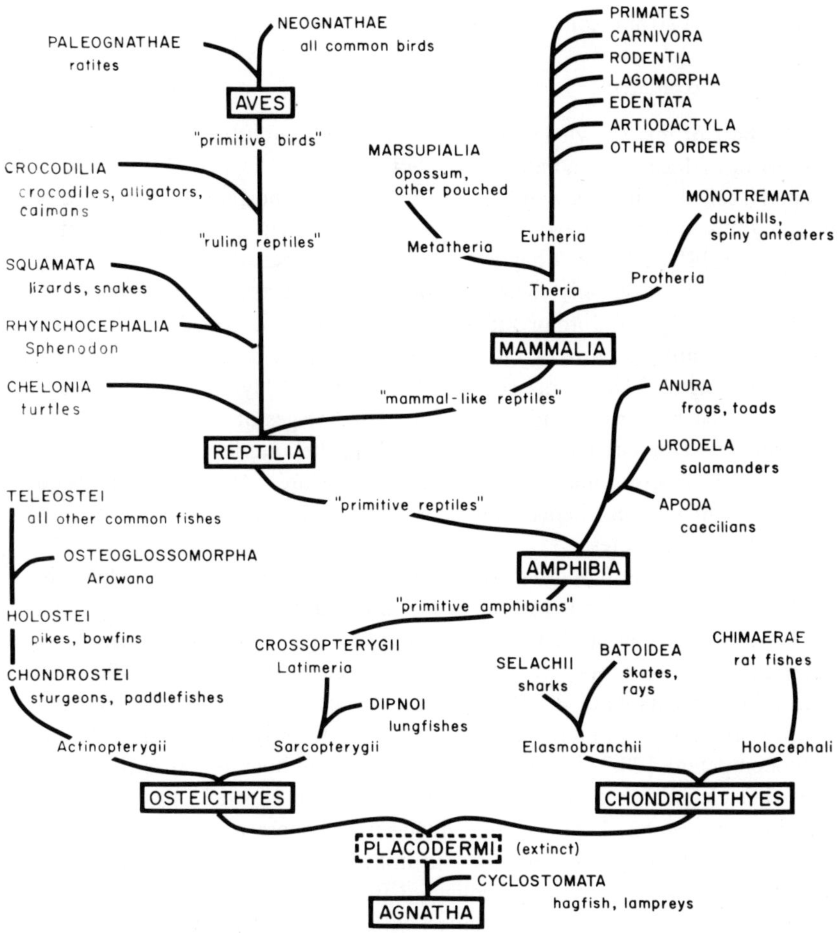

FIG. 1. Scheme of vertebrate evolution.

II. Immunologically Relevant Lymphoid Tissues and Cells of Ectothermic Vertebrates

A. Class Agnatha

Agnathans are the most primitive of all known vertebrates. Members of the subclass Ostracodermi exist only in the fossil records of the Ordovician and Devonian periods. Members of the subclass Cyclostomata are not in the direct line of evolution of land vertebrates and have been known as early as the

Devonian (Fig. 1). Living cyclostomes are classified in the orders Myxinoidea (hagfish) and Petromyzontidae (lampreys).

1. *Order Myxinoidea*

To the best of my knowledge, no investigator has published a description of any organ or focal accumulation of cells in the adult hagfish that can be properly called a thymus gland. Indeed, all those who refer to the question of a thymus in hagfish have explicitly stated that such a structure does not exist [7,23,24]. Although hagfish also lack any organs that are structurally comparable to the spleens of more advanced ectotherms and endotherms, Good et al. [24] and Jordan and Speidel [25] have described hematopoietic foci in the lamina propria of the gut wall which they designate as a primitive splenic precursor. These foci consist of small round "lymphocyte-like" cells, large reticular blast cells, and all developmental stages of erythrocytes. According to Holmgren [26] and Fänge [27], the anterior pronephros, or head kidney, is also a major hematopoietic structure. As shall be discussed in subsequent sections, hematopoiesis is associated with the kidneys of most ectothermic vertebrates.

The peripheral blood and (other?) hematopoietic "organs" of hagfish contain a small round cell with a scant rim of basophilic cytoplasm [24,25, 28-30]. Since Good et al. [24] could identify cell types intermediate between these cells and thrombocytes, they have referred to them as lymphoid hemoblasts (i.e., precursors of diverse blood cell types [25]). However, Hildemann and his associates, who have demonstrated conclusively that hagfish are immunocompetent [28-31], call such cells small lymphocytes. It is this cell type that characterizes the infiltrate of hagfish skin allografts that are exhibiting chronic rejection [28] and that divides in response to an in vitro confrontation with allogeneic cells [31] in mixed lymphocyte culture (MLC). Moreover, when such cells were collected from hagfish that were actively synthesizing antibody and then stained with a fluorescent antihagfish serum, specific fluorescence was seen [29]. In the face of such morphologic and highly suggestive functional criteria, whether such cells should be called lymphocytes no longer seems a moot point.

Despite extensive in vitro immunization of hagfish that results in antibody synthesis and secretion or in graft rejection, no plasma cells or medium and large lymphocytes have been seen. However, hagfish do possess macrophages, granulocytes, and blast cells, in addition to small lymphocytes [30].

2. *Order Petromyzontidae*

Larval (ammocetes) and adult lampreys appear to have a primitive thymus [24,32-34]. Just where it is, and whether it deserves the appellation of a thymus, is another matter. Schaffer referred to small aggregates of lymphoid cells in the submucosa near the external openings of the pharyngeal pouches of ammocetes as thymic tissue [32]. Wallin felt that seven placodes located on the epipharyngeal fold constituted the thymic homolog [33], while Finstad et al. felt that in the newly transformed adults, the thymus is represented by foci of lymphoid cells that develop in the gill region from epithelial cells within or just beneath the pharyngeal gutter between the second and fifth pharyngeal pouches [24,34]. However, Sterba's [35] analysis of lamprey anatomy led him to the conclusion that a thymus does not exist in the species. Part of this confusion may stem from the fact that different investigators were examining larval and adult forms and that changes in the "primitive" thymus, such as those associated with involution, might occur with age [36]. Clearly, if the previously described cellular accumulations are thymic homologs, there are no functional studies to support their being analogs.

Fichtelius et al. [37] indicate that the lamina propria and epithelium of the gut wall of the lamprey contain only a few lymphocytes. However, Good et al. refer to an accumulation of cells in an invagination of the anterior gut of the adult as a "primitive spleen." In addition to its being a site of erythropoiesis, thrombopoiesis, and granulopoiesis, this accumulation of cells contains small foci of lymphocytes and, as such, appears to be involved in lymphopoiesis. No immunologic role has been attached to this "organ." Indeed, after antigenic stimulation that results in a demonstrable immune response, no changes in this tissue, such as proliferation or an increase in size, have been recorded.

There is no literature that indicates whether any concentration of lymphocytes is present in the lamprey kidney. However, the protovertebral arch in adults of this order has been assigned a hematopoietic function. Moreover, after antigenic stimulation with *Bacillus* Calmette-Guérin (BCG) in complete Freund's adjuvant, proliferation of cells in this site has been visualized by the in vivo uptake of tritiated thymidine [38]. The nature and function of the large mononuclear cells in the protovertebral arch (which has been called a primitive bone marrow) are unknown.

As in hagfish, no mammalian-type plasma cells have been seen in lampreys. Clawson [39], however, has described a proliferating pyroninophilic cell which bears an ultrastructural resemblance to plasma cells of fishes and higher vertebrates. There are also significant functional and morphologic data that lampreys have cells which can properly be called small lymphocytes. In a preliminary report [40], Olson indicated that lamprey cells divide in response to phytohemagglutinin (PHA). Similarly, cells from lampreys immunized with complete Freund's adjuvant also proliferate after an in vitro challenge with old tuberculin. Far more definitive and quantitative data on the in vitro behavior of lymphocytes were presented by Cooper, who, in a light microscope study, determined the number of cells undergoing blast cell transformation in response to specific and nonspecific mitogens [41]. His major observations are worth summarizing, because they indicate that, even at the primitive level of the lamprey, basic properties of mitosis and antigen discrimination are characteristics of the lymphocyte. First, about 70% of the peripheral blood cells from ammocetes (about 80% of the peripheral blood leukocytes of ammocetes are lymphocytes) transform into blast cells during a dose-dependent response to PHA. Although a similar transformation occurred in response to staphylococcal filtrate, no reactions to allogeneic cells were seen in an MLC. These cultures were maintained for only 4 days at 15°C, a temperature which delays in vivo manifestations of immunity in all ectotherms [1,7,8]. Although these two technical considerations might be associated with MLC negativity, PHA, but not staphylococcal filtrate, potentiated an MLC response. Potentiation in this sense means that the percentage of blast cell transformation was higher in cultures that contained allogeneic cells plus PHA than it was in cultures with PHA and a comparable number of leukocytes from just one animal. Cooper hypothesized that PHA potentiated the MLC reaction because of its leukoagglutinating properties.

Cooper also immunized larval lampreys with trichloroacetic acid-precipitated insoluble hapten-serum conjugates [41]. Sixteen days after the second injection, the lymphocytes were exposed to homologous or heterologous haptens conjugated to a soluble carrier. Respectable hapten-specific blast cell transformations were seen after 3 days in culture. Although carrier-specific responses were not demonstrable in this experimental series (probably due to the degraded nature of the carrier used for the in vivo immunizations), both carrier and hapten specificities were noted in another series in which orthanilic acid was conjugated directly to guinea pig serum. In such a system, the highest percentage of blast cell transformation was obtained after an in vitro exposure to the specific hapten-serum conjugate, rather than in response to the hapten or carrier itself.

3. *Comments*

I interpret the literature on agnathan immunology as indicating that, even by the least stringent mammalian criteria, hagfish and lampreys lack organized lymphoid tissue that can be called a definitive thymus or spleen. My interpretation would be altered if I were to be confronted with new data that indicated, for example, that juvenile hagfish do have a recognizable thymus which involutes with age, and thereby becomes undetectable in the laboratory, or that those "tissues" which have received the appellation of "primitive" or "precursor" organs are, indeed, both analogous and homologous with the thymus and spleen of higher vertebrates. However, without such new information, but with the fact that when they are judged even by mammalian criteria, agnathans are immunocompetent creatures, I am forced to adopt the iconoclastic viewpoint that in vivo cellular and humoral immune responses can be effectively mounted in the absence of well-organized lymphoid tissue. Thus, it is the small lymphocyte that appears to be primarily, if not totally, responsible for the range of immune capabilities displayed by these so-called primitive animals.

B. Class Chondrichthyes

As seen in Fig. 1, one of the two evolutionary offshoots of the Agnatha leads to the Chondrichthyes, a group of vertebrates which includes the rat fishes (Holocephali) and the sharks and rays (Elasmobranchii). It is commonly but erroneously assumed that because of their cartilaginous skeleton, sharks and rays are more primitive than the bony fish who possess a cartilaginous supporting structure only during larval life. We now understand that elasmobranchs have nothing directly to do with the evolution of bony fish. Indeed, bony fish appear earlier in the fossil record than do sharks, which have been found no earlier than the middle Devonian. Chondrichthyes are not on the main line of evolutionary progression to terrestrial vertebrates.

1. Subclass Holocephali

There are no data on the immune response capacity of rat fishes, and only the most minimal information regarding their lymphoid tissues is available. We know that chimaeroids do have both a thymus gland and a very prominent lymph glandlike organ in the cranial region which may serve a hematopoietic function [42,43]. Fänge [27] has briefly described a vascular organ in the orbit, but it is unclear whether it is lymphopoietic. Unlike most chondrichthyes, chimaeroids appear to lack lymphoid accumulations in their excretory organs [44].

2. Subclass Elasmobranchii

So-called primitive rays (guitar fish) and sharks (horn shark) and advanced rays (spotted eagle ray, sting ray) and sharks (leopard and nurse shark) have a definitive and well-organized lymphoid system that is comparable in its complexity to the lymphoid system of representative Osteichthyes and urodele amphibians. All species that have been studied have an encapsulated thymus which is characterized by cortical and medullary differentiation, small, medium, and large lymphocytes, and "primitive" Hassall's corpuscles. Age-related thymic involution occurs in the higher forms but does not in those which have been designated as less advanced [24]. Regardless of their phylogenetic position in the subclass, all elasmobranchs have a spleen with a distinctive red and white pulp. Lymphoid accumulations in the gut and in the parenchyma of the gonads have also been described. Although lymphoid foci are seen in the kidneys of certain elasmobranchs, they do not appear in the renal tissue of the advanced leopard sharks [24]. All elasmobranches that have been investigated have, in addition to a family of small, medium, and large lymphocytes, large pyroninophilic lymphoid cells. Good et al. [24], however, only found true mammalian-type plasma cells in advanced sharks and in just one of the three species of advanced rays they examined. Whether there is an evolutionary progression in the phylogeny of plasma cells within the elasmobranchs will not be known until the ultrastructure of lymphoid cells from more species is analyzed.

Shark immunoglobulins are restricted to the IgM class, but they exist in monomeric 7S and pentameric 19S forms. The monomer does not appear to be a precursor or a degradation product of the pentamer. In an attempt to determine whether the monomer and pentamer are products of the same or different cells, Clem and his coworkers prepared one antiserum with specificity toward both the monomer and the pentamer and a second antiserum directed against only the pentamer [45]. The latter reagent was made in guinea pigs that had been rendered tolerant to the 7S monomer. Both antisera were fluorescein labeled and were used to stain the cytoplasm of cells in the lymphoid tissues of nurse and dogfish sharks. Very few antibody-containing cells were found in the kidney, thymus, or liver. Quantitative counts of the spleen and peripheral blood, however, indicated a 3:1 ratio of anti-immunoglobulin (stains both 19S and 7S producers) to antipentamer (stains 19S producers only) fluorescing cells. This ratio suggests that 7S producers outnumber 19S producers by at least two to one. The fundamental question of whether 19S-producing cells also make 7S IgM cannot be answered until the appropriate specific antimonomer antisera become available.

In a preliminary report, Olson indicated that lymphocytes from sting rays proliferate in vitro when exposed to PHA, pokeweed mitogen, or streptolysin 0 [40]. In vitro behavior of peripheral leukocytes from nurse sharks has been more thoroughly examined by Sigel and his associates [46-48], and their exciting findings are worth summarizing. After in vivo immunization of sharks with bovine gamma globulin (BGG), polio virus, or extracts of sheep erythrocytes, their leukocytes manifested increased rates of thymidine incorporation in the presence of the specific antigen. Despite their use of optimal culture conditions to support mitosis and cell growth, these investigators never observed reactivity of shark lymphocytes that had been confronted with allogeneic cells [46]. Whether PHA can potentiate such a response, as it apparently can in the lamprey MLC, is unknown.

It is also significant that although unpurified shark peripheral blood cells can be stimulated by comparatively large amounts of concanavalin A (con A), the same cells are unresponsive to a wide dose range of PHA. Purification of peripheral cells on a Ficoll-Isopaque gradient resulted in the localization of cells in three separate bands and in a sediment. Cells from all fractions were stimulated by con A. PHA responsiveness was now demonstrable, but mitotic activity was restricted to those cells in the sediment. It is most provocative that the proliferative responses of this population of cells were inhibited by the addition of leukocytes from the other layers [46]. This observation suggests that there exists a suppressor population of cells.

3. *Comments*

In mammals, there is considerable evidence for functional and structural heterogeneity, not only between B and T cells but among the T cells themselves. In mice, the existence of distinct subsets of T cells has been demonstrated with respect to the graft-versus-host (GVH) reaction [49-51], distribution and recirculation pathways [49,50], density of surface alloantigenic markers [51], and turnover times [50,52]. Stobo and Paul [53] have also demonstrated that, in mice, one population of T cells responds equally well to con A and to PHA, while another responds mainly to con A [53]. It is still unclear whether these differences are reflections of the properties of two separate lines of T cells or whether they mirror activity of T cells of the same line that happen to be at different stages in their differentiation [53]. The experiments of Lopez et al. [47,48] on shark peripheral blood cells indicate that one subset of leukocytes responds to PHA and con A, while others proliferate only in response to con A. These data argue strongly by analogy that lymphocyte heterogeneity evolved at least as early as the Elasmobranchii. Shark lymphocyte heterogeneity is also suggested by the observations that the response to PHA by one subset of cells is inhibited when this population is mixed with another subset of cells prior to the addition of the mitogen. The nature of this suppressor activity is totally unknown.

In mice, MLC responsiveness has been associated with the subset of T cells that responds to both PHA and con A [53]. Thus, if an analogous population of lymphocytes is responsible for MLC reactivity in sharks, the lack of shark MLC reactivity may be due to the limited availability of cells with these properties. It is unknown, however, whether a subset of lymphocytes can respond in MLC as they can to PHA, but (like the cells that respond to PHA) their reactivity is somehow suppressed by other lymphocytes. Further comments on the evolution of MLC reactivity and PHA responsiveness will be presented after I review the lymphoid complex of the teleostei.

C. Class Osteichthyes

The class, Osteichthyes, is comprised of all living bony fish. The first known Osteichthyes from the lower Devonian and the present day forms are divided into two subclasses, the Actinopterigyii (ray-finned fishes) and the Crossopterygii (lungfish and lobefins). Although representatives of a side-branch of the fossil lobefins are still with us today and are of great phylogenetic importance because of their phylogenetic relationships with the Amphibia and higher vertebrates, we know very little about their immune system, except that adult *Latimeria* have a well-developed lobulated thymus which shows no involution with age (see Ref. 2). Modern lungfish are more diversified and are represented by three genera. We know the structure of their immunoglobulins [54] and that their liver, pancreas, and gonads are lymphopoietic (see Ref. 2). Although they lack true plasma cells, lungfish do possess lymphoid accumulations along the gut tract and have a spleen which is clearly divided into a red and white pulp. In the region of the intestinal valve, abundant lymphoid tissue has also been noted [24].

Actinopterygii are derived from either the placoderms or the ancient Choanichthyes and are not on the line of evolutionary progression that leads to tetrapods (Fig. 1). They are the largest vertebrate group, with about 30,000 living species. We are going to be concerned with the lymphoid organs and cells in the three major superorders, Chondrostei, Holostei, and Teleostei. We are indebted to Good and his colleagues for nearly all of our information on the immune system of representatives of the first two superorders [24].

1. Superorder Chondrostei (Paddlefish, Sturgeons)

The thymus of the paddlefish is organized into lobes and lobules [24]. Primitive Hassall's corpuscles and small, medium, and large lymphocytes are seen in this organ, which involutes with age. The spleen is also well developed, and there is a clear dissociation into a red and white pulp. The white pulp has dense collections of lymphocytes, in addition to "true" plasma cells, in the mantle region. Nodules of lymphocytes have also been described in the region of the ileocecal valve and in the gut. There is no bone marrow per se, but there is an abundance of hematopoietic tissue, which overlies the base of the heart and extends down over the atrium and ventricle. According to Good et al. [24], the organization of this tissue is similar to that of mammalian bone marrow. Like the spleen, it contains lymphocytes and plasma cells.

The kidney of the paddlefish, like that of the higher teleosts, is a lymphoid organ [55]. The kidney extends throughout the entire length of the body cavity and beyond the cavity anteriorly. Posteriorly, it forms a single thickened mass, which contains urinary tubules and intertubular lymphoid accumulations. This mass is continued anteriorly as two narrow strands of lymphoid tissue, which end up as a thick mass of lymphoid tissue which lacks tubules. This mass is generally termed the head kidney. In the paddlefish, it is divided into more or less complete lobules by connective tissue trabeculae, which are derived from the capsule. According to Downey, this tissue contains a full family of lymphoid cells [55].

Extensive immunization of paddlefish results in a marked increase of plasma cells in the spleen and in the pericardial hematopoietic tissue [24]; if any changes occur in the head kidney, they have not been described. An electron microscope analysis by Clawson et al. [56] has disclosed that the plasma cells and small lymphocytes of this species are ultrastructurally similar to those of mammals. Two populations of lymphocytes were noted. One had a primarily polyribosomal organization, whereas the other had a preponderance of free ribosomes. It has been suggested that these distinctions are similar to those made for the B and T lymphocytes of birds [55].

There have been no in-depth studies on the in vitro behavior of lymphocytes from any chondrostean. However, Olson did mention that lymphocytes from an immune paddlefish responded to the specific immunizing antigen and to PHA with two- to fivefold and three- to eightfold increases, respectively, in thymidine incorporation [40].

2. *Superorder Holostei (Bowfin, Gar Pike)*

The thymus of the bowfin (which does not involute) has a lesser degree of cortical and medullary differentiation than that of chondrosteans or elasmobranchs [24]. The discrete spleen of the bowfin has a red and white pulp and a full range of lymphocytes and plasma cells [24]. The kidney of this or other holostean fish has not been investigated.

3. *Superorder Teleosteii*

The histology, anatomy, and function of the lymphoid cells and organs (thymus, spleen, pharyngeal accumulations, pronephros) have been described for several species. The paired thymuses of the adult Mozambique mouth breeder are attached to the inner surface of the branchial epithelium at the junction of the operculum and the dorsal body musculature. The thymus is completely surrounded by a capsule of collagen fibers and consists of outer, inner, and middle zones [57]. According to Sailendri [57], the middle and inner zones are comparable to the cortex and medulla of the thymus of endotherms, while the homology of the outer zone is conjectural. Sailendri has also described a loose aggregation of small, medium, and large lymphocytes at the anterior end of the thymus, but whether this aggregation corresponds to the lymphoid accumulations in the pharyngeal submucosa of the bluegill is unclear [58]. Involution of the thymus of the mouth breeder is associated with the appearance of cysts and epithelial islands, as well as with infiltrations of muscle, adipose, and connective tissues [57].

As part of her comprehensive analysis of the immune responses of teleosts, Sailendri has also described the ontogeny and function of the thymus gland of the mouth breeder [57]. The pair of rudiments first appear 2 days before hatching as a spherical mass of epithelial cells attached to the second, third, and fourth pharyngeal pouches. With the formation and proliferation of lymphoblasts during the next few developmental stages, the rudiment increases in size. It subsequently detaches, and cortical-medullary differentiation occurs at the early postlarval stages. During postlarval life, the rudiment assumes the shape and cellular organization typical of the mature gland. Subsequent maturation involves the development of the outer zone, Hassall's corpuscles (which are lacking in the bluegill [58]), and blood vessels. The thymus attains lymphoid maturation at the juvenile stage.

The thymus of the mouth breeder plays a key role in the development of immunocompetence. Scale allografts on 1.5-month-old fish survived nearly twice as long as did grafts on 4.5-month-old animals, which were rejected with the rapidity typical of teleost alloimmune responses [1]. Yet, thymectomy of 4-month-old (but not older) immunocompetent fish resulted in the extended survival of test scale grafts. Two-month-old fish were unable to make antibodies to sheep red blood cells (sRBC), as tested for by the Jerne plaque assay, whereas 2.5-month-old animals could. Thymectomy of 2-month-old (but not older) animals totally suppressed the immune reactivity to a subsequent challenge with sRBC [57].

The head kidney or pronephros is a major lymphoid organ in many, but not all, teleost species (see Ref. 27). Sailendri described the head kidney of the mouth breeder as a highly organized tissue with lymphoid follicles, a hilus-like area, and lymphatic vessels. Plasma cells, monocytes, lymphocytes, and granulocytes are found in this structure, as well as in the spleen [57]. In the bluegill, the pronephros is primarily composed of lymphoreticular tissue that is arranged in cords that radiate toward a central vessel. Smith et al. found two zones in this organ. One was a reticular zone close to the renal epithelial cells; the second was more distal and was filled with lymphocytes [58].

The transformation of the pronephros of the mouth breeder into a lymphoid head kidney occurs during postlarval stages of development [57]. The pronephros first becomes erythroid, and then lymphoid accumulations are found among the urinary tubules. The transition is completed at the juvenile stage by the reduction in the number of tubules and by the appearance of a few sinuses. At the mid and late postlarval stages, the thymus and the head kidney are connected by a "lymphoid bridge."

The splenic rudiment of the mouth breeder appears as a mesenchymal thickening in 1-day-old hatchlings and develops into an erythroid structure during late prelarval life [57]. Large lymphoid cells are evident at the postlarval stage, and the red and white pulp differentiate in the juvenile period [57]. The white pulp of the adult spleen is devoid of lymphoid centers, and the red pulp is primarily erythroid.

There are several in vivo and in vitro studies that indicate that the spleen and head kidney are major sites of antibody synthesis. Yu et al. studied the effects of splenectomy on the immune response of the blue gourami to infection with pancreatic necrosis virus and found that it reduced antibody levels to undetectable amounts [59].

Ortiz-Muniz and Sigel [60] harvested and cultured fragments of spleen, thymus, and head kidney from groupers and snappers that had been immunized with BGG or bovine serum albumin (BSA). De novo in vitro synthesis of antibody in all three organs was determined by passive hemagglutination. Titers were highest in the spleen, lower in the thymus, and lowest in the pronephros. The kinetics of antibody production, however, were the same for each organ. Antibody-forming cells (AFC) in each tissue were demonstrated by immunofluorescence. These fundamental observations that AFC are found in the thymus, spleen, and anterior kidney have been confirmed in the mouth breeder with the Jerne plaque assay [57]. Others used this assay [58,61], or the immunocytoadherence test [62], to demonstrate AFC in the spleen and kidney of the bluegill [58], and in these organs plus the peripheral blood and the middle and posterior kidney of the trout [62]. The thymus of these two species, however, was not examined for AFC. Phase-contrast and electron microscope analyses indicated that rosette-forming cells (RFC) in trout were lymphocytes, plasma cells, blastlike cells, macrophages, and eosinophil-like cells [61].

Sigel and Lee [63] recently reported that peripheral leukocytes, spleen, and thymus cells from grey snappers that had been immunized with rubella virus (RV) responded to RV in vitro with an increased tritiated thymidine uptake, whereas normal cells did not. Specificity was determined by inhibiting the response with an anti-RV antibody. Antigen-antibody complexes, however, were not stimulatory. Unlike elasmobranches, unpurified leukocytes from the spleen and peripheral blood of the snapper showed a 20-fold increase in [^{3}H] thymidine incorporation when they were exposed to PHA. However, these teleost cells, like those from sharks, did not respond in an MLC reaction [46,63].

Clem and his colleagues, Yocum and Cuchens, have presumptive evidence that the helper function of T cells that is characteristic of the mammalian immune response is also necessary for secondary antihapten responses in teleosts [64]. Sea robbins were primed with either BSA, BGG, DNP_{30}-BSA, or DNP_{45}-BGG. Three to 4 weeks later, they were restimulated with either the homologous or heterologous carrier-DNP conjugate.

Antibody responses to the hapten were determined by the DNP-modified bacteriophage neutralization test. Maximal neutralization constants for the primary antihapten responses averaged around 20; those for the secondary response in animals primed and restimulated with the same DNP-carrier conjugate averaged around 200. Fish primed with carrier alone and restimulated with DNP conjugated to the homologous carrier exhibited neutralization constants of 150; secondary stimulation with DNP conjugated to the heterologous carrier elicited the much lower constants of two to 20 that were characteristic of a primary response. The nature of the carrier-responsive population is not known.

4. *Comments*

After the first reading, it may seem that the living Osteichthyes are far more immunologically sophisticated than the Chondrichthyes. While this assumption may, indeed, be true, such a distinction could well be illusory, simply because of the relatively abundant and recent detailed literature on the lymphoid system of the teleosts. Therefore, I should remind the reader that at least some elasmobranchs, like teleosts, have plasma cells, lymphocytes, well-organized spleens and thymuses, and renal lymphoid tissues. Moreover, like elasmobranchs, the immunoglobulin class of teleosts is restricted to IgM [4,6], and all fish can synthesize antibodies to a wide range of antigenic determinants.

Extensive amounts of lymphoid tissue in the kidney are characteristic of elasmobranchs and (perhaps more so) of teleosts. If one is searching for selective pressures relevant to the evolution of organized lymphoid structures, it is provocative that aggregates of lymphoid cells are found in or near sites where potentially pathogenic microorganisms may be concentrated and trapped. Such locations include not only the kidney but also the pharynx of fish [58], the opercular region of larval frogs and toads [65], along the gastointestinal tract of many vertebrates [66], and in the bladder of frogs [67,68] and turtles [68,69].

A role of the teleost thymus gland in cellular and humoral immunity has been elegantly and classically demonstrated by ablation experiments [57]. The observation that there is a slow maturation of immunity in the mouth breeder vis-á-vis mammals and that thymectomy is effective in abrogating the subsequent development of immunity during this period are facts that will be echoed in the next sections that deal with the Amphibia and Reptilia and shall be commented on at that time. It is unknown whether thymectomy in teleosts impairs humoral immunity to sRBC by deleting T helper cells. This key point might be resolved, and insights into the organ derivation of putative B-cells might be obtained, if inbred strains of fish [70] were utilized in the way in which inbred strains of mice and rats have served to resolve this question in mammals. A significant start in furthering our understanding of the evolution of lymphocyte heterogeneity has been provided by the observations of Yocum et al. [64], which, by analogy with murine systems, indicate that in teleosts, two cell populations are involved in generating antihapten responses.

The ability of unpurified leukocytes from teleosts (but not sharks) to respond to PHA [47,48] is made more puzzling by the previously discussed results of Cooper's experiments, which revealed exemplary PHA-induced transformation of peripheral blood leukocytes from larval lampreys [41]. One simplistic resolution of these species discrepancies might be that the population of lymphoid cells which functions in a suppressor capacity in sharks is lacking in agnathans and teleosts. If so, the nature of this suppression and of the PHA response itself is of at least equal importance in understanding the evolution of lymphocyte function.

There are many intriguing explanations (all untested) of the negative MLC reactions in teleosts and sharks [47,48] and the positive reactions in toads [71]. Prior to our awareness of the fine structure of the *H-2* complex [22,72], I proposed that the chronic rejection reactions which characterize the transplantation alloimmune responses of many classes or orders of vertebrates, including the Agnatha [1,8,28], Elasmobranchii [1,8], Chondrosteii [1,8], Urodela [1,8,73,74], and all Reptilia [1,8,74,75], are due to extensive intraspecific antigen sharing and to the absence of a major *H-2* type or *HL-A* type of histocompatibility complex [21,74,76]. That is, chronic rejection is a function of only weak histoincompatibility interactions. On the other hand, the acute reactions of advanced anurans [74] and teleosts [38] are due to the presence of a major H locus. Based on the phylogenetic relationship among species which reject allografts chronically, subacutely, and acutely, it seemed natural to further hypothesize that these differences were reflections of histocompatibility gene evolution [21]. By extrapolating from the mammalian data that MLC reactivity is either nonexistent or comparatively weak when the donors of the allogeneic lymphocytes are histoincompatible only at that species' minor loci [77,78], I predicted that MLC of the chronically rejecting sharks would be negative and that MLC of the acutely rejecting toads would be positive. Although these predictions have been verified, the observation that teleosts, which reject scale allografts even more rapidly than murine recipients of the most histoincompatible grafts [1], are also MCL negative [46,48] has forced me to consider additional explanations as to why MLC reactivity can be independent of the rapidity of skin graft rejection. We now appreciate that, at least in man and mouse, MLC reactivity appears to be under genetic control and that the so-called MLC locus is separate from but closely linked to the *H-2* or the *HL-A* genes which code for the serologically definable H alloantigens [79]. It may be either that teleosts and elasmobranchs lack the MLC locus or that the diverse products of the MLC genes they do possess are antigenically indistinguishable by their lymphocyte receptors. If either possibility is true, MLC reactions would not be expected to bear any relationship to the rapidity of graft rejection. Another possible (untested) explanation of MLC negative reactions is that a subset of lymphocytes in some way suppresses the proliferative response of other lymphocytes to allogeneic cells. Additional explanations of a lack of MLC reactivity also suggest themselves. It may be that fish lymphocytes lack receptors for the MLC gene products. It may also be that they have the appropriate receptors but that the number of cells that bear such specific recognition units in unimmunized fish is far lower than the 1 to 3% found in mammals [80]. Reciprocal immunization of the donors used in the MLC test might resolve this point. Still another possibility is based on the observations that although allogeneic mixes of lymphocytes from lampreys are MLC negative, the addition of PHA to mixed cell cultures potentiates a response that is somewhat greater than when PHA is added to an equal number of cells from only one individual [41]. If unpurified PHA were also to effect a similar potentiation of an MLC response in fish, while highly purified PHA that lacks leukoagglutinating activity [81] could not, it would suggest that MLCs without the addition of PHA are negative because the complementary stimulatory and response units on the allogeneic cells are unable to contact each other. Such structures may be present on the cell surface either in a very dispersed fashion or in a very low density. The observations that more mouse lymphocytes proliferate when a threshold number of sites have been triggered by a mitogen [82] and that it takes a comparatively large amount of PHA or con A to trigger mitosis in shark lymphocytes may be circumstantial evidence for a low density of other receptor structures.

D. Class Amphibia

The transition from lobefins to amphibians occurred late in the Devonian. These earliest land dwellers appeared in the world at a time when ostracoderms were still present and when acanthodians and arthrodires (placoderm ancestors of the Osteichthyes and Elasmobranchii, respectively) were common. Sharks had not yet reached their maximum abundance, and there were no teleost fish. During the late Paleozoic, there was a rapid radiation of many lines of Amphibia. Most of these early amphibians are known as labyrinthodonts. It now seems probable that frogs (Anura) and salamanders (Urodela) originated from a relatively primitive and semiaquatic group of labyrinthodonts called Rhactitomi. Although frogs and salamanders may have had a common ancestry, they are quite different immunologically. Frogs have IgM and IgG classes of immunoglobulins [15,16], whereas salamanders have only IgM [13,14]; frogs have lymph nodes, a lymphopoietic bone marrow, and lymphoid accumulations in the bladder, whereas salamanders do not; and representatives of at least four families of salamanders reject skin allografts chronically, while acute rejection is typical of the more advanced families of frogs [74]. It is partly because the Amphibia appear to be a key group in the evolution of immunity that they will be considered in depth in this review. Amphibians will also be emphasized, since they have provided and will continue to provide a powerful model for the study of immunologic problems that know no phylogenetic restrictions.

1. Order Urodela (salamanders)

a. Structure of Lymphoid Organs. The thymus of the salamander is not heavily encapsulated and, at least in the three species that have been examined, does not possess a clearly demarcated cortex and medulla [83-85]. In the common spotted newt (*Notophthalmus viridescens*), stromal cells and lymphocytes are distributed throughout the thymus. Lesser numbers of erythrocytes, granulocytes, and melanocytes are also seen [83]. Plasma cells have been seen in the thymus of nonimmunized postmetamorphic *Pleurodeles* [84]. Hassall's corpuscles are absent in *Notophthalmus* [83] and in axolotls [86], but they have been seen in larval stages of the Spanish newt, *Pleurodeles waltlii* [85]. Cowden and Dyer indicate that thymic involution occurs in all salamanders [86], a point that has not been substantiated by Hightower's observation on *Notophthalmus* [87].

The splenic red pulp of the newt* is lymphopoietic, thrombopoietic, and erythropoietic and consists of reticular fibers (which extend inward as trabeculae to join the reticular network), reticular cells, and fixed macrophages which form a framework within which erythropoiesis occurs. The inner region, or white pulp, is not clearly separated from the red pulp and consists of a reticular framework that contains predominantly lymphocytes [83,86, 88-91]. As with higher vertebrates, the disposition of the splenic lymphoid tissue mainly follows the arterial vasculature [85,86]. Hightower and St. Pierre [83], an active group of French investigators [84], and I and my associates have never seen Malphigian corpuscles or follicles in unimmunized newts. However, Cowden and Dyer make the significant and frequent observation of variable numbers of lymphoid nodules ("in the sense of germinal centers") in the spleens of field collected *Amphiuma* [86]. These nodules contain small, medium, and large lymphocytes, in addition to lymphoblasts and macrophages. To the best of my knowledge, the histology of the spleen from deliberately immunized animals has not been reported.

---

*It is important to note that all newts are salamanders, but not all salamanders are newts.

In this regard, it is noteworthy that plasma cells in the spleens of normal animals are quite rare. Houillon et al. have never seen them [84]; Tooze and Davies have seen only a few in their electron microscope analyses [90,91]; and Cowden and Dyer make the cautious statement that "only infrequently could a cell be encountered which might be described as a plasma cell" [86]. Nevertheless, in animals stimulated with allogeneic tissues, a limited number of plasma cells have been seen in other sites [92].

Although the spleen and the thymus are the major organized lymphoid tissues in salamanders, other focal accumulations of lymphocytes have been seen in the buccal area [85,93] and, at least in some species by some authors, in a thick layer of tissue that surrounds the liver [83,94]. According to other authors, however, this perihepatic area is exclusively granulopoietic [84,87,88]. Both Cowden and Dyer [86] and Ruben et al. [94] indicate that a minor component of the intertubular tissue of salamanders is lymphoid but that its predominant function is in myelopoiesis. In representatives of the family, Plethodontidae, the bone marrow has a granulopoietic function [95], while in other families, it is not at all hematopoietic and contains fat and fibroblasts [83].

Good et al. [24] described the abundant presence of plasma cells in the lamina propria of the *Necturus* gut. Cowden and Dyer [86], however, indicate that in *Ambystoma, Desmognathus, Notophthalmus* [83], *Amphiuma,* and *Siren,* lymphoid accumulations in the gut are minimal and that the number of plasma cells is quite low. *Necturus* may be unusual, or the animals that were examined may have been immunized. The meningeal region of the giant salamander appears to be a site of lymphopoiesis [86], but this region has not been examined in other species.

b. Function of Lymphoid Organs and Cells. Thymectomy of larval tiger salamanders [96], alpine newts [97], and Spanish newts [98] totally or significantly delays the rejection of skin allografts transplanted in adult life. This procedure causes only one of the species to undergo a significant wasting disease 1 to 2 years postsurgery. Tournefier [97] has studied the ontogeny of the lymphoid organs in the alpine newt relative to the age when thymectomy ceases to be effective. Both the thymus and the spleen become lymphoid slowly, so that at the time of hatching, when the larvae become free-swimming, these organs are far from fully developed. The thymus becomes lymphoid before the spleen (as has been reported for other amphibians [65]), and it is only by 10 weeks of age (about 2 weeks prior to metamorphosis) that these organs assume the structure and cellularity of the adult tissue. Nearly three-fourths of the larvae thymectomized during this 10-week period were unable to reject skin allografts that were transplanted as long as 18 months later. About half of the remaining larvae that rejected these grafts did so more chronically than did intact controls and were found to have thymic remnants that resulted from either incomplete thymectomy or thymic regeneration. Although a few animals that were completely thymectomized did reject grafts, a later study by Tournefier indicates that even when thymectomy is performed during the first few weeks after metamorphosis, at least some newts can be rendered incapable of graft rejection [84].

The ability of the larval tiger salamander to partially or completely destroy a single skin allograft, the ability of bilateral thymectomy to interfere with this reaction, and the time it takes for grafts to be rejected in intact and thymectomized premetamorphic animals are the outcome of a complex interplay between many variables. These factors include the age of the recipient at the time of transplantation and/or thymectomy (i.e., the "maturity" of the lymphoid complex), the age of the transplant donor (i.e., the immunogenicity of its H antigens), the extent to which H antigens are shared between the donor and host, and the strength of the histocompatibility barrier [74,96].

When thymectomy is performed at a time when it impairs destructive transplantation reactions, it also significantly reduces a RFC response to normally immunogenic doses of sRBC [85,99]. The urodele also has a factor in its blood which behaves like mammalian thymosin [85,100]. That is, it can restore azathioprine sensitivity and antilymphocyte serum susceptibility to lymphocytes from neonatally thymectomized mice. This factor is lost after thymectomy of the salamander.

The roles of the thymus, spleen, and liver in the immune responses of adult salamanders have been demonstrated by reconstitution and GVH experiments. Murakawa removed either the thymus, spleen, or a small fragment of liver from Japanese newts [101]. He then exposed these animals to a dose of whole body irradiation that was sufficient to abrogate transplantation immunity in intact controls. After he separately autografted each organ to the irradiated animals, the ability to reject grafts was restored. Spleen grafts caused the most rapid rejection, while those of the thymus caused the slowest. However, allograft rejection by these reconstituted animals was always less rapid than that of unirradiated controls. That the spleen is a source of immunocompetent cells was further demonstrated when Murakawa gave x-irradiated newts allogeneic spleen cell suspensions or intact allogeneic spleens and observed lethal GVH reactions. Although liver could extend the life of lethally irradiated animals, it did not cause GVH disease. The spleen also seems to be a source of memory cells. Spleens from skin-grafted newts were transplanted to x-irradiated animals. These x-irradiated recipients were subsequently challenged with a skin graft from the newt which had also been used to immunize the spleen donors. Rejection of the original donor test skin graft was significantly more rapid than was the rejection of a third-party test graft. Liver also adoptively immunized newts, but the rapidity of test graft rejection on such animals was less than when a spleen was used [101].

Tournefier utilized the immunocytoadherence assay to determine that the type of RFC changes with the immune status of the animal. A single injection of sRBC resulted in RFC that were predominantly all lymphocytes, two injections elicited medium and large RFC, and more than two injections resulted in a preponderance of blast cells [99].

Ruben used newts and the immunocytoadherence assay to define the organ sources of AFC, to determine the kinetics of such responses in intact and in splenectomized animals, and to provide evidence of cellular cooperation in the generation of antibody at this phylogenetic level [94]. Spleen, liver, or kidney cells from newts that received a single injection of chicken or toad erythrocytes coupled to the hapten trinitrophenyl (TNP) did not form rosettes when they were incubated with TNP-coated noncross-reactive horse red blood cells (hRBC). However, when newts were first immunized with only the carrier erythrocytes and were then injected with the carrier-hapten conjugate, cells from the aforementioned organs did display anti-TNP activity. Carrier specificity was indicated by the fact that to generate the anti-TNP response, the carrier used to prime the newts and the carrier coupled to the hapten in the second injection had to be the same. Hapten specificity was in part demonstrated by the observation that when cells from the carrier-primed and carrier-hapten-challenged animals were first incubated with 2,4,6-trinitrophenyl (TNP) coupled to human serum albumin, the number of RFCs directed against the TNP-coated RBC dropped markedly.

In another series of experiments, Ruben compared the responses of unpurified cells from the spleen, liver, and kidney to primary and secondary immunizations with HRBC. Secondary responses were determined in animals injected 21 days after the first immunization and were assayed for RFC 3 days later. At the peak of the primary response (between Days 8 and 12), a 51-fold increase in RFC over background was noted in the spleen, a 24-fold increase in the liver, and a 19-fold increase in the kidney. These observations are very puzzling in view of the fact that the minimal hematopoietic tissue in the liver and kidney of this species is thought to be primarily myelopoietic [86,94]. In other words, in a starting preparation of the same number of unpurified cells from each of these three organs, I would expect to find a vastly greater number of lymphocytes, potential anti-sRBC RFCs, in the spleen than in either the liver or kidney. Yet, the number of RFC in the spleen at the peak of the response was only about two and one half times that of the liver and about six times that of the kidney. Ruben then splenectomized a group of animals prior to a primary immunization and found that the numbers of RFCs from the kidney and liver of these animals were similar to those found in intact controls. These data suggest either that RFCs developed locally in the liver and kidney or that if they migrated into these organs after being stimulated, they did not originate in the spleen.

PHA reactivity of *Necturus* lymphocytes has been reported by those interested in karyotypes of salamanders rather than in the structural evolution of the lymphocyte membrane [102]. Collins and I have recently studied *Necturus* lymphocytes in vitro, and our preliminary observations indicate that, although they do proliferate when exposed to PHA, their stimulation indexes are less than those reported for an anuran [71]. Further detailed studies are in progress.

2. *Order Anura (frogs and toads)*

Various immunologic phenomena that relate to immunoglobulin class, the cellular basis and kinetics of antibody formation, tolerance, cell-mediated immunity, and the structure and function of an extensive lymphoid complex have been more extensively studied in larval and adult anurans than in any other order of ectothermic vertebrates. This wealth of data has been accumulated in a limited number of "favorite" species, such as *Rana pipiens* (leopard frog), *Rana catesbeiana* (bullfrog), *Bufo marinus* (marine toad), *Xenopus laevis* (clawed toad), and *Alytes obstetricans* (midwife toad). Despite the small sample of species, a perusal of this extensive literature of anuran immunology reveals many significant but somewhat confusing differences between the immune system of adults and larvae of the same species and among adults and larvae of these five different animals. To avoid making as yet unwarranted generalizations concerning the immune responses of *all* anurans, and to minimize the confusion that might arise from these specific and ontogenetic differences, I will separately review the literature that deals with the structure and function of the lymphoid complex and its component cells in adult representatives of each of the three families that have been well studied. I will then discuss the development of these lymphoid tissues and their role in the maturation and maintenance of immune competence in representatives in each family. Finally, I will comment on how amphibians have served and will continue to serve as unique models for exploring immunologic problems of general, rather than phylogenetic, interest.

a. *Structure and Function of Lymphoid Organs in Adult Anurans*

(1) The Ranidea. The thymus glands of sexually mature adult bullfrogs are structurally similar to those of postmetamorphic juveniles or tadpoles that are older than 6 months. However, with increasing age, there is a corresponding decrease of lymphoid cells in the cortex, an increase in the collagenous connective tissue in the medulla, and an overall greater vascularity of the organ [103]. The thymus is surrounded by a connective tissue capsule composed of collagen fibers and fibroblasts. The connective tissue penetrates deeply into

the parenchyma of the gland and serves to separate the cortex and the medulla into many small lobules. The cortex contains the greatest number of lymphocytes, while the medulla contains reticular cells and Hassall's corpuscles, in addition to thymocytes [103].

Although thymic involution has been reported, such degenerative changes might have been confused with the dramatic structural alterations of the thymus gland that occur during each of the four seasons [104,105]. These seasonal changes have been well described for *Rana esculenta* [105] and are presented in some detail as a warning to the investigator who might plan experiments with frogs while he continues to think of them as mice. The thymus of *R. esculenta* collected during the summer months has a clear demarcation between its cortical and medullary regions. In the cortex, the thymocytes are so numerous and mitotically active that they mask the cells of the reticulum. The vascular system of the thymus is well developed, and the blood vessels are arranged radially. No thymocytes are found in the lumen of these vessels in the thymuses of "summer frogs." The thymuses of frogs sacrificed in October contain substantially fewer thymocytes than do the thymuses of "summer frogs." The limits between the cortical and medullary areas of the gland are less sharp than in the "summer gland," but some mitosing thymocytes are still seen. In the medulla, the cells of the reticulum are similar to those seen during the summer. In the blood vessels of the thymus, there was a ratio of one thymocyte for every four erythrocytes. It is most significant, however, that the ratio of lymphocytes to erythrocytes in a blood smear made from the peripheral circulation was radically different, about 2:65 to 100. Thus, the significant relative number of thymocytes in the thymic vessels of frogs sacrificed in autumn implies a migration of lymphoid elements either to or from the gland. Since the total number of thymocytes in "autumn frogs" is less than that seen in "summer animals," it appears that the migration pathway leads from the thymus. During the winter period, when the frog is hibernating, the thymus is very small and yellowish. The number of thymocytes is decreased even further, and many of the cells exhibit degenerative changes. Very little proliferation is seen, and the demarcation between the cortex and medulla is vague. The thymus of frogs sacrificed in the spring is intermediate in size between that of winter and summer animals. The cortex and medulla become more clearly separated, and the number of thymocytes in the cortex increases, as does the number of mitotically active cells. At this period, there is no evidence for the immigration of cells from the periphery into the thymus. Thus, the increased number of thymocytes during the spring and summer months appears to be due primarily, if not exclusively, to localized mitotic activity. These observations are in complete agreement with those made by Turpen et al. on the contributions of thymocytes in the developing frog thymus to the lymphoid populations of the peripheral lymphoid tissues of adults [106,107].

Unlike the other vertebrates discussed thus far, adult frogs (but not tadpoles) have a bone marrow which is both lymphopoietic and myelopoietic and erythropoietic [108,109]. Lymphocytes appear in significant quantities in both the intravascular and extravascular spaces, and, like the situation in mammals, no nodular arrangements have been seen. According to Campbell [109], the ultrastructure of the plasma cells in the marrow of the leopard frog is similar to that of mammalian plasma cells, but frog cells have conspicuous cytoplasmic granules which are larger and more abundant than those in the mammalian plasma cells. These granules resemble lysosomes, but their function in frog cells is unknown. Cooper and Schaeffer [110] found that bone marrow from lead-shielded femurs can restore transplantation immune responsiveness to leopard frogs which would have otherwise been rendered immunoincompetent by a large dose of x-irradiation. However, animals which were thymectomized and then given the same amount of x-irradiation without shielding were unable to reject skin allografts after they were implanted with their own thymus glands [111].

In addition to the thymus, spleen, and bone marrow, adult bullfrogs have a variable number of paired lymph nodelike organs in their ventral neck region [103,112-115]. According to Baculi and Cooper, these organs in this species appear to filter blood but not lymph. Basically, these organs are encapsulated aggregates of lymphoid cells which are separated into lobules by sinusoids that are lined with reticuloendothelial elements. The so-called jugular bodies are found in all adult bullfrogs and are located ventral and lateral to the sternohyoid muscle. The parenchyma of these structures is characterized by a dense central accumulation of cells, small lymphocytes (70-90%), plasma cells (1-6%), granulocytes (1-4%), and monocytes (1-3%) [114]. The propericardial body is located on either side of the larynx. In some animals it is encapsulated, while in others it is not. It too contains lymphocytes, some plasma cells, blasts, and granulocytes. It is noteworthy that the number and size of this organ vary in different animals. Indeed, it does not appear in all animals of the same species. Likewise, the procoracoid body (located anterior to the truncus arteriosus) may not always be found, but when it is, it is covered by a thick capsule, is highly vascular, and contains primarily lymphocytes and plasma cells. A fourth lymphomyeloid organ, the epithelial body, may also be found near the parathyroids. When it is present, it is smaller and less complex than the aforementioned lymphomyeloid organs, and according to Cooper, it may be a satellite of the jugular body [103].

The variability in number and actual presence of these lymphoid organs in bullfrogs is echoed by the variable appearance of certain organs of this complex in other anuran species. Baculi and Cooper [113] compared the lymphoid complex of *R. catesbeiana* with that of other genera and species. Just the jugular body was seen in two Ranidae. Likewise, this was the only nodelike organ seen in representatives from two other genera. Only the jugular body and the procoracoid bodies were found in a *Hyla,* while *B. marinus* had these two structures plus another unnamed organ. In an additional three genera (two of which were *Bufo*), no organs were seen in the ventral neck region. *Xenopus* (which will soon be discussed at length) also had no lymph nodelike structures, but Baculi et al. [115] did describe a structure that resembled a hemal node.

This lymphoid complex in the neck region of anurans has also been described for *R. pipiens* by Horton [116]. The bilateral jugular bodies are the largest nodelike organs in this species, and procoracoid bodies are also seen. The presence of the propericardial bodies is variable. It is interesting that in the leopard frog, the anlagen of the jugular and procoracoid bodies appear during and just before metamorphosis, respectively. The jugular body develops from a scattered array of lymphocytes and granulocytes in and around several capillaries medial to the parathyroids and jugular veins.

(2) The Bufonidae. Evans et al. [118] indicated that while most of the thymuses of the adult *B. marinus* they examined were atrophic, those that were not had a clearly delineated cortex and medulla. The medulla contained hyalinized cells suggestive of those seen in Hassall's corpuscles, but definitive Hassall's corpuscles were not seen. They also noted an occasional plasma cell in the thymuses of immunized animals.

The marine toad has from four to 10 thinly encapsulated lymph nodelike organs located along the great vessels at the base of the heart and along their branches in the neck and axilla [118-120]. These structures lack the trabecular arrangement of mammalian nodes, but in some animals, the fact that lymphocytes are less dense in the subcapsular area suggests a cortical and medullary organization. Although the smaller nodes have the appearance of a single germinal center of a mammalian node, they are more loosely organized.

The function of these nodes and other lymphoid tissues in the immune responses of adult Ranidae has not been extensively analyzed. In one study, Cowden and Dyer [86] immunized adult leopard frogs with various dilutions of a pure culture of *Aeromonas hydrophilia,* a normal pathogen. The spleens of all animals that had detectable serum antibody levels were considerably enlarged. At higher dilutions, cysts in the spleen and increases in white pulp were noted. Dilutions of bacterial culture that elicited humoral anitbody production and substantial splenic enlargement failed to affect the intertubular hematopoietic tissue. Ambrosius and Hanstein [117] studied the dynamics of the plague-forming colony (PFC) response to sRBC in *R. esculenta* and found two maxima, one around the 10th day postimmunization and a second near the 20th day. The kinetics of the PFC response in the spleen, kidney, and jugular body were the same. However, more PFC were found in the spleen than in the jugular body, and these organs contained more PFC than did the kidney. The procoracoid and the propericardial had the fewest PFC. Although there were five classes of PFC, more than one half of the cells actively synthesizing antibody were small lymphocytes. According to Diener and Nossal [120], these nodes filter lymph and therefore appear to be different from the jugular bodies of the bullfrog [113].

The spleen of *B. marinus* has a relatively thick capsule. It is not divided by trabeculae; rather, there is only an irregular network of reticular fibers within the splenic pulp. The spleen lacks a sharp demarcation into a red and white pulp [121] or marginal zone [120] typical of the mammalian spleen. The amount of white pulp is variable and consists of small and medium lymphocytes that are in association with the major artery. The red pulp is composed of reticulum fibers, fixed macrophages, and lymphocytes. Primitive hemoblasts are rarely seen.

Wong et al. have described gut-associated lymphoepithelial tissue in the esophagous, stomach, duodenum, and rectum of another toad, *Bufo melanosticum* [122]. There are multiple aggregates in the esophageal region of sexually mature adults, while in juvenile forms, there is only a single collection in the submucosa. Different lymphoepithelial relationships were noted [123]; at least one involved the complete infiltration of the surface epithelium by lymphocytes. These structures are only rarely lobulated and are not distinguished by cortical and medullary zones or by germinal centers. They contain a preponderance of lymphocytes, with an occasional plasma cell [123]. Goldstine and Manickaval, in my laboratory, have observed a vast array of clearly defined lymphoid nodules along the entire length of the gut of *B. marinus* and of *R. pipiens.* These organs have been visualized by the in situ acetic acid fixation technique of Cornes [124]. An additional site of lymphoid accumulation is the mucosa of the bladder of not only *B. marinus* but also of *R. pipiens* [67,68].

The immunocytoadherence assay and immunofluorescence have revealed AFC in the thymus, spleen, lymph nodes, and kidneys of marine toads that were immunized with BSA [86,118,121,125] or *Salmonella adelaide* flagella [120,126-128]. After an extensive immunization with BSA (with and without complete Freund's adjuvant), the nodes of *B. marinus* were characterized by an increased number of lymphoblasts, by increased mitotic activity, and by the presence of AFC. When toads were injected with ^{125}I-labeled flagella, autoradiography indicated that the antigen became widely distributed in the nodes shortly after it was administered [120]. Clumps of antigen were found in reticular cells, and antigen was also localized in a stringlike pattern in or on other reticular cells. There was no follicular concentration of antigen, and, except for a gradual loss of label, there were no changes in antigen localization with time. By 5 days postimmunization, primitive pyroninophilic cells were scattered randomly throughout the nodes. These cells multiplied and differentiated into plasma cells, which became grouped in small clusters. No germinal centers were seen.

The increased spleen size of toads hyperimmunized with BSA was due primarily to an increase of the compact lymphocyte-containing area referred to by Evans et al. [118] as a primary lymphoid follicle. Pyroninophilic cells were seen mainly at the periphery of this "follicle," as were AFC. After 3 hr, radiolabeled flagellin was localized in the red rather than in the white pulp. After 24 hr, it became located around the white pulp, but there was no increase in the white pulp itself.

The kidneys of unimmunized *B. marinus* contain pockets of lymphocytes. Immunization with BSA causes an increase in this intertubular tissue. Many blasts and plasma cells are seen, and they appear more numerous in this site than in either the spleen or nodes of the same animals [120]. Autoradiographs of the kidney [120] of ^{125}I-labeled flagella revealed labeled cells scattering singly or in small clusters. By 3 to 7 days, there was an increase in the number of pyroninophilic cells, a cell type that is relatively uncommon in the kidney of unstimulated animals.

The immunocytoadherence assay has been used in conjunction with analyses of tritiated thymidine uptake, equilibrium density centrifugation, microscopic measurements, and sedimentation velocity separation to follow the differentiation of AFC in the spleens of *B. marinus* immunized once with polymerized flagellin [126-128]. AFC were detected in the spleen and peripheral blood as early as 3 days postimmunization, providing that the animals were in good nutritional state [127] and were kept at 37°C. Two peaks of AFC were seen in the spleen, one at Day 5 and another at Day 7. After Day 7, there was a gradual decline in the numbers of AFC. It is noteworthy that the total number of AFC in peripheral blood was higher than in the spleen. The kidneys and jugular bodies were not considered. The early AFC have been characterized as a relatively homogeneous light-density population that contains very large cells. These immature cells consisted of several size populations and were almost all actively engaged in cell division. Data suggest that these large cells undergo a series of halving divisions before they enter a division growth cycle. As the response developed, an additional dense population of AFC appeared. These cells, identified as small lymphocytes, became the predominant class of cells in the later responses. Throughout the response, there were always some immature large forms, an observation that suggests there is some continual recruitment of immunocompetent cells.

Cowden et al. originally described the ultrastructure of plasma cells from *B. marinus* as being totally comparable to that of mammalian plasma cells [125]. In a subsequent report, they not only described these plasma cells with their abundant rough endoplasmic reticulum, well-developed Golgi, and normally distended Golgi, but they also pointed out another, even more common, cell type that displayed considerable intracisternal enlargement with an accumulation of intracisternal material and a less complex Golgi. They suggested that such an ultrastructure could be compatible with a mature cell which is storing a greater amount of immunoglobulin than is normally found in mammalian plasma cells [86].

(3) The Pipidae. Animals in this family are phylogenetically more primitive than those previously discussed. The major lymphoid tissues of the adult clawed toad, *X. laevis,* are the thymus, bone marrow, spleen, and kidney [129-131]. They lack the nodes described for *Rana* and *Bufo.*

The white pulp of the spleen is comprised of several lymphoid follicles that are separated from the red pulp by a narrow boundary layer of cells [128,129]. In spleens from unimmunized animals, the white pulp still has a considerable number of small lymphocytes. These cells are also present in the red pulp either as a "cuff" around the white pulp or as a part of more rounded accumulations. There are no germinal centers in immunized or unimmunized animals.

There are only a few large and small pyroninophilic cells in the spleens of normal toads [129,131]. The fine structure analysis of these large pyroninophilic cells indicates a more saclike than lamellar endoplasmic reticulum, free or aggregated ribosomes, and a poorly defined Golgi [129].

Intertubular foci of lymphocytes are located along the entire length of the *Xenopus* kidney. These foci are associated with renal blood sinuses, and in some animals, large numbers of cells similar to those in the foci are found in the blood vessels that supply the kidney. The foci contain a predominance of small lymphocytes, but the larger pyroninophilic cells, comaprable to those just described in the spleen, are also present. In addition to the spleen, thymus, kidney, and bone marrow, small irregular accumulations of lymphocytes that lack follicular organization have been seen in the skin, liver, and gut [129,130,132].

The spleen of *Xenopus* is a source of cells that are active in cell-mediated immunity. Clark and Newth made adult *Xenopus* unresponsive to allogeneic tissues by grafting them during their embryonic life [133]. The spleen from the original donor toad was then implanted in the tolerant animal, and GVH reactivity was observed.

Immunization of adult *Xenopus* with human gamma globulin (HGG) in complete Freund's adjuvant resulted in a marked increase in splenic weight, in proliferation of pyroninophilic cells, and in the appearance of adjuvant-induced vacuoles in the white and red pulp [128,134]. Injecting the particulate antigen sRBC also resulted in proliferation, but it was primarily restricted to the periphery of the follicles of the white pulp. Plasma cells typical of those seen in mammals were rare in immunized and in normal toads. Booster injections elicited good antibody production but effected very little change in splenic histology. There was no reappearance of large pyroninophilic cells that were so characteristic of the primary response [134].

In an attempt to determine the relative importance of lymphoid tissues other than the spleen in humoral immunity, Turner splenectomized toads before he immunized them with HGG or sRBC [130]. Antibody titers and kinetics of antibody formation were similar in sham-operated and in splenectomized animals. Moreover, splenectomy alone, or splenectomy plus immunization with sRBC, caused no compensatory changes in the lymphoid component of the kidney. Although these data indicate that both the kidney and the animal's antibody-forming capabilities appear to be unaffected by removal of a major lymphoid organ, differences were found between the kidneys of toads that had been given HGG in adjuvant and the kidneys of those given either nothing or sRBC. HGG-injected animals had kidneys which were significantly larger and contained greater amounts of intertubular tissue [130]. The other focal aggregates in splenectomized immunized animals did not differ from those with an intact spleen. Thus, in the absence of the only organized lymphoid tissue other than the thymus, *Xenopus* were able to maintain normal immunologic function.

b. Some in Vitro Manifestations of Cellular and Humoral Immunity in Adult Anurans. At least three criteria that serve to define mammalian lymphocytes as T cells have been met with anuran lymphocytes. Whether these cells also satisfy the mammalian criteria of B cells is unknown. Splenic lymphocytes from adult *B. marinus* undergo blastogenic conversion in vitro in response to PHA and to allogeneic splenocytes [72]. At 26°C, the maximum incorporation of tritiated thymidine occurs on Day 3 in response to PHA and on Day 7 in MLC. The response to PHA is concentration dependent, and the maximum responses to PHA and to alloantigens vary from toad to toad. Recent experiments in my laboratory indicate that toad spleen cells also proliferate in response to con A, but the critical responses to lipopolysaccharides have yet to be studied. Gebhardt also demonstrated mitotic reactivity of small lymphocytes purified on a BSA gradient to PHA and to antilymphocyte serum. In vivo administration of the latter reagent caused prolonged graft survival, lymph node and spleen hypoplasia, and reduction of peripheral blood lymphocytes [135]. Mixed lymphocyte reactivity of spleen cells from *X. laevis,* a species that normally rejects skin allografts more chronically than do *Bufo* and *Rana* [136], has recently been reported [137]. That this reaction is under the control of a single genetic region is suggested by a comparison between the percentages of negative MLC between siblings (22%) and unrelated individuals (3%), by the distribution of MLC identical individuals into four different classes in two distinct sibships; and by a clear-cut haplotype effect.

In two recent reports, Ambrosius and Drossler [138,139] defined the conditions under which *Bufo bufo, Rana esculenta,* and *Rana temporaria* could be immunized with BCG, so that when their peritoneal exudates or spleen cells were cultured in the presence of purified protein derivative (PPD) and macrophages, inhibition of macrophage migration (MIF) occurred. Goldstine, Hoffeld, and I have recently confirmed MIF activity in lymphocytes from *B. marinus* that had been immunized in a similar fashion. Attempts to demonstrate delayed hypersensitivity of these animals by skin testing have been unsuccessful.

Several examples of the application of in vitro assays to enumerate the dynamics and cellular basis of antibody production in various organs of adult frogs have already been presented [117,120,126-128]. Two other studies will now be discussed. Amirante simultaneously immunized adult *Xenopus* with rabbit and chicken erythrocytes and noted a 1:1:1 ratio of pure antichicken RFC:pure antirabbit RFC:mixed antichicken and antirabbit RFC in the immunocytoadherence assay [140]. Since these two antigens did not appear to be cross reactive when tested with immune *Xenopus* serum, the high percentage of mixed cell rosettes indicates either that the number of individual cells capable of synthesizing antibodies with more than one specificity is greater in the toad than in the mammal, or that serum antibodies of both specificities had cytophilically bound to a lymphocyte or a macrophage. The former exciting possibility can only be considered after the morphology of the RFC is critically evaluated and after serum from these doubly immunized animals is incubated with nonimmune lymphoid cells which are then analyzed for mixed rosettes.

Auerbach and Ruben [141] simultaneously exposed spleen fragments of normal *Xenopus* to sRBC and mouse red blood cells (mRCB) and successfully initiated a primary immune response that could be evaluated by agglutination and localized hemolysis in gel. The kinetics of these in vitro responses, in which no cross reactivity could be demonstrated on a cellular lvel, paralleled the development of immunity in vivo. It is noteworthy that the sequential exposure of a primary culture to sRBC, followed 1 week later by an incubation with mRBC, led to the sequential appearance of antigen-specific PFC. It is also interesting (but as yet unexplained) that the number of PRCs that resulted from the simulataneous exposure of a spleen culture to both antigens was two to four times that which resulted when twice as many spleen cells were exposed to either antigen alone. The development of these techniques that allow for the initiation of an in vitro primary response with as few as 5×10^4 spleen cells, plus the fact that such cultures can be maintained for several weeks, opens the door for investigating a variety of contemporary immunologic problems in ectotherms, such as the clonal theory of selection, stem cell renewal, and tolerance.

c. Differentiation, Structure, and Function of Larval Lymphoid Organs.

(1) The Ranidae. *Rana* tadpoles lack the bone marrow and the nodelike jugular and procoracoid bodies seen in adults. However, in addition to the

thymus, spleen, intertubular, and gut-associated lymphoid tissues, they also have discrete organs called lymph glands and a variable number of ventral cavity bodies. The lymph glands and ventral cavity bodies disappear during metamorphosis at the time when the jugular and procoracoid bodies begin to differentiate [116].

The larval lymph gland of bullfrogs [102] and leopard frogs [116,142] is an encapsulated structure located bilaterally in the branchial chamber near the developing anterior limb. No true trabeculae are seen, and the organ is not divided into lobules. The support of the walls of the sinusoids and the parenchymal cords is provided for by collagen and reticular fibers. The cellular composition of the parenchyma is primarily lymphoid (all sizes of cells), although a few granulocytes and plasma cells have also been seen. Baculi and Cooper did not find any lymphatics in the bullfrog lymph gland [113], while Horton noted that in *Rana clamitans, R. catesbeiana* [116,142], and *R. pipiens,* the gland develops in and projects into the anterior lymphatic channel. Thus, it appears that this structure does filter lymph and blood. The lymph gland disappears shortly after metamorphosis. In vitro studies with bullfrog larval lymph glands indicate that in the presence of thyroxine, they undergo dramatic and degenerative changes [143]. The effects of this hormone on other lymphoid structures which do not degenerate during the metamorphic period have not been determined.

Ventral cavity bodies are located in the branchial cavity of bullfrog and leopard frog larvae [113,142]. Each of these structures is smaller than the lymph gland and appears to be a replica of one of its lobules. Based on gross dissection, Baculi and Cooper [113] originally reported only three pairs of ventral cavity bodies in bullfrog tadpoles. Horton, however, histologically examined the branchial region of larval bullfrogs and green frogs and found six or more pairs of large ventral cavity bodies. Indeed, there can be up to 30 such organs in the leopard frog [116,142].

Cooper has outlined the early development of the bullfrog thymus [112]. Five to 10 days posthatching, large lymphocytes and lymphoblasts are seen. By the end of the first week, cortical and medullary differentiation has begun; by Day 8, lobulation is seen; and by Day 9, the demarcation between cortex and medulla is sharp. Between Days 36 and 51, the capsule, cortex, and medulla are well established, and the organ has assumed the structure of the adult gland.

Thymus development and the ontogeny of other lymphoid structures have been detailed for the more rapidly developing *R. pipiens* by Horton [116, 142] and others [144,145]. For reference purposes, the Roman numeral staging system of Taylor and Kollros will be used [146]. The thymus has already been determined in the gill bud region of 72-hr-old embryos [106]. As early as 1 week after fertilization (stage 1), the thymus rudiment is seen as a small epithelial proliferation from the dorsal surface. At this early stage, anlagen of other lymphoid organs are not seen. Although the pronephros is present, the intertubular tissue is strictly erythropoietic. By the end of the second week postfertilization (stage II), the free-swimming tadpole has a thymus that is remarkably well differentiated. The ventral cavity bodies and the lymph glands appear about this time, but it should be stressed that lymphocytes appear in the thymus before they are found in any other tissues of the larval lymphoid complex. Between Days 16 and 19 (late stage II), the cortex and medullary areas of the thymus begin to be distinguishable, and the lymph gland has become differentiated into cords of lymphocytes (all sizes) with intervening sinuses. Lymphocytes are also found in the intertubular tissues of the pronephros and are beginning to populate the mesonephros and spleen. During stage III (Days 20-27) and stage IV (Days 30-35), the thymus, ventral cavity bodies, lymph glands, and kidneys continue to differentiate and grow, so that by the end of stage IV, they resemble the comparable organs of older animals. It should be noted that the lymphoid development of the spleen lags significantly behind that of the other lymphoid organs. By stage V and later, lymphoid accumulations are found in close association with the epithelium along the gastrointestinal tract from the oral cavity to the cloaca. These dorsal accumulations in the oral and pharyngeal cavity of the leopard frog may be the same accumulations found in the lingual region of adults [147].

There have been several studies in which the development of the thymus and lymphoid complex has been correlated with the maturation of destructive transplantation immunity, with the number of peripheral blood small lymphocytes [148], and with the ability of thymectomy to abrogate or to delay graft rejection [116,150]. Skin allografts placed on stage-IV leopard frog tadpoles were rejected with the timing characteristic of adults, while grafts placed on the less mature stage-III animals were rejected somewhat more slowly [149]. It is noteworthy that at stage III, lymphocytes are already present in all lymphoid tissues. Grafts exchanged during early embryonic life showed the earliest signs of lymphocytic infiltration at stage II and had a more marked infiltration by stage III [116]. Larvae thymectomized during stage II and early stage III exhibited prolonged allograft retention [116,150]. Those animals, which eventually did reject their grafts, were shown on autopsy to have a small bit of thymic tissue that had apparently resulted from the marked regenerative powers of this tissue. Thymectomy at later stages failed to affect graft rejection.

Early thymectomy of bullfrogs during the first month of their larval life also delayed the rejection response [151,152]. Cooper originally reported that removal of the thymus gland both from young and from 3- to 4-month-old tadpoles markedly impaired their antibody responses to goldfish serum [152].

He later reinterpreted these data and now suggests that, instead of removing the thymus gland, he extirpated the lymph gland [3,153].

Cooper has investigated the antibody-related functions of the lymph gland, spleen, and thymus of bullfrog tadpoles. In his first series of experiments, immunocompetent 6- to 9-month-old tadpoles failed to make any detectable antibodies following multiple injections of BSA after they had been bilaterally "lymph glandectomized" [154]. Unilateral extirpation was ineffective, and bilateral extirpation had no effect on graft rejection. It is unfortunate that the titers of antibodies in control animals never exceeded 1:64 [154]. In another series of experiments, Baculi and Cooper examined the antibody responses to lobster hemocyanin in tadpoles that ranged in age from 6 to 12 months [155]. My interpretation of their data is that neither total extirpation of the lymph glands nor splenectomy resulted in significantly decreased antibody titers, as measured by passive hemagglutination. However, the simultaneous removal of both the spleen and the lymph glands from the same tadpoles did seem to result in antibody titers that were lower than those obtained for controls. While they claim that late larval thymectomy was actually associated with an increase in antibody synthesis, the variability of the antibody responses among individual control and experimental animals makes such a conclusion rather tenuous. There is, however, no doubt that cells in the larval lymph glands do synthesize antibody. Moticka et al. immunized old bullfrog tadpoles with sRBC and observed significant numbers of PFC in the spleen, lymph gland, and thymus [156]. Based on the number of PFC/10^6 cells, the PFC response in the spleen was about three times that of the lymph gland but only 1.2 times that of the thymus. These authors also studied the histologic changes in these organs induced by immunization with sRBC [154]. In the thymus, the numbers of plasma cells and mitotically active cells increased from basically zero to significant numbers. In the lymph gland, the number of mitotic figures also increased, as did that of blast cells and plasma cells. In the spleen, antigenic challenge did not result in an increase in blast cells, and mitoses were rare. However, there was a slight increase in the number of plasma cells in this organ. The importance of the larval spleen in the immunologic competence of the bullfrog is suggested by observations that when it was removed from an animal that then received sufficient x-irradiation to immunosuppress normal animals and was then reautografted, the reconstituted larvae made agglutinins to sRBC, destroyed allografts, and had a restored hematocrit [157]. Moreover, when the autografted spleens were subsequently removed from animals that had been immunized with sRBC, they contained PFC [158].

(2) The Pipidae. The rapidly developing embryos and larvae of *X. laevis* have provided an exceptionally fine animal model for the descriptive and experimental analyses of the ontogenesis of immunity, a model which

has been systematically and profitably exploited by Manning, Horton, and Turner in England [159-163] and by Du Pasquier and his associates in Switzerland [164-167]. *X. laevis* has a spleen, thymus, and ventral cavity bodies. Accumulations of lymphocytes and granulocytes are also seen in the subcapsular area of the liver and along the medial wall around the nephrostomes of the metanephros [159]. *Xenopus* tadpoles are unlike *Rana* larvae in that they have only three pairs of ventral cavity bodies (compared with upwards of 30) and that they lack lymph glands and discrete and reproducible lymphocyte accumulations along the gut. Moreover, they do not have lymphoid tissue in the pronephros or between the tubules of the kidney [159].

The thymus [168] is the first lymphoid organ to develop in *Xenopus* [159], as it is in *R. pipiens* [116]. The anlage appears during the third day of life. By 8 days, it measures 0.1 mm, has about 1,000 cells, and is encapsulated but is not divided into a cortex and medulla. Small lymphocytes appear around Day 11, when the medullary and cortical demarcation is clear. At this time, there are large- or medium-sized cells in the splenic white pulp, and the anlagen of the ventral cavity bodies are present. Around 14 days postfertilization, the spleen and ventral cavity bodies have undergone greater differentiation, and within another day of development, small lymphocytes are found in both organs. At this time, the cortex of the thymus contains many small lymphocytes, and the formation of Hassall's corpuscles has begun. In some animals examined at this time or later, extrathymic accumulations of lymphocytes were seen near the subthymic and branchial veins [159,168]. Between Days 17 and 19, the thymus becomes fully differentiated, as do all of the other lymphoid tissues. The number of cells in the thymus increases to about 8×10^5 by about 5 weeks postfertilization [166]. This number remains constant for another 2 weeks and then suddenly decreases, so that by the end of metamorphosis (about 9 weeks postfertilization), the total number of thymocytes is about 2 to 3×10^5. The ventral cavity bodies are lost at this time. The thymus then begins to undergo a second period of growth, and it reaches its maximum size 15 to 16 weeks after fertilization. The average cell number at this time is about 4×10^7. When the animal reaches sexual maturity at the end of its first year, involution of the thymus begins. The small thymus of a fully grown adult is located in a mass of adipose tissue and consists of 2 to 4×10^6 cells [166].

Horton's analysis of the ontogeny of transplantation immunity in *Xenopus* [160] reveals that the extent of lymphocytic infiltration in a skin allograft correlates with the developmental state of lymphoid organs at the time of grafting. He found that when the lymphoid complex was either undeveloped or newly developed, lymphocyte infiltration was delayed, and graft survival was prolonged. Grafts transplanted after the complex was fully differentiated were rejected with the timing characteristic of adults.

Manning [161] studied the effects of larval thymectomy on the subsequent histogenesis of the larval lymphoid complex. Thymectomy performed at Day 11, when small lymphocytes are present only in the thymus (but large and medium lymphocytes are in the spleen), resulted in a moderate to severe depletion of lymphocytes in the ventral cavity bodies. The spleen was smaller in these thymectomized animals than it was in the controls, but this size difference became insignificant as the larvae grew older. Although thymectomy resulted in a fall in the number of the lymphocytes in the red pulp, there was an increase in the reticulomyeloid elements of the red pulp. The lymphoid differentiation in the white pulp remained unaffected by early thymectomy, as did the accumulation of lymphocytes in the liver and the kidney. If one believes that during ontogeny the amphibian thymus seeds lymphocytes to the peripheral organs [106,107], these data suggest that thymectomy may have been carried out too late to prevent the appearance of lymphocytes in the spleen but, nevertheless, early enough to delete the lymphocyte population in the ventral cavity bodies.

In a later study [162], Horton and Manning thymectomized larvae at several developmental stages and test grafted them either 2 to 3 weeks later or shortly after metamorphosis. Regardless of when they were thymectomized, no wasting disease was observed. Early thymectomy at 8 days of age dramatically impaired the ability of animals to reject skin allografted during the larval or the adult period. However, some larval grafts did show delayed and mild lymphocytic infiltration, and *some* of the grafts made during adult life were chronically rejected. Later thymectomy performed at a time when the lymphocytes were just beginning to appear in the spleen (11 days) also delayed and "weakened" the alloimmune responses of the subsequently grafted animals. Indeed, some animals thymectomized as late as 14 days, a time when lymphocytes were present in all of the lymphoid organs, were still unable to reject their grafts in the relatively vigorous manner characteristic of sham-operated animals. However, thymectomy performed between Days 17 and 19 was basically ineffective in altering graft rejection. Preliminary studies indicate that thymectomized animals can be immunologically reconstituted with grafts of thymus but not of spleen [163]. Unpublished observations of Horton also indicate that animals which had been thymectomized at 8 days, and which therefore took an unusually long time (6-14 weeks) to reject their first-set grafts, rejected second-set grafts with the timing typical of control second sets [163]. In other words, immunologic memory can develop in the absence of a thymus. Finally, Manning et al. [163] have recently found that thymectomy during the first 2 weeks of life can also impair the animals' humoral immune responses to human γ globulin. The normal localization of this antigen in the splenic white pulp does not occur in thymectomized animals [163].

It is not surprising that thymectomy dramatically impairs allograft immunity when it is performed at a developmental stage (8 days) when lymphocyte differentiation is just beginning in the thymus, the spleen contains fewer than 1,000 cells (just a few of which are medium and large lymphocytes), and only a few lymphocytes are present in the granulopoietic metanephros. What is intriguing is that this procedure quantitatively delays and minimizes rather than totally eliminates the alloimmune reaction. One explanation of the quantitative, rather than the qualitative differences, after very early thymectomy is that some seeding from the thymus had already occurred by 8 days of age and that this seeding was interrupted by thymectomy. Thus, a delay in rejection and the reduced numbers of cells infiltrating the graft would be attributed to a decrease, rather than to an elimination, of a population of cells that are capable of subsequently interacting with histocompatibility alloantigens. Although we do know that virtually all of the lymphocytes in the spleen, kidney, and bone marrow of the adult leopard frog are derived from a population of cells that originally self-differentiated from the thymus anlagen (Refs. 106 and 107; Sec. II.D.3.a), we do not know just when this colonization process is initiated. If this "interrupted seeding" explanation is valid, it also implies that only the shortest period of residence of a small number of cells in or in contact with the developing thymus is sufficient to sustain immunologic function of thymus-derived cells in later life. This assumes, of course, that like mammalian cells, frog lymphocytes do assume certain unique properties by virtue of a thymic influence. On the other hand, if it could be proved that thymectomy had been performed prior to any seeding, and if it could be confirmed in normal intact *Xenopus* that peripheral lymphocytes are ontogenetically derived from the thymus, the absence of a thymus but the present of immunologically active cells would suggest a compensatory source of lymphocytes, a compensatory nonthymic signal for the acquisition of T-cell function, and alternate pathways of lymphocyte differentiation.

3. Comments

While there are comparative immunologists who are actively studying the "anatomy of immunity" in nonmammalian species, there are also comparative immunologists who are attacking in ectotherms the very same frontier questions that are now being intensively investigated in mammalian systems. Aside from the very substantial "kickback" of fundamental phylogenetically relevant information, the major reason that some of these questions are being explored with amphibians is that these animals provide an excellent biologic tool. If you are interested in the structure of an antibody-combining site or in elucidating fundamental immunogenetic principles, you work with myeloma proteins or inbred strains of mice or rats. Similarly, if your interests include the origin of antigen-sensitive cells and their migration pathways during development or the earliest appearance of antibody and the generation of antibody diversity, you could work with mice and be hampered by a lack of easily acquired and maintained embryos and by maternal-fetal obfuscations, or could use the developing embryos and larvae of an amphibian and explore these problems with the whole slow developmental period at your surgical and intellectual disposal. Therefore, while a common (and perhaps valid) explanation of why one uses lower vertebrates is "to provide a 'simpler' system to shed light on one that is more complex," it is important to realize that there is an increasing number of immunologists who are simply using the best animal material to answer complicated immunologic questions that know no phylogenetic restrictions. Some of the fundamental knowledge that has been generated in anuran models in response to such questions will now be reviewed.

a. During Development, Do Thymic Lymphocytes Arise in Situ and Then Seed the Peripheral Lymphoid Tissues? The ontogeny of lymphocytes in the thymus and in other lymphoid tissues has been the subject of extensive investigation and of equally intensive controversy for many years [174]. That during embryogenesis the lymphoid population of the thymus arises from extraembryonic sources in birds (i.e., a blood-borne stem cell from the yolk sac) is strongly suggested by studies of parabiosed chick embryos [175]. On the other hand, the extensive in vitro and transplantation experiments with 12-day-old mouse thymic rudiments by Auerbach [176] supported the theory that lymphocytes develop directly from the epithelial component of the thymic anlage after an indictive stimulus from the mesenchyme. However, subsequent cytologic analyses of the 11- to 12-day-old mouse thymic rudiment suggested that lymphocyte precursors were already present in the thymus at the time it was explanted or transplanted [177]. Recently, Turpen et al. have reinvestigated the question of the thymic versus the extrathymic origin of lymphocytes in the developing thymus and peripheral lymphoid organs of the leopard frog [106,107]. The embryo of this species has provided us with a model with which we have been able to identify the presumptive thymic tissue, label it by inducing triploidy in the egg, remove it from a 72-hr-old embryo whose vascular system and blood islands are still undifferentiated, and orthotopically and bilaterally transplant it to a diploid embryo of the same developmental stage. We can then raise these triploid-diploid chimeras through metamorphosis and quantitatively determine the relative percentage of donor and host cells that populate the differentiated thymus transplant and the lymphoid organs of the host. Our experiments reveal that thymic lymphocytes arise in situ from components in the presumptive thymus area rather than from blood-borne stem cells that migrate into the thymic rudiment. During or after thymic differentiation, these lymphocytes or their descendants then leave the thymus and colonize the spleen, kidney, and bone marrow of adults. Moreover, in adult life, there is no indication of a significant inward afferent stream of lymphocytes entering the intact thymus. In other words, during adult life, the population of lymphocytes within the thymus is self-perpetuating.

b. During Ontogeny, Are Antigen-binding and Antibody-forming Cells Multipotential or Unipotential? Du Pasquier investigated the ontogeny of spontaneous antigen binding RFC [173] and of antibody-forming RFC and PFC [2,172] in larval *Alytes* [169-171] during a developmental period when the number of splenic lymphocytes increases from about 5×10^2 to 10^4 cells. Although no background PFC were seen, there were thymus-dependent [173] RFC to human red cells (huRBC) and sRBC which increased during development from about five to 10 per spleen to 50 to 100 per spleen. However, since the total number of spleen cells also increased during the period, there was really a relative decrease in the percentage of RFC and huRBC from about 0.8% in spleens that contained between 500 and 1,000 cells to about 0.1% in spleens with approximately 10,000 cells. Since the absolute number of RFC remained constant after the spleens reached this number of cells, the relative number of spontaneous RFC decreased even more during subsequent development.

Injections of huRBC or sRBC into larvae with fewer than 6×10^3 spleen cells did not increase the number of RFC significantly above the highest background; nor did it result in the appearance of PFC. However, immunization of animals during the first 2 months of larval life that had between 6×10^3 and 12×10^3 spleen cells did elicit an immune response in some spleens. Immunity *always* occurred when the spleens contained more than about 12×10^3 cells. Similarly, spleens from *Rana temporaria* that had been immunized in vitro with phage or in vivo with *Salmonella* or phage began to respond when they contained about 15×10^3 cells [2]. These observations that such a population of spleen cells can synthesize antibodies in tadpoles whose total number of lymphocytes has been estimated as about 10^6 cells are difficult to reconcile with the unipotentiality of the lymphocyte that is implied by the clonal theory of selection and with the estimates that a mammal can synthesize specific antibodies to a minimum of 10^6 antigenic specificities [178,179]. In other words, if we assume that a tadpole with 10^6 lymphocytes has no more than 10^4 or, at the most, 10^5 potential clone-forming lymphocytes (reduced from 10^6, because not all lymphocytes have immunoglobulin on their membrane at the time of antigen confrontation, and some of the lymphocytes are part of the same clone), this animal can synthesize antibody to no more than 10^4 or 10^5 specificities. Therefore, either serum antibodies or receptor sites must be cross-reactive, or the lymphocyte must be multipotential at the level of its receptor site, or the estimate of 10^6 possible antibody specificities of Jerne [178] and Haurowitz [179] must be revised downward for tadpoles. Haimovitch and Du Pasquier [165] found that bullfrog tadpoles (with an estimated 1-2 $\times 10^6$

lymphocytes) produced noncross-reactive hapten-specific antibodies to TNP- and 2,4-dinitrophenyl (DNP)-conjugated bacteria or protein. Similarly, Du Pasquier and Panijel [2] found that tadpole antibodies to tobacco mosaic virus and T4 (and to T4 and T uneven phages) are not cross reactive. These data argue against the possibility that the large number of antigenic determinants which tadpole lymphocytes can recognize is due to extensive cross reactivity of a limited number of specificities. These considerations have also forced Du Pasquier to advocate that, at least during larval life, the lymphocyte is multipotential [2,165,172]. If this notion is true, it is still unknown whether multipotentiality exists at the level of the receptor site and/or whether there is a restriction in potentiality during development that may be antigen driven.

c. Are Membrane Immunoglobulins Synthesized by Thymocytes? Whether the mammalian thymocyte contains membrane immunoglobulin (Ig) is a major area of immunologic controversy [20,22]. However, we now know that not only are there a large number of Ig-positive thymocytes in *Xenopus* tadpoles but also that such cells can be detected by immunofluorescence as early as 1 week postfertilization (i.e., before small lymphocytes are found in the spleen and other lymphoid organs). That such immunoglobulins are actively synthesized by the cell has been confirmed by observing the sequence of cap formation, endocytosis, and reformation of a cap [164].

d. Do Thymocytes Lose Membrane Immunoglobulins During Development? It will be recalled that during development, the number of thymocytes increases, plateaus, and then decreases, so that by the end of metamorphosis, it is about 3×10^5 [166]. The thymus then undergoes a second period of growth and reaches its maximum size by 15 to 16 weeks postfertilization. Du Pasquier and Weiss have followed the development of the thymocyte population during this period with respect to changes in membrane Ig [166]. Immunoglobulins on the cell surface were detected by two methods. One, the spot technique, is carried out in the presence of sodium azide and measures fluorescence when it is spread over the entire cell surface. The more sensitive cap test is carried out in the absence of sodium azide and measures the fluorescence at one pole of the cell. Between Days 8 and 14 postfertilization, the percentage of Ig-positive cells increases. It peaks around 3 weeks of age at 80%. From 3 weeks through early postmetamorphic life, the percentage of Ig-positive cells remains at about 70%. When the sensitive cap test was used to follow Ig-positive cells, they remained at about 70% after metamorphosis. However, the less sensitive spot test recorded a diminution in the percentage of Ig-bearing cells that started about 1 week after metamorphosis. This is the time that the second growth phase of the thymus occurs. The decrease in Ig-positive cells reached its nadir at a time when the thymus contained its greatest number of cells. At that time, it is still speculative as to whether the different results obtained with the cap and spot test mean that the percentage of Ig-positive cells does remain constant throughout this period but that the number of Ig molecules on each cell decreases. The resolution of this point bears a key relationship to the induction of self-tolerance during the metamorphic period [2,166].

e. Does the Thymus Play Any Regulatory Role on Immunoglobulin Synthesis? Weiss et al. [167] demonstrated with the sensitive capping technique that thymectomy of 6- to 8-day-old *Xenopus* larvae resulted in a permanent increase in the percentage of Ig-positive cells in the spleen, in addition to an increase in the amount of Ig per spleen cell. Serum Ig levels also increased permanently. These data suggest that the thymus exerts an inhibitory effect on the production of membrane-associated and serum Ig. The nature of this control mechanism is unknown.

f. Dissociation of the Molecular Events Involved in Antigen-driven Maturation of Immunocompetent Cells. It has been known for many years that humoral and cellular immunities are suppressed when ectotherms are kept at low ambient temperatures but can be initiated when immunized cold-treated animals are placed in a warmer environment [1,4,8]. Recently, Cone and Marchalonis have used temperature as a tool to study the maturation of the response of *B. marinus* to hRBC [180]. Animals immunized and maintained at 37° and at 20°C have the same number of RFC in their spleens by Day 3. These rosettes can be inhibited with a rabbit antitoad IgM antibody. At 20°C, but not at 37°C, the number of RFC decreases until Day 6, when it again begins to increase. Likewise, the appearance of circulating hemagglutinins is delayed or suppressed at 20° relative to 37°C. Shifting immunized animals from 20° to 37°C or from 37° to 20°C on the third day postimmunization causes corresponding increases or decreases in the number of RFC and in the antibody titer at Day 6. These data indicate that the immune response to hRBC is separable into two phases. The initial RFC response is independent of temperature but proportional to the antigen dose. These RFC may be the precursors of antibody-secreting cells, but whether they are equivalents of T or B cells is not clear. The second step results in the production of circulating antibody and is dependent on both the amount of antigen and on the temperature. These observations, plus those that indicate that antigen priming in Amphibia is independent of temperature [181], make ectotherms an excellent model with which to dissect and analyze the molecular events which control discrete steps in the immune response.

E. Class Reptilia

The first reptiles (Cotylosaurs) evolved from primitive labyrinthodont amphibians nearly 300 million years ago during the Carboniferous period. All modern reptiles, with the exception of Crocodilia, are direct descendants of these Cotylosaurs. These stem reptiles also gave rise to other lines. One of these lines, the Therapsids, led to the mammals; another one, the Thecodonts, led to the crocodilians and modern birds. Since modern avian and mammalian species originally evolved from reptilian stock, modern-day reptiles might offer significant clues to the origins of certain facets of the immune response. It is unfortunate, therefore, that only a limited number of representatives from two of the four reptilian orders, the Chelonia and the Squamata, have been immunologically evaluated in any depth [75].

1. Order Chelonia (turtles and tortoises)

The lymphoid complex of the snapping turtle consists of a thymus, spleen, lymph nodelike structures, and accumulations of lymphocytes in the pharynx, intestine, lung, kidney, cloaca, and bladder. No lymphocytes have been seen in the liver or bone marrow [69,182,184]. The adult thymus is composed of several small lobes, each of which is divided into lobules by trabeculae that extend into the cortex from the dense collagenous capsule. The cortex is densely packed with small lymphocytes, while the medulla is dominated by myeloid cells but also contains some lymphocytes and an occasional reticular cell [182]. The large almost spherical spleen is encapsulated by dense irregular collagen. The red pulp is present throughout the parenchyma and consists of a system of sinusoids that contain blood cells. The white pulp is more extensive than that of a mammalian spleen, but it lacks typical splenic nodules and germinal centers. In the white pulp, numerous dense aggregates of lymphocytes (follicles) each surround a central arteriole [182,183].

The spleen of the snapping turtle contains cells that can effect GVH reactions either in vitro [184] or in vivo [185]. In a recent study, Borysenko and Tulipan made use of the fact that for the first few months of life, snapping turtles are immunoincompetent [185]. Thus, intraperitoneal injections of adult allogeneic spleen cells into turtle hatchlings resulted in acute GVH disease at 30°C but in more chronic reactions at 20°C. No GVH activity with the kidney was noted [185].

Small lymph nodelike organs were located in the axillary and inguinal areas of some, but not all, of the snapping turtles examined by Borysenko and Cooper [182]. These heavily encapsulated structures appear to filter lymph and blood and are composed in part of large aggregates of lymphocytes which are separated from each other by collagen and fibroblasts. Smaller diffuse aggregates of lymphocytes are found throughout the small and large intestines. In the cloacal region, the alimentary canal also contains many large aggregates of small lymphocytes that often distend portions of the lamina propria [182,184]. Borysenko and Cooper [182] described still another large accumulation of lymphocytes in the tracheal wall of the pharynx.

Recently, LeFevre et al. [69] described numerous lymphoid nodules in the bilobed bladder of *Pseudemys scripta.* Such structures have also been seen in the bladder of the snapping turtle by Goldstine and Manickavel in my laboratory. In *Pseudemys,* these nodules consist of masses of dense lymphocytes that range in size from 0.004 to 0.52 mm^2. They are usually located immediately beneath the epithelial layer and often cause the epithelium to bulge into the lumen. In many instances, the epithelium over the nodules shows thinning or marked interruption. Occasional groups of lymphoblasts are seen, but no germinal centers exist. Additional diffuse lymphocytic infiltrations, in addition to a few pyroninophilic cells, have been seen in the epithelial and connective tissue layers of the bladder. It is noteworthy that since the ureters of the turtle enter the cloaca, urine is briefly exposed to cloacal contamination before it is stored in the bladder. Therefore, both the cloaca and the bladder are sites where a natural exposure to antigens can be expected with regularity.

In vitro procedures have permitted the enumeration of AFC in the spleen and peripheral blood of turtles but not in their kidney, thymus, or intestine [184-187]. The role of the liver as a source of AFC is questionable [187,189]. In a recent ultrastructural analysis of PFC in the spleen and peripheral blood of the tortoise, Ambrosius and Hoheisel indicated that nearly half of the PFC were mature plasma cells, while the remainder were immature blast cells in various stages of differentiation [188]. Only a few antibody-forming small lymphocytes were noted. There appear to be many noteworthy differences between the plasma cells of mammals and tortoises [188-191]. The tortoise AFC contains very little dense chromatin. The cisternae of the rough endoplasmic reticulum are distended and form small irregular storage sacs. The large confluent vacuoles typical of mammalian plasma cells are not seen. The Golgi of these reptilian cells consist primarily of stacks of flat cisternae, and these cisternae are often irregular and distended. The pinching off of Golgi vesicles is uncommon, and no such vesicles were in evidence in the periphery of the cell. Thus, it appears that reverse pinocytosis is not the predominant method of antibody secretion. Since Ambrosius and Hoheisel have observed that the membranes of the sacs of the endoplasmic reticulum can be in contact with the cell membrane, they have proposed an eccrine type of secretion [188].

2. Order Squamata (lizards and snakes)

The lymphoid complexes of only a few species of lizards have been examined in any depth. The bobtailed lizard (*Tiliqua rogosa*) is a member of the family

Scincidae, which probably originated during the Triasic period from a group that had already given rise to the stock of the Rhynchocephalia [192]. Its primary and anamnestic responses to *Salmonella,* heterologous erythrocytes, and BSA have been described [192]. The bloodsucker lizard, *Calotes versicolor*, has been intensively investigated by Muthukkaruppan and his students, and its lymphoid system has received special attention [183,193-195]. The red and white pulp of the spleen of *Tiliqua* is clearly demarcated [192], while that of *Calotes* is not [183]. Indeed, the splenic red pulp in this latter species is represented only by narrow strands of blood spaces distributed in the white pulp. In both species, as well as in the snapping turtle [182], the white pulp consists of numerous follicles or aggregates of lymphocytes. Each follicle consists of a reticular area with a central artery that is surrounded by lymphocytes. At least in *Calotes,* these follicles form a continuous phase of lymphoid tissue throughout the spleen. Despite intensive immunization schedules, no germinal centers have been seen. This basic architecture characterizes the spleens of two other species [183].

One of the most striking findings in some species of lizards has been the presence of lymph nodelike structures. In the bobtailed lizard, a 1- to 2-mm bean-shaped lymphoid organ was located close to the ventral surface next to the forelimb. This lymph node contained sinuses and large numbers of lymphocytes of varying sizes. It is not clear whether these structures are homologous to the perivascular accumulations of lymphocytes seen in geckos [196]. In these lizards, these bilateral accumulations are found where the lateral vein passes through the axillary sinus. Under the endothelium of this vessel, there are connective tissue cells and a fine network of reticular fibers that support a large number of lymphocytes, the most common of which is the small lymphocyte. There are no germinal centers or trabeculae associated with these or other accumulations which have been noted in the veins that drain the body wall at a point where they cross the axillary sinus and join the lateral vein. Kotani has also found lymphoid tissue in the wall of the cardinal lymphatics of a snake [197]. At present, no such structures have been seen in *Calotes.* In this species, however, there are cloacal accumulations of lymphoid tissue that have not yet been described for other lizards [183].

Neither splenectomy nor thymectomy of adult *Calotes* alters the survival of skin allografts [198]. Splenectomy, however, does have an effect on the PFC and hemagglutinating antibody responses to sRBC [194], as well as on the humoral response to BSA [183]. When animals were immunized either 7 days after or 2 hr before splenectomy, no antibody was detected. In the latter situation, no reconstitution with autologous spleen cells could be obtained. These observations, which indicate that, at least in this reptile, the spleen is the major source of AFC, are in contrast to data derived from splenectomized *Xenopus* [130]. Confirmation [193] of the importance of the spleen in antibody production is derived from the fact that PFC have been found in the spleen and blood of normal sRBC-immunized animals but not in the cloacal accumulations, thymus, bone marrow, and lungs. Fluorescent antibody staining of liver cells from desert iguanas immunized with BSA has, however, been recorded [189].

A potentially valuable reagent for discerning lymphocyte heterogeneity in lizards is a rabbit antiserum directed against *Calotes* thymocytes. Parenteral administration of this antiserum results in a profound lymphopenia and in aplasia of the thymus and spleen. It also suppresses allograft rejection, but its effects on humoral immunity are unknown [198].

3. *Orders Crocodilia and Rhynchocephalia*

Crocodilians have big teeth and have been neglected by immunologists. Limited investigations, however, do indicate that the alligator has a thymus, pharyngeal and gut-associated aggregates of lymphocytes, a lymphatic plexus rather than discrete nodes, and significant accumulations of lymphoid tissue in the cloaca [24,184,199].

Ancestors of the tuataras (*Sphenodon punctatum*) deviated from the stem reptiles in the Triassic period. They are the sole surviving members of the Rhynchocephalia, and they live in New Zealand under strict governmental protection. It is for this reason that the only information we have on the lymphoid system of the tuatara comes from a vigorous analysis of two immunized adults [200]. No thymus, nodes, or lymphoid accumulations in the liver, kidney, and intestine were seen. The only organized lymphoid tissue that was found is the spleen. Like that of other reptiles, it consists of lymphoid follicles that surround a central artery. Although the red and white pulps were clearly separated, there were no marginal zones or germinal centers. It seems highly unlikely that tuataras do not have a thymus. Whether it was undetected because of age-related involution or because of difficulty in locating the proper area for histologic analysis is unknown.

4. *Comments*

Whereas the Amphibia have been a veritable and heavily exploited gold mine of immunologic information, the Reptilia are an untapped resource. For example, the multiple aggregates of lymphoid tissues in the cloacal region of the alligator [184], turtle [184], and lizard [183], and the presence of significant amounts of lymphoid tissue in the bladder [70], represent an opportunity to determine the phylogenetic origins of the bursal system of birds. In this regard, it is significant that alligators and modern birds share a common origin from the Thecodonts.

The inability of turtle hatchlings to reject skin allografts or make circulating antibodies for the first 3 months of life has not yet been correlated with a stage of differentiation of the thymus or other lymphoid tissues. Yet, these observations raise the enigmatic question (as they do in free-swimming tadpoles) of how immunoincompetent young ectotherms survive in an antigenically hostile environment. Whether they rely on the passive transfer of maternal immunity or whether they possess an undiscovered alternate system of defense is a virgin area for research.

It is evident that the immunoincompetence of the snapping turtle hatchling is not the hallmark of all reptiles. Kanakambika and Muthukkaruppan revealed the immunocompetence of hatchling lizards when they enumerated PFC in spleens of animals that had been immunized within 24 hr after hatching and by the observation that the parenteral administration of adult spleen cells into young animals did not induce a GVH reaction [194]. The fact that when they immunized an ainmal whose spleen contained about 8×10^5 cells, they obtained as many as 1.6×10^3 PFC a few days later reminds me of Du Pasquier's contention that the lymphocyte may be multipotential [1,172,173].

III. Final Comments

The title of this chapter is presumptuous, because without a fossil record that allows us to examine both soft and hard tissues of animals that have been extinct for millions of years, we can only assume that comparative immunology tells us something about the phylogenetic emergence of lymphoid tissues and cells. The following remarks are predicated on the validity of this assumption.

Despite their phylogenetically primitive status, agnathans possess small lymphocytes that synthesize antibody and participate in the destruction of allografts [28-30]. Small lymphocytes from hagfish and lampreys share additional key properties of the mammalian small lymphocyte, such as proliferation in vitro in response to phytomitogens [40,41], histoincompatible cells [31,41], and haptenic groupings to which the lymphocyte donor has been previously exposed in vivo [41]. To generalize, lymphocytes from agnathans, like lymphocytes from all vertebrates that have thus far been examined, are capable of rather subtle discriminatory recognition of nonself and of duplicating or amplifying themselves as a result of such a recognition event. Since lampreys and hagfish lack organized lymphoid tissues, these observations on the immunologically relevant in vivo and in vitro behavior of their lymphocytes imply that the phylogenetic origin of the lymphocyte preceded the origin of lymphoid organs. We do not know whether these membrane-associated properties of recognition and responsive proliferation evolved in concert or independently. We are also ignorant as to whether they first appeared during agnathan evolution or prior to the phylogenetic emergence of this class of vertebrates. I would speculate, however, that their origins are to be found in the Invertebrata. The extensive studies of the defense systems of a multitude of invertebrate species [201] have laid a suitable groundwork for proving or disproving this simple speculation. Now, we must explore in immunologic terms, and with all available technical expertise, the nature of the invertebrate cells that synthesize opsonins, agglutinins, and lysins and are involved in the recognition and destruction of tissue allografts and xenografts [202-204]. Similarly, we must define in invertebrates the molecular and cellular events that are involved in the initiation of these effector mechanisms.

One obvious change that has occurred during the evolution of the lymphocyte is an increase in the number of differentiated cell types that constitute the lymphoid series. For example, although agnathans have small lymphocytes, they lack large lymphocytes and plasma cells. Plasma cells, which first appear in the Elasmobranchii, have themselves undergone certain structural modifications during evolution [86,109,125,129,188,191]. Critical questions about the evolution of plasma cells must focus on whether these structural differences bear any discernible relationship to functional dissimilarities. Such problems are already being investigated by Ambrosius and Hoheisel [188], who suggest that the mechanism of antibody secretion in tortoises involves the fusion of the membrane of the endoplasmic reticulum with the cell membrane (eccrine secretion) and not reverse pinocytosis.

Although there are data that indicate that lymphocyte subsets exist in sharks [47,48] and that cell cooperation is involved in the synthesis of antibody by fishes [64] and salamanders [94], such markers of lymphocyte diversity have not yet been looked for in representative species from each vertebrate order. Thus, with only bits and pieces of the phylogenetic puzzle at hand, it is presently impossible to know the extent to which the evolution of the small lymphocytes has been marked by changes that involved structural and functional heterogeneity. I should point out that future studies designed to detect and analyze T- and B-cell equivalents in ectotherms will provide more than just descriptive data. For example, if cell cooperation does occur in hagfish, the ontogeny of two or more populations of lymphocytes in a species that lacks a definitive thymus raises many provocative questions. So do the observations that, regardless of the heterogeneity of anuran lymphocytes, all lymphocytes in an adult frog are originally derived from the cells in the developing thymus [106]. Clearly, now is the time to study the biology of lymphocytes from more than just a restricted number of mammalian species.

Whereas the evolutionary origins of the lymphocyte will probably be found in the Invertebrata, it appears that the organization of these cells into organs evolved somewhat later. The phylogenetic roots of the lymphoid system are mirrored by the foci of hematopoietic elements in the pharynx and gut of the agnathans. The basic pattern of the lymphoid system, a definitive well-organized thymus and spleen plus focal accumulations of lymphocytes, first appears in living Chondrichthyes. It is unknown whether the immunologic role of the thymus evolved concurrently with the appearance of this tissue, since the most "primitive" species in which a relationship between the maturation of the immune response and the presence of the thymus has been demonstrated is a teleost. On the other hand, the spleen of all vertebrates tested is a significant source of antibody-forming cells and of lymphocytes that participate in cell-mediated immunity. A lymphopoietic bone marrow and encapsulated lymph nodelike structures first appear in anuran amphibians. It is of phylogenetic interest that the lymph and blood-filtering "nodes" in frogs are lacking in the adult representatives of less advanced families. Bone marrow and "nodes" are perpetuated in at least some reptiles. However, the homology of such structures in ectotherms with the nodes of birds and mammals will be satisfactorily determined only when more reptilian species are analyzed.

Although focal accumulations of lymphocytes remain as constant features throughout the vertebrate series, the number and size of such foci, their location, and their immunologic importance may be different in various species. For example, accumulations of lymphocytes are associated with the excretory system of nearly all vertebrates. In terms of its abundance and perhaps its role, kidney-associated lymphoid tissue reaches its zenith in the Osteichthyes. It is still present and functionally important in amphibians, but it reaches its apparent nadir in the Reptilia, where the spleen seems to assume a greater relative importance in antibody synthesis [194]. Similarly, some gut-associated lymphoid accumulations are found in all vertebrates higher than the Agnatha, but in ectotherms, this structure is probably best represented in the Anura. Whether there is an association between gut-associated lymphoid tissue and the emergence of IgA is under investigation. Bladder- and cloaca-associated lymphoid accumulations are found in frogs and turtles, but it is unknown whether they are analogous with the avian bursa of Fabricius.

Two additional points should be emphasized because of their applicability throughout the whole phylogenetic series of ectothermic vertebrates. First, complex highly organized lymphoid organs are not prerequisites for a complex immune response. Thus, splenectomy of the primitive frog, *Xenopus,* eliminates the only lymphoid organ other than the thymus, but it does not alter the humoral antibody response of the animal [129,130]. Similarly, simultaneous removal of the spleen, gut, and thymus from adult salamanders does not impair their ability to reject skin allografts [205]. Thus, lymphocytes in the kidney, peripheral blood, and elsewhere are fully capable of handling the immunologic defenses of these animals, at least on a short-term basis. Second, even with the repeated immunization of an assortment of ectotherms with many different antigens, no germinal centers have ever been seen in any of their lymphoid tissues, organized or not. It has been suggested that, among their other attributes [206], germinal centers are primary sites for the development of immunologic memory [207].

Yet, there are substantial data which indicate anamnesis in anurans [34,208] and reptiles [75,209].

We all accept that birds and mammals are the most highly evolved animals. We sometimes tend to equate this evolutionary position with maximum complexity. Indeed, relative to the immune system, this seems to be the case. However, such complexity is not necessarily synonymous with a superior survival value. We must appreciate that, regardless of its complexity, the immune system of each vertebrate species that I have discussed in this chapter is in sufficient equilibrium with other physiologic processes to permit this species to flourish in its own ecologic niche.

Acknowledgments

I would like to express my appreciation to my fellow scientists whose collective curiosity has provided me with the literature that I have attempted to summarize. I apologize for any omissions of relevant studies but must add that the fact that such omissions have no doubt occurred is testimony to the wealth of information available on just one aspect of immune phylogenesis. Particular thanks are due to my colleagues who provided me with as yet unpublished data from their laboratories and with the benefit of their wisdom. In phylogenetic order (of the species they have studied), they include: Drs. Tripp, Wittig, Cheng, McKay, Hildemann, Clem, Sigel, Sailendri, Hightower, Houillon, Charlemagne, Tournefier, Manning, Horton, Turner, Du Pasquier, Ambrosius, and Muthukkaruppan.

Research cited from my laboratory and the preparation of this manuscript were supported by Grants A1-08784 and HD-07901 from the National Institutes of Health. I am a recipient of Research Career Development Award AI-70736.

Note Added in Proof

In the interval between submission and publication of this chapter, there have been several significant advances in the understanding of the phylogenetics emergence of lymphoid tissues and cells. These include: the in vitro delineation of T and B cell-type heterogeneity at the level of anuran amphibians [210-212], the absence or presence of strong proliferative responses of lymphocytes from urodele amphibians which have been cultured with T or B cell mitogens, respectively [213]; and the clear cut responsiveness of teleost [214,215] and alligator [215] lymphocytes to both T and B mitogens. An alternative pathway of lymphopoiesis in thymectomized tadpoles has also been described [216], as has the very early localization of the precursors of thymocytes (and peripheralized lymphocytes) in the endodermal germ layer of frog embryos [212]. Readers interested in updating their knowledge of these and other facets of immune phylogenesis should peruse the several recent books [218-220] and journal issues [221] exclusively devoted to this subject.

References

1. W. W. Hildemann, in *Transplantation Antigens; Markers of Biological Individuality* (B. D. Kahan and R. A. Reisfeld, eds.), Academic, New York, 1972, Chap. 1.
2. L. De Pasquier, in *Current Topics in Microbiology and Immunology,* Springer-Verlag, New York, 1973, Vol. 61, pp. 37-88.
3. E. L. Cooper, in *Contemporary Topics in Immunology* (A. J. S. Davies and R. L. Carter, eds.), Plenum, New York, 1973, Vol. 2, Chap. 1.
4. H. Grey, in *Advances in Immunology* (F. J. Dixon and H. G. Kunkel, eds), Academic, New York, 1969, Vol. 10, pp. 51-104.
5. R. T. Smith, P. A. Miescher, and R. A. Good (eds), *Phylogeny of Immunity,* University of Florida, Gainesville, 1966.
6. L. W. Clem and G. A. Leslie, in *Immunology and Development* (M. Adinolfi and J. Humphrey, eds.), Lavenham, Suffolk, England, 1969, pp. 62-88.
7. R. A. Good and B. W. Papermaster, in *Advances in Immunology,* (F. J. Dixon and J. H. Humphrey, eds.), Academic, New York, 1964, Vol. 4, pp. 1-115.
8. W. H. Hildemann and E. L. Cooper (eds.), Transplant. Proc. 2, 179 (1970).
9. J. J. Marchalonis and G. M. Edelman, J. Exp. Med. **122**, 601 (1965); J. J. Marchalonis and G. M. Edelman, Science **154**, 1567 (1966).
10. L. W. Clem and P. A. Small, Jr., J. Exp. Med. **125**, 893 (1967); L. W. Clem, F. De Boutand, and M. M. Sigel, J. Immunol. **99**, 1226 (1967).
11. R. T. Acton, W. Niedermeier, P. F. Weinheimer, L. W. Clem, G. A. Leslie, and J. C. Bennett, J. Immunol. **109**, 371 (1972).
12. G. A. Leslie and L. W. Clem, J. Immunol. **108**, 1656 (1972).
13. J. J. Marchalonis and N. Cohen, Immunology **24**, 395 (1973).
14. M. Houdayer and M. Fougereau, Ann. Inst. Pasteur **123**, 3 (1973).
15. R. T. Acton, E. E. Evans, P. F. Weinheimer, W. Niedermeier, and J. C. Bennett, Biochemistry, **11**, 2751 (1972).
16. J. J. Marchalonis and G. M. Edelman, J. Exp. Med. **124**, 901 (1966).
17. J. J. Marchalonis, Immunology **20**, 161 (1970).
18. F. W. Putnam, G. Florent, C. Paul, T. Shinoda, and A. Shimizu, Science **182**, 287 (1973).
19. P. W. Kincade and M. D. Cooper, Science **179**, 398 (1973).
20. G. Möller (ed.), Transplant. Rev. **14**, 210 (1973).
21. N. Cohen and M. Borysenko, Transplant. Proc. **2**, 333 (1970).
22. H. D. McDevitt and M. Landy (eds.), *Genetic Control of Immune Responsiveness,* Academic, New York, 1972, p. 469.
23. C. P. Stockard, Anat. Anz. **29**, 91 (1906).
24. R. A. Good, J. Finstad, B. Pollara, and A. E. Gabrielsen, in *Phylogeny of*

Immunity (R. T. Smith, P. A. Miescher, and R. A. Good, eds.), University of Florida, Gainesville, 1966, Chap. 15.
25. H. E. Jordan and C. C. Speidel, Amer. J. Anat. **46**, 355 (1930).
26. N. Holmgren, Acta Zool. **31**, 234 (1950).
27. R. Fänge, in *Phylogeny of Immunity* (R. T. Smith, P. A. Miescher, and R. A. Good, eds.), University of Florida, Gainesville, 1966, Chap. 14.
28. W. H. Hildemann and G. H. Thoenes, Transplantation **7**, 506 (1969).
29. D. S. Linthicum and W. H. Hildemann, J. Immunol. **105**, 912 (1970).
30. G. H. Thoenes and W. H. Hildemann, in *Developmental Aspects of Antibody Formation and Structure* (J. Šterzl and I. Řiha, eds.), Academic, New York, 1970, Vol. 2, pp. 711-726.
31. W. H. Hildemann and L. Reddy, Private communication, 1973.
32. J. Schaffer, S.-B. Akad. Wiss. Wien, Math.-Naturwiss. **103**, 149 (1895).
33. I. E. Wallin, Amer. J. Anat. **22**, 1 (1917).
34. J. Finstad and R. A. Good, J. Exp. Med. **120**, 1151 (1964).
35. G. Sterba, Wiss. Z. Friedrich-Schiller-Univ. Jena Math.-Naturwiss. **2**, 239 (1953).
36. J. Salkind, Arch. Zool. Exp. Gen. **55**, 81 (1915).
37. K. E. Fichtelius, J. Finstad, and R. A. Good, Lab. Invest. **19**, 339 (1968).
38. J. Finstad and R. A. Good, in *Phylogeny of Immunity* (R. T. Smith, P. A. Meischer, and R. A. Good, eds.), University of Florida, Gainesville, 1966, Chap. 16.
39. C. C. Clawson, Fed. Proc. **26**, 357 (1967).
40. G. B. Olson, Fed. Proc. **26**, 357 (1967).
41. A. J. Cooper, in *Fourth Leucocyte Culture Conference* (O. R. McIntyre, ed.), Appleton-Century-Crofts, New York, 1971, p. 137.
42. C. Farenholz, Anat. Anz. **66**, 349 (1929).
43. T. Fujita, Z. Zellforsch. **60**, 147 (1963).
44. H. P. Stanley, J. Morphol. **112**, 99 (1963).
45. D. E. Yocum, M. A. Cuchens, and L. W. Clem, in preparation (1973).
46. M. M. Sigel, G. Ortiz-Muniz, J. C. Lee, and D. M. Lopez, in *L'Etude Phylogènique et Ontogènique de la Réponse Immunitaire et Son Apport à la Théorie Immunologique,* Colloque Organisé par La Société Française d'Immunologie, Paris, 1972.
47. D. M. Lopez, M. M. Sigel, and V. Esquenazi, Fed. Proc. **32**, 1017 (1973).
48. D. M. Lopez, M. M. Sigel, and J. C. Lee, Cell. Immunol. **10**, 287 (1974).
49. R. E. Tigelaar and R. Asofsky, *J. Exp. Med.,* **137**, 239 (1973).
50. H. Cantor, in *Cell Interactions, 3rd Lepetit Colloquim* (L. G. Silvestri, ed.), North-Holland, Amsterdam, 1972, p. 172.
51. H. Cantor, Cell. Immunol. **3**, 461 (1972).
52. J. F. Dardenne and M. Dardenne, Cell. Immunol. **6**, 394 (1973).
53. J. D. Stobo and W. F. Paul, J. Immunol. **110**, 362 (1973).
54. J. J. Marchalonis, Aust. J. Exp. Biol. Med. Sci. **47**, 405 (1969).
55. H. Downey, Folia Haematol. **8**, 415 (1909).
56. C. C. Clawson, J. Finstad, and R. A. Good, Lab. Invest. **15**, 1830 (1966).
57. K. Sailendri, Ph.D. Thesis, Madurai University, Madurai, India, 1973.
58. A. M. Smith, M. Potter, and E. B. Merchant, J. Immunol. **99**, 876 (1967).

59. M. J. Yu, J. Filazzola, D. A. Sarot, and A. Perlmutter, Life Sci. **9**, 749 (1970).
60. G. Ortiz-Muniz and M. M. Sigel, J. Reticuloendothel. Soc. **9**, 42 (1971).
61. J. M. Chiller, H. O. Hodgins, R. S. Weiser, J. Immunol. **102**, 1202 (1969).
62. J. M. Chiller, H. O. Hodgins, V. C. Chambers, and R. S. Weiser, J. Immunol. **102**, 1193 (1969).
63. M. M. Sigel and J. C. Lee, 3rd Annu. Meeting, Amer. Soc. Microbiol., Miami, Fla., May 1973, Abst. p. 119.
64. D. E. Yocum, M. A. Cuchens, and L. W. Clem, J. Immunol. **114**, 925 (1975).
65. M. J. Manning and J. D. Horton, J. Embryol. Exp. Morphol. **22**, 265 (1969).
66. K. E. Fichtelius, Lymphology **1**, 50 (1970).
67. M. E. LeFevre, U. Reincke, and J. F. Gennaro, Biophys. J. **12**, 201a (1972).
68. S. N. Goldstine, V. Manickavel, and N. Cohen, Amer. Zool. **15**, 107 (1975).
69. M. E. LeFevre, U. Reincke, R. Arbas, and J. F. Gennaro, Anat. Rec. **176**, 111 (1973).
70. K. D. Kallman, Transplant. Proc. 2, 263 (1970).
71. S. J. Goldshein and N. Cohen, J. Immunol. **108**, 1025 (1972).
72. J. Klein and D. C. Schreffler, Transplant. Rev. **6**, 3 (1971).
73. N. Cohen, J. Exp. Zool. **167**, 37 (1968).
74. N. Cohen, Amer. Zool. **11**, 193 (1971).
75. N. Cohen, J. Amer. Vet. Med. Ass. **159**, 1662 (1971).
76. N. Cohen and W. H. Hildemann, Transplantation **6**, 208 (1968).
77. R. J. Mangi and M. R. Mardiney, Jr., Transplantation **11**, 369 (1971).
78. D. G. Colley and C. W. DeWitt, J. Immunol. **102**, 107 (1969).
79. F. H. Bach, M. L. Bach, P. M. Sondel, and G. Sundharadas, Transplant. Rev. **12**, 30 (1972).
80. D. B. Wilson, J. C. Howard, and P. C. Nowell, Transplant. Rev. **12**, 30 (1972).
81. M. L. Goldberg, W. Rosenau, and G. C. Burke, Proc. Nat. Acad. Sci. USA **64**, 283 (1969).
82. G. Möller, Immunology **19**, 583 (1970).
83. J. A. Hightower and R. St. Pierre, J. Morphol. **135**, 229 (1971).
84. C. Houillon, J. Charlemagne, and A. Tournefier, Private communication, 1973.
85. H. Klug, Z. Zellforsch. **78**, 388 (1967).
86. R. R. Cowden and R. F. Dyer, Amer. Zool. **11**, 183 (1971).
87. J. H. Hightower, Private communication, 1973.
88. H. E. Jordan and C. C. Speidel, Amer. J. Anat. **33**, 485 (1924).
89. H. E. Jordan and C. C. Speidel, Amer. J. Anat. **46**, 55 (1930).
90. J. Tooze and H. G. Davies, J. Cell Sci. **2**, 617 (1967).
91. J. Tooze and H. G. Davies, Amer. J. Anat. **123**, 521 (1968).
92. J. Charlemagne, Z. Zellforsch. **123**, 224 (1972).
93. B. F. Kingsbury, Anat. Anz. **42**, 593 (1912).
94. L. N. Ruben, A. v.d. Hoven, and R. W. Dutton, Cell. Immunol. **6**, 300 (1973).
95. W. C. Barrett, Jr., Folia Haematol. **54**, 165 (1936).
96. N. Cohen, in *Recent Results in Cancer Research, Supplement, Biology of Amphibian Tumors* (M. Mizell, ed.), Springer-Verlag, New York, 1969, p. 153.

97. A. Tournefier, J. Embryol. Exp. Morphol. **29**, 383 (1973).
98. J. Charlemagne and C. Houillon, C. R. Acad. Sci. (Paris) Ser. D **267**, 253 (1968).
99. A. Tournefier, C. R. Acad. Sci. (Paris) Ser. D **275**, 2443 (1972).
100. J. F. Bach, M. Dardenne, A. L. Goldstein, A. Gruha, and A. White, Proc. Nat. Acad. Sci. USA **68**, 2734 (1971).
101. S. Murakawa, SABCO J. **4**, 17 (1968).
102. T. Seto, Jap. J. Genet. **39**, 268 (1964).
103. E. L. Cooper, in *Ontogeny of Immunity* (R. T. Smith, R. A. Good, and P. A. Miescher, eds.), University of Florida, Gainesville, 1967, Chap. 12.
104. A. von Braunmühl, Leitschr. Mikrosk. Anat. Forsch. **4**, 635 (1926).
105. P. C. Balduzzi, Private communication, 1973.
106. J. B. Turpen, E. P. Volpe, and N. Cohen, Science **182**, 931 (1973).
107. J. B. Turpen, E. P. Volpe, and N. Cohen, Amer. Zool. **15**, 51 (1975).
108. H. E. Jordan, Amer. J. Anat. **25**, 437 (1919).
109. F. R. Campbell, Amer. J. Anat. **129**, 329 (1970).
110. E. L. Cooper and D. W. Schaeffer, Proc. Soc. Exp. Biol. Med. **135**, 406 (1970).
111. M. L. Mandell and E. L. Cooper, Amer. Zool. **5**, 731 (1965).
112. E. L. Cooper, J. Morphol. **122**, 381 (1967).
113. B. S. Baculi and E. L. Cooper, J. Morphol. **123**, 463 (1967).
114. B. S. Baculi and E. L. Cooper, J. Morphol. **126**, 463 (1968).
115. B. S. Baculi, E. L. Cooper, and B. A. Brown, J. Morphol. **131**, 315 (1970).
116. J. D. Horton, Amer. Zool. **11**, 219 (1971).
117. H. Ambrosius and R. Hanstein, Acta Biol. Med. Ger. **27**, 771 (1971).
118. E. E. Evans, S. P. Kent, R. Bryant, and M. Moyer, in *Phylogeny of Immunity* (R. T. Smith, P. A. Meischer, and R. A. Good, eds.), University of Florida, Gainesville, 1966, Chap. 20.
119. S. P. Kent, E. E. Evans, and M. H. Attleberger, Proc. Soc. Exp. Biol. Med. **116**, 456 (1964).
120. E. Diener and G. J. V. Nossal, Immunology, **10**, 535 (1966).
121. R. R. Cowden, B. M. Gebhardt, and E. P. Volpe, Z. Zellforsch. **85**, 196 (1968).
122. W. C. Wong, K. H. Sit, K. K. F. Ng, and K. N. Chin, Acta Anat. **80**, 82 (1971).
123. W. C. Wong, Acta Anat. **83**, 461 (1972).
124. J. S. Cornes, Gut **6**, 225 (1965).
125. R. R. Cowden, R. F. Dyer, B. M. Gebhardt, and E. P. Volpe, J. Immunol. **100**, 1293 (1968).
126. E. Diener and J. J. Marchalonis, Immunology **18**, 279 (1970).
127. N. Kraft, K. Shortman, and J. J. Marchalonis, Immunology **20**, 919 (1971).
128. N. Kraft and K. Shortman, J. Cell Biol. **52**, 438 (1972).
129. R. J. Turner and M. J. Manning, J. Exp. Zool. **183**, 21 (1973).
130. R. J. Turner, J. Exp. Zool. **183**, 35 (1973).
131. S. Mitsuhashi, S. Kurashige, S. Mishima, N. Yamagushi, and K. Fukai, Tohoku J. Exp. Med. **103**, 7 (1971).
132. I. Hadji-Azimi and M. Fischberg, Rev. Suisse Zool. **74**, 641 (1967).
133. J. C. Clark and D. R. Newth, Experientia **28**, 951 (1972).
134. M. J. Manning and R. J. Turner, Comp. Biochem. Physiol. **42**, 735 (1972).

135. B. M. Gebhardt, Fed. Proc. **29**, 698 (1970).
136. J. D. Horton, Transplant. Proc. **2**, 282 (1970).
137. L. Du Pasquier and V. C. Miggiano, Transplant. Proc. in press (1974).
138. H. Ambrosius and K. Drossler, Acta Biol. Med. Ger. **29**, 437 (1972).
139. K. Drossler and H. Ambrosius, Acta Biol. Med. Ger. **29**, 441 (1972).
140. G. A. Amirante, Experientia **24**, 1059 (1968).
141. R. Auerbach and L. N. Ruben, J. Immunol. **104**, 1242 (1970).
142. J. D. Horton, J. Morphol. **134**, 1 (1971).
143. H. B. Riviere and E. L. Cooper, Proc. Soc. Exp. Biol. Med. **143**, 320 (1973).
144. M. Fabrizio and H. A. Charipper, J. Morphol. **68**, 179 (1941).
145. S. K. Curtis, E. P. Volpe, and R. R. Cowden, Z. Zellforsch. **127**, 323 (1972).
146. A. C. Taylor and J. J. Kollros, Anat. Rec. **94**, 7 (1946).
147. M. A. Myers, J. Morphol. **45**, 399 (1928).
148. W. H. Hildemann and R. Haas, in *Mechanisms of Immunological Tolerance* (M. Hašek, A. Lengerová, and M. Vojtišková, eds.), Academic, New York, 1962, p. 506.
149. A. M. Bovberg, J. Exp. Zool. **161**, 69 (1966).
150. S. K. Curtis and E. P. Volpe, Develop. Biol. **25**, 177 (1971).
151. E. L. Cooper and W. H. Hildemann, Transplantation **3**, 446 (1965).
152. E. L. Cooper, W. Pinkerton, and W. H. Hildemann, Biol. Bull **127**, 232 (1964).
153. E. L. Cooper, B. A. Brown, and B. S. Baculi, in *Morphological and Fundamental Aspects of Immunity* (Lindahl-Kiessling, Alm, and Hanna, eds.), Plenum, New York, 1971, p. 1.
154. E. L. Cooper, Anat. Rec. **162**, 453 (1968).
155. B. S. Baculi and E. L. Cooper, J. Exp. Zool. **183**, 185 (1973).
156. E. J. Moticka, B. A. Brown, and E. L. Cooper, J. Immunol. **110**, 855 (1973).
157. B. A. Brown, E. J. Moticka, and E. L. Cooper, Amer. Zool. **12**, 310 (1972).
158. B. A. Brown and E. L. Cooper, in *Abstracts of the Fourth International Congress of the Transplantation Society,* San Francisco, 1972, p. 32.
159. M. J. Manning and J. D. Horton, J. Embryol. Exp. Morphol. **22**, 265 (1969).
160. J. D. Horton, J. Exp. Zool. **170**, 449 (1969).
161. M. J. Manning, J. Embryol. Exp. Morphol. **26**, 219 (1971).
162. J. D. Horton and M. J. Manning, Transplantation **14**, 141 (1972).
163. M. J. Manning, J. D. Horton, and R. Turner, Private communication, 1973.
164. L. Du Pasquier, N. Weiss, and F. Loor, Eur. J. Immunol. **2**, 366 (1972).
165. J. Haimovitch and L. De Pasquier, Proc. Nat. Acad. Sci. USA **70**, 1898 (1973).
166. L. Du Pasquier and N. Weiss, Private communication, 1973.

167. N. Weiss, J. D. Horton, and L. Du Pasquier, in *L'Etude Phylogènique et Ontogènique de la Rèponse Immunitaire et Son Apport à la Thèorie Immunologie,* Colloque Organisè par la Sociètè Française d'Immunologie, Paris, 1972, p. 165.
168. G. Sterba, Abhandl. Saechs. Akad. Wiss. Leipzig Math.-Naturwiss. Kl. **44**, 1 (1950).
169. L. Du Pasquier, Ann. Inst. Pasteur **114**, 490 (1968).
170. L. Du Pasquier, C. R. Soc. Biol. (Paris) **161**, 1974 (1967).
171. L. Du Pasquier, C. R. Acad. Sci. (Paris) Ser. D **261**, 1144 (1965).
172. L. Du Pasquier, Immunology **19**, 353 (1970).
173. L. Du Pasquier, Transplant. Proc. **2**, 293 (1970).
174. D. Metcalf and M. A. S. Moore, *Haemopoietic Cells,* North Holland, Amsterdam, 1971, pp. 172-271.
175. M. A. S. Moore and J. J. T. Owen, J. Exp. Med. **126**, 715 (1967).
176. R. Auerbach, Develop. Biol. **3**, 336 (1961).
177. J. J. T. Owen and M. A. Ritter, J. Exp. Med. **129**, 431 (1961).
178. N. K. Jerne, Proc. Nat. Acad. Sci. USA **41**, 849 (1955).
179. F. Haurowitz, Cold Spring Harbor Symp. Quant. Biol. **32**, 559 (1967).
180. R. E. Cone and J. J. Marchalonis, J. Immunol. **108**, 952 (1972).
181. A. Macela and A. Romanovsky, Folia Biol. (Prague) **15**, 157 (1969).
182. M. Borysenko and E. L. Cooper, J. Morphol. **138**, 487 (1972).
183. P. Kanakambika and V. R. Muthukkaruppan, Proc. Indian Acad. Sci. Sect. B **78**, 37 (1973).
184. Y. A. Sidky and R. Auerbach, J. Exp. Zool. **167**, 187 (1968).
185. M. Borysenko and P. Tulipan, Transplantation in press (1973).
186. L. F. Kassin and L. A. Pevnitskii, Bull. Exp. Biol. Med. (USSR) (Engl. Transl.) **67**, 287 (1969).
187. F. Rothe and H. Ambrosius, Acta Biol. Med. Ger. **21**, 525 (1968).
188. H. Ambrosius and G. Hoheisel, Acta Biol. Med. Ger. in press (1973).
189. E. E. Evans, Fed. Proc. **22**, 1132 (1963).
190. H. M. Grey, in *Phylogeny of Immunity* (R. T. Smith, P. A. Miescher, and R. A. Good, eds.), University of Florida, Gainesville, 1966, Chap. 21.
191. H. Ambrosius and G. Hoheisel, Experientia **25**, 1177 (1969).
192. J. D. Wetherall and K. J. Turner, Aust. J. Exp. Biol. Med. Sci. **50**, 79 (1972).
193. P. Kanakambika and V. R. Muthukkaruppan, J. Immunol. **109**, 415 (1972).
194. P. Kanakambika and V. R. Muthukkaruppan, Experientia **28**, 1225 (1972).
195. P. Kanakambika and V. R. Muthukkaruppan, Proc. Soc. Exp. Biol. Med. **140**, 21 (1972).
196. M. R. L. Johnston, J. Morphol. **139**, 431 (1973).
197. M. Kotani, Acta Scholoe Med. Univ. Kyoto Jap. **36**, 121 (1959).
198. V. Manickavel, Ph.D. Thesis, Annamali University, Tamilnadu, India, 1972.

199. W. J. McCauley, Amer. J. Anat. **99**, 189 (1956).
200. J. J. Marchalonis, E. H. M. Ealey, and E. Diener, Aust. J. Exp. Biol. Med. Sci. **47**, 367 (1969).
201. M. R. Tripp, in *Immunity to Parasitic Animals* (G. J. Jackson, R. Herman, and I. Singer, eds.), Appleton-Century-Crofts, New York, 1969, Vol. 1, p. 111.
202. W. H. Hildemann and T. G. Dix, Transplantation **15**, 624 (1972).
203. R. K. Hostetter and E. L. Cooper, Immunol. Commun. **1**, 155 (1972).
204. E. L. Cooper, in *Proceedings, Third International Colloquium on Invertebrate Tissue Culture* (J. Rahecek, D. Blaskovic, and W. F. Hink, eds.), Slovak Academy of Sciences, Bratislava, Czechoslovakia, 1973, p. 381.
205. N. Cohen, Unpublished observations, 1972.
206. H. Cottier, N. Odartchenko, R. Schindler, and C. C. Congdon (eds.), *Germinal Centers in Immune Responses,* Springer-Verlag, New York, 499 pp.
207. G. J. Thorbecke, E. B. Jacobson, and R. Asofsky, J. Immunol. **92**, 734 (1964).
208. H. H. Lin, B. E. Caywood, and D. T. Rowlands, Immunology **20**, 373 (1971).
209. H. Ambrosius, J. Hemmerling, R. Richter, and R. Schimke, in *Developmental Aspects of Antibody Formation and Structure* (J. Šterzl and I. Řiha, eds.), Academic, New York, 1970, Vol. 2, pp. 727-744.
210. L. DuPasquier and J. D. Horton, Immunogenetics **3**, 105 (1976).
211. M. J. Manning, N. Donnelly, and N. Cohen, in *Phylogeny of T and B Cells* (R. K. Wright and E. L. Cooper, eds.) North Holland, Amsterdam, in press (1976).
212. N. Donnelly, M. J. Manning, and N. Cohen, in *Phylogeny of T and B Cells* (R. K. Wright and E. L. Cooper, eds.) North Holland, Amsterdam, in press (1976).
213. N. H. Collins and N. Cohen, in *Phylogeny of T and B Cells* (R. K. Wright and E. L. Cooper, eds.) North Holland, Amsterdam, in press (1976).
214. H. M. Etlinger, H. O. Hodgins, and J. M. Chiller, J. Immunol. **116**, 1547 (1976).
215. M. Cuchens, E. McLean, and L. W. Clem, in *Phylogeny of T and B Cells* (R. K. Wright and E. L. Cooper, eds.) North Holland, Amsterdam, in press (1976).
216. J. B. Turpen and N. Cohen, Ann. Institut Pasteur (Paris), in press (1976).
217. J. B. Turpen and N. Cohen, Cell Immunol. **24**, 109 (1976).
218. W. H. Hildemann and A. A. Benedict, eds., *Immunologie Phylogeny,* Adv. Expt. Med. Biol. 64, Plenum Press, New York (1975).
219. R. W. Wright and E. L. Cooper, eds., *Phylogeny of T and B Cells,* North Holland, Amsterdam, in press (1976).
220. M. J. Manning and R. J. Turner, *Comparative Immunology,* Blackie, Glasgow, 1976.
221. Amer. Zool. **15**, 1, 3 (1975).

SECTION III

Physical Separation of Lymphocytes

CHAPTER 5

Physical Separation of Lymphocytes

Richard G. Miller

Ontario Cancer Institute
Toronto, Ontario, Canada

and

Department of Medical Biophysics
University of Toronto
Toronto, Ontario, Canada

Under the light microscope, the lymphocyte is a rather nondescript object best described as a small round cell with a large, nearly round nucleus. Although microscopists have divided lymphocytes into various categories, they failed completely to recognize the division of these cells into two main groups, B and T lymphocytes, which were, in fact, first recognized on the basis of differences in function. The human eye is a remarkably sensitive instrument for detecting small physical differences. Thus, we might expect any differences to be either very small or of a type not obvious to the eye.

Real progress in fractionation of lymphocytes has been made almost entirely in the last 5 years. The physical differences observed are, for the most part, quite small and require very careful standardization of techniques to obtain reproducibility. Superficially identical protocols in different laboratories may give quite different results because of small differences in lymphocyte subpopulations have now been established and may be used either as the basis of characterization or separation of lymphocyte subpopulations.

Lymphocyte separation is usually performed with one of two objectives: either to obtain a population of lymphocytes depleted of other cells, such as granulocytes, i.e., as essentially a preparative procedure, or to measure (and perhaps separate) lymphocyte populations as a function of some physical variable, such as size, density, or surface charge, i.e., as essentially an analytic procedure. Traditionally, cell separation has been used to obtain a cell population enriched for lymphocytes, i.e., in the former sense. The basic problem with such procedures is that they give little information about the actual physical properties of the cells and are essentially recipes which work only under a given set of circumstances. They can be generalized to other situations only with difficulty, if at all. This chapter will be concerned primarily with analytic procedures. Such procedures have recently been reviewed in more detail [1].

Physical properties which have been successfully exploited for analytic separation of cells to date are differences in average chemical composition, size, and surface characteristics. Each procedure can yield frequency distributions of lymphocytes in terms of the separation variable.

The following sections each describe one analytic separation method: first, in terms of the physics of the system and, then, in terms of the biologic meaning of different values of the separation variable. Next, some of the technical problems in the application of the method are discussed. Finally, the physical properties of lymphocytes as ascertained by the method will be discussed. The examples given are illustrative rather than being an exhaustive survey of the literature.

I. Density Separation

Separation of cells on the basis of differences in buoyant density has been the most extensively applied procedure for physical separation of cells. The density differences are small; the total range is typically no more than 1.05 to 1.10 g/cm^3. They reflect variations both in the chemical composition of a cell and in its local environment. Cell membranes are readily permeable to water, so that cells approach osmotic equilibrium with a new environment very rapidly (in less than 1 min) as the result of loss or gain of water but are less permeable to electrolytes and impermeable to high-molecular-weight solutes [2]. Following Anderson et al. [3], the concept of reduced density (RD), defined as $\rho - 1$ (ρ being the cell density), is useful for considering variations in cell density. They show that

$$\mathrm{RD} = \frac{m_{\mathrm{d}}}{V} (1 - \Phi_{\mathrm{d}}) \tag{1}$$

where m_d and V are the dry mass and volume of the cell, respectively, and Φ_d is the apparent specific volume of the dry matter (i.e., volume per gram dry mass). Note that m_d and Φ_d are almost independent of the environment but that V can vary widely as material, primarily water, is taken up or lost to maintain osmotic and hydrostatic equilibrium. Differences in density among cells can be due to independent variations in each of the parameters. One special case is worthy of note. For at least some established cell lines in tissue culture, Φ_d is a constant, and m_d is proportional to V, so that density is a constant independent of position in the cell cycle [3,4]. These cell lines form a single narrow peak when analyzed on a density gradient. The same might be expected for a lymphoid cell population if it is truly a homogeneous population.

There are a large variety of ways in which density separation can be applied. The most powerful are the analytic procedures, in which one obtains not only separation of different cell classes but also a direct measurement of the density profile of each class. The first truly analytic procedure was that of Leif and Vinograd [5,6], who used continuous bovine serum albumin (BSA) gradients at neutral pH to study the buoyant density distribution of human erythrocytes and found that erythrocyte density was correlated with the age of the cell. The most extensive studies on lymphocytes have been performed with a BSA gradient procedure devised by Shortman et al. [7,8].

There are several technical problems which must be overcome. The most critical one involves the choice of a suitable gradient material and its preparation before use. The material should be nontoxic to cells and have a high molecular weight. A common problem is that the density gradient may also be a tonicity gradient, either because the gradient material itself is light (e.g., sucrose) or because the gradient material used contains a significant amount of water or salt impurity. Thus, if the material contains salt impurities, as a cell moves into a region of higher density, it also moves into a region of higher tonicity. Osmotic forces will cause the cell to shrink, which, in turn, will increase its density, and so on. In the extreme case, the cells will all be pelleted at the bottom of the tube.

The most popular choice for the gradient material has been BSA. The results obtained depend critically upon the procedure used to prepare the BSA; different treatment procedures tend to give different and often not very reproducible results. Shortman et al.'s procedure [7,8] results in a strictly isotonic gradient and is highly reproducible but does not give completely satisfactory results on a rebanding experiment; i.e., cells of a particular density on a first separation do not return to precisely the same position if reseparated on a second gradient. Rebanding appears to be significantly better if the tonicity of the medium used is strictly iso-osmotic with respect to the species of origin of the cells [8]. Leif's procedure [6] gives satisfactory rebanding for human erythrocytes but has not been tested for other cells. Ficoll gradients, if properly deionized, appear to give satisfactory rebanding results [9], but these gradients are not isotonic at high Ficoll concentrations, probably due to interactions of Ficoll with water [8].

Both BSA and Ficoll tend to enhance cell aggregation. This problem can be reduced by lowering the pH or by the use of a dispersing agent such as 2-naphthol-6,8-disulfonic acid [7]. Initial dispersion of the cells throughout the gradient reduces the probability of aggregation and also reduces both wall effects and cell streaming, which can be serious problems when the cells are loaded on top of the gradient.

Discontinuous step gradients have been widely used for density separations; two of the more popular procedures are those of Dicke et al. [10] and Raidt et al. [11]. These procedures have several intrinsic disadvantages compared to a continuous gradient: (a) the number of cells that can be processed before there is aggregation at the step interfaces is much lower than on a continuous gradient; (b) unless the number of steps is very large, one does not obtain a measure of the density profile of the cell of interest; (c) even if one's aim is solely to achieve high enrichment of the cell of interest, optimization of enrichment requires a large number of experiments with different density increments; and (d) a procedure suitable for one application is difficult to generalize to another.

A popular preparative procedure for obtaining enriched populations of lymphocytes from blood is the "Ficoll-Hypaque" method, originally developed by Böyum [12], in which a diluted suspension of whole blood is layered over a mixture of sodium diatrizoate (Hypaque) and Ficoll and is spun to equilibrium. Lymphocytes (contaminated with platelets) collect at the interface, whereas all other cells are found in the bottom layer. This procedure may be thought of as a two-step density gradient, although tonicity probably also plays a role.

The most extensive analytic studies of density separation of lymphoid tissue have been made by Shortman and associates, who have investigated lymphoid cells from various organs of the mouse, rat, and toad. All lymphoid tissues studied show a complex density distribution that consists of many narrow peaks and shoulders spread over a broad density range. When replicate separations are performed on the same tissue from apparently identical animals (e.g., thymocytes from 5-week-old male BALB/c mice [13]), quite different density profiles can be obtained. Some peaks appear to recur in many different separations, which suggests that the profile seen is a composite of a large number of usually unresolved peaks, each of variable magnitude. Such peaks can often be resolved by using a gradient that covers a smaller density range and that therefore has a higher resolution.

Lymphocyte density is correlated with lymphocyte size. As a rough rule, large lymphocytes are less dense than small lymphocytes, presumably because of a smaller nuclear/cytoplasmic ratio. There are many exceptions to this rule.

Injection of cortisone into mice 10 hr before analysis leads to a large involution of the thymus and to a large increase in the apparent density heterogeneity of the remaining cells. This heterogeneity could either be due to specific lysis of the most frequent cells in the central-density region, thus enhancing the relative importance of other cells already there, or could be due to the production of new peaks, i.e., new populations of cells. In either case, variable release of corticosteroids as a result of stress could be the explanation for the observed animal to animal variation [13]. In support of this conclusion, the density profiles of rat and mouse thymus cells 10 to 21 days after adrenalectomy were less variable from animal to animal; adrenalectomy did not affect the reproducibility of the fine structure peaks, which could still be seen [13].

Marked heterogeneity in density is also typically seen when a functionally homogeneous class of cells is analyzed. As an extreme case, cells in the rat that make antibody against sheep erythrocytes can be resolved into 12 distinct peaks [14]. Differences in biologic function can be partially correlated with this heterogeneity. Tissue-fixed and circulating antibody-forming cells (AFC) had different profiles. A mitotic inhibitor had a different effect on different peaks. Later studies of the immune response of the toad against POL (polymerized flagellin protein from *Salmonella adelaide*) also showed pronounced density heterogeneity in the AFC [15,16]. Early in the response, AFC were almost all of low density. As time passed, additional peaks of higher density developed, until by Day 21, most AFC were in a single peak at high density. As AFC density increased, AFC size decreased.

The cells of mouse thymus, all T cells in the sense that they carry θ antigen, can be divided into two groups by a variety of criteria. The majority (approximately 85%) have high levels of surface θ antigen, low levels of surface H-2 alloantigen, and appear to be the population sensitive to corticosteroid hormones. The remainder have low levels of surface θ antigen and high levels of surface H-2 alloantigen. These two populations can be partially separated on the basis of density [17-20], in that the minority population is markedly enriched in the low-density region of the gradient. This minority low-density population appears to contain all of the immunologically competent cells in the thymus.

When detailed density profiles are measured, it is found that high-θ and low-θ cells in thymus each form broad overlapping distributions that contain complicated but reproducible peaks and shoulders [18]. Low-θ thymocytes from CBA and C57BL/6 mice have quite different density profiles, although for each, one gets enrichment for low-θ cells at low density. Phytohemagglutinin (PHA) is is believed to selectively stimulate T cells [21]. Only the minority low-θ population in thymus respond to it [17,20]. The profile of T cells that respond to PHA in spleen is quite different; it resembles more closely the profile of the major, unresponsive population of cells in the thymus. This finding has led to interesting speculations about the relationship between the low-θ and high-θ cells in thymus and to the development of peripheral T cells [18,19].

Gorczynski et al. [22], by use of linear Ficoll density gradients, were able to obtain separation of B and T cells in a study of C3H mouse spleen cells taken from previously unimmunized mice. The fractionated cells were tested for immunocompetence by their ability to restore the response of lethally irradiated mice to sheep erythrocytes. A response is obtained only if the fraction being assayed contains both B and T cells. The initial observation was that the sum of the activity obtained by assaying all fractions separately was much less than in an equivalent unfractionated control. Substantial synergism could be obtained on mixing appropriate fractions, which further suggested a separation between B and T cells.

B cells, identified by their ability to form rosettes with sheep erythrocytes, were in a narrow peak in the central region of the gradient. Activity in a transplantation assay was obtained from regions on either side of the B-cell peak and was interpreted as resulting from the overlap of the B-cell peak with two T-cell peaks, one on each side of the B-cell peak. The synergistic response obtained on mixing appropriate fractions was consistent with this view.

As further confirmation, gradient fractions were mixed with either bone marrow cells (as a source of B cells) or thymus cells (as a source of T cells) and assayed for immunocompetence. Addition of thymus cells produced additional activity in the region of the B-cell peak, and addition of bone marrow cells produced additional activity, consistent with there being two T-cell peaks at either end of the gradient.

The above studies differ from those of Shortman et al. (see, e.g., Ref. 18) in two respects. First, Gorczynski et al. saw no fine structure, probably because the density increments of their individual fractions were too large to detect small density differences. Second, Shortman et al. have failed to obtain significant separation of B and T cells. Their studies [18] were of CBA and C57BL/6 spleen cells. The B- and T-cell distributions were very different in each case; there was almost complete overlap in CBA spleen but a considerable excess of T cells at both high and low densities in C57BL/6 spleen. The spleen of the C3H mouse studied by Gorczynski et al. would appear to be an extension of this trend and was an extremely fortuitous choice for the study.

II. Sedimentation Separation

The concept of the separation is very simple. A thin layer of cell suspension is put on top of a fluid column, and the cells are allowed to settle through the column, under the action of either the earth's gravitational field or of the larger forces available in a centrifuge. The sedimentation rate is given by

$$s = \frac{2}{9\eta} (\rho - \rho') g r^2 \qquad (2)$$

where s is the sedimentation rate, g is the acceleration due to gravity (1 g separation) or the centrifugal acceleration (centrifugal separation), ρ is the density of the cell, ρ' is the density of the supporting fluid column, and r is the radius of the cell. Typically, ρ' has a value of about 1.01 g/cm^3, whereas ρ ranges from 1.05 to 1.10 g/cm^3. Thus, density variations alone will produce about a twofold variation in sedimentation rate. For lymphocyte populations (including large progenitors and progeny) r may vary from 3 to 10 μm. Thus, size variations may produce up to a 10-fold variation in sedimentation rate, and sedimentation produces separation primarily on the basis of differences in cell size. For lymphoid populations separated gravitationally at 4°C in a fluid column whose physical properties are similar to those of water, Eq. (2) reduces approximately to

$$s = \frac{r^2}{4} \qquad (3)$$

where s is the sedimentation rate in millimeters per hour, and r is the radius of the cell in microns [23]. Within limits, the sedimentation rate is independent of cell chape [23].

The major technical problems are three in number. The first concerns the fluid column through which the cells sediment. Clearly, this must be primarily an isotonic saline solution to prevent osmotic effects. In addition, to prevent the column from being unstable to either convection or small mechanical disturbances, the column must contain a mild density gradient, constructed such that $(\rho - \rho')$ is as large and nearly constant as possible throughout the column. Under these conditions, separation remains based primarily on differences in size. The same problem in choice of material as that discussed in Sec. I will apply here. However, the problems will be much less acute, since the amount of gradient material required to achieve the necessary stabilization is about 10-fold less than that needed for density separation.

The second problem involves a poorly understood phenomenon called "streaming." If the concentration of cells in the starting band exceeds a certain critical concentration, called the streaming limit, local density inversions apparently occur, and small sections of the starting band sediment into the underlying fluid column, carrying the cells with them at very high sedimentation rate. Below the streaming limit, all cells appear to sediment individually according to Eq. (2). Above the streaming limit, useful separation is seldom achieved. For mouse lymphoid cells, the streaming limit is about 5,000,000 cells/ml, but this limit can be increased by appropriate design of the gradient shape [23]. The resolution of the separation will be largely determined by the thickness of the starting cell band. Thus, to process large numbers of cells and achieve good resolution, one must use a starting band of large area. This is one major advantage of using the earth's gravitational field as the sedimenting force; it is simple to provide a uniform force over a large area.

For 1-*g* separation, the third technical problem concerns a method for forming a thin layer of cells on top of the fluid column. This problem has been solved by appropriate design of the sedimentation chamber, with appropriate procedures for filling and emptying it. The first seccessful system is that of Mel [24], which can also be used for electrophoresis. However, most work has been done with the systems of Peterson and Evans [25] or Miller and Phillips [23], which appear to give better resolution and are simpler to use. Another alternative is provided by the system of MacDonald and Miller [4]. In these systems, sedimentation times of 2 to 4 hr are typically used, and the separations are performed at 4°C.

Centrifugation in tubes or in a zonal centrifuge may also be used for sedimentation separation [26-29]. However, at the present level of development, it appears that the 1-*g* systems mentioned above can both process larger numbers of cells and produce higher resolution.

Most work on lymphoid cells has been done by use of 1-*g* sedimentation under conditions equivalent to those defined by Miller and Phillips [23]. The technical problems and applications of this method have been recently reviewed in detail [30]. The following discussion will be limited to this situation.

Separations are very reproducible. Thus, for example, mouse erythrocytes reproducibly sediment at a rate of 2.00 ± 0.05 mm/hr. Note that sedimentation rates (*s* values) can be accurately calculated only after appropriate correction for the geometry of the sedimentation chamber [30]. Different lymphoid tissues give different and characteristic sedimentation profiles, which vary little from mouse strain to mouse strain. In fact, the shape of the sedimentation profile for a given tissue varies little among different mammalian species (species tested: mouse, rat, guinea pig, and man), although the absolute magnitudes of the sedimentation rates do change.

The B cells in suspensions of either mouse bone marrow or spleen sediment in a well-defined peak centered at 3 mm/hr [31,32]. Within 24 hr of immunization, B cells in mouse spleen specific for the immunizing antigen undergo blast transformation and are found centered in a peak around 6 mm/hr [33,34]. This peak occurs for both thymus-independent and thymus-dependent antigens [POL and sheep red blood cells (sRBC)]. Specific antigen-binding cells are associated with the peak at 6 mm/hr [34]. At long times after immunization, immunocompetent cells are again found in the 3-mm/hr region. At the height of a secondary immune response to sRBC, 7S AFC in mouse spleen have maximum frequency at s = 4.4 mm/hr [35]. The AFC sedimentation profile sedimentation profile can be analyzed as one population of cells in an active growth and division cycle and a second population of cells that are not dividing. In this study, enrichments of AFC producing antibodies against sRBC of up to 110-fold and purities of up to 28% were obtained.

The development of B cells into AFC seemsto be a blastogenic response; it also involves both division and differentiation. It appears to be followed quite closely by changes in the sedimentation profile. A similar, but more complicated, situation is seen in the toad, in which sedimentation analysis suggests a blastogenic response, followed by a series of divisions which successively halve the cell volume before the cells enter growth and division cycles [16].

The development of T cells into cytotoxic lymphocytes (CL [36] has been studied by MacDonald et al. [37] and follows a similar pattern. The progenitor T cells sediment in a well-defined peak centered at 3.5 mm/hr in both thymus and spleen. In spleen, this profile is similar to the profile of cells that carry the θ antigen. The CL early in the response are large cells with a peak frequency at s = 6.5 mm/hr. Late in the response, most CL seen are small cells, somewhat smaller than their progenitors. The sedimentation profiles throughout the response are complex, which suggests either several intermediate states in the development of CL or several different classes of CL. A basically similar picture has been reported by Andersson and Häyry [38]. Shortman et al. [39] have studied the same response by use of density separation and also obtain results consistent with the above interpretation.

Sedimentation separation has been extensively used to study the stem cells responsible for generating lymphocytes in mice. It has been suspected for some time that the hematopoietic stem cell (CFU) is also the stem cell for lymphoid cells. The most direct demonstration is that of Edwards et al. [40]. They produced mice whose entire hematopoietic system was repopulated by the progeny of a single CFU that carried a unique radiation-induced chromosome marker. These mice were immunized with sRBC, and at the peak of the secondary immune response, a suspension of their spleen cells was made. A significant fraction of the cells in this suspension are rosette-forming cells (RFC); i.e., they have specific surface receptors that enable them to bind large numbers of sRBC, forming objects called rosettes. Rosettes were made in the suspension and, by virtue of their much larger size, could be readily separated by sedimentation from other cells in the suspension by use of a sedimentation chamber designed specially for this purpose. It was found that some (but not necessarily all) RFC contained the unique chromosome marker and were therefore differentiated from CFU. These RFC are probably of the B-cell lineage, a conclusion strengthened by the subsequent work of Elliott and Haskill [41] on the sedimentation analysis of rosettes and RFC.

Lafleur et al. [42-44] have studied the CFU to the B-cell differentiation pathway. By use of sedimentation separation, they found a B-cell precursor (PB cell) which sediments much more rapidly than do B cells. This cell appears to have antigen-specific surface receptors and to be already specificity restricted, although it is incapable of interacting with antigen and T cells to give rise to AFC. On transplantation into irradiated mice, it can give rise to significant numbers of B cells within 3 days. This cell is presumed to be well along the differentiation pathway from CFU to B cells. There is, presumably, a more primitive precursor in which specificity is acquired, since CFU appear not to be specificity restricted.

Worton et al. [45] measured the sedimentation profile of CFU in mice and found that they form a disperse peak with maximum height at 3.9 mm/hr, but significant numbers were obtained at much higher sedimentation velocities. In the same mice, both B cells [31] and cells capable of producing graft-versus-host (GVH) disease [46] sediment as narrow well-defined populations centered at 3.0 mm/hr in both spleen and bone marrow. Thus, it is possible to obtain a pool of fractionated cells that contains CFU but is strongly depleted in both B and GVH cells. Phillips and Miller [46] utilized this fact to obtain successful allogeneic bone marrow transplantation in mice. The identical sort of separation appears to be possible in human bone marrow, but its clinical application has been less successful than in mice [47]. A possible explanation [47a] is that the human bone marrow samples separated had a higher number of GVH cells than that for mouse. In both cases, the separation procedure removed the same percentage (about 95%) of GVH cells, but this percentage leaves a much larger absolute number of GVH cells contaminating the stem cell pool in the human case.

III. Electrophoretic Separation

A cell placed in an electric field will migrate in the direction of the field at a uniform rate determined by its electrophoretic mobility, μ. Assume the cell to be spherical, of radius r, and to have surface charge density σ. If one neglects all interactions of the cell with the suspension medium, one finds that

$$\mu = \frac{2}{3} r \cdot \frac{\sigma}{\eta} \tag{4}$$

where η is the viscosity of the supporting medium.

This expression is unrealistic, since the suspension medium will contain ions which will, at least in part, neutralize the surface charge, so that Eq. (4) is an upper limit to the actual mobility. In particular, a negatively charged cell will have excess positive ions in its neighborhood, with a total charge equal to that on the cell surface. In the simplest model, it can be shown (see, e.g., Ref. 48) that all of these charges can be assumed to be on a concentric shell, at a distance d from the cell surface, and that, under these conditions, the mobility is given by

$$\mu = d\frac{\sigma}{\eta} \qquad (5)$$

The parameter d is inversely proportional to the square root of the ionic strength of the suspending medium, so that electrophoretic mobility will increase as the salt concentration is lowered. Note the perhaps surprising result that μ is independent of cell size. It can also be shown [48] that, within broad limits, it is also independent of cell shape.

All cells studied to date have a net negative surface charge, which appears to be primarily due to the presence of sialic acid on the cell membrane [49]. Treatment of lymphocyte populations with *Vibrio cholerae* neuraminidase, an agent which specifically removes exposed sialic acid groups, greatly reduces their electrophoretic viability [50]. Thus, the number of exposed sialic acid groups would appear to be the major factor in determining lymphocyte electrophoretic mobility. In addition to mobility variation between B and T cells, discussed in detail later, there are, in mice, significant strain to strain variations in the mobility of a given class of lymphocyte [51,52].

The technical problems encountered in attempting to fractionate cells by electrophoresis largely result from the necessity of performing the separation in a free fluid layer in the absence of a carrier, such as paper or gel, as commonly used in protein electrophoresis. Special precautions must be taken to stabilize the fluid layer against thermal convection and to overcome the effects of gravitational settling of the cells. These problems have been most successfully overcome in an instrument developed by Hannig [53], which is now being used by several laboratories throughout the world. In this instrument, cells are introduced at one point in a layer of fluid that flows vertically between two glass plates and are dispersed horizontally across the layer, according to electrophoretic mobility, by an electric field applied perpendicularly to the direction of fluid flow. Gravitational effects are overcome by having the fluid flowing vertically. Effects of thermal convection are overcome in two ways, First, the electrical conductivity of the buffer medium has been reduced by reducing its ionic strength, thus reducing the current flow. Isotonicity is maintained by addition of neutral molecules, such as glucose. The reduction in ionic strength has the added advantage of increasing d in Eq. (5) and thus the electrophoretic mobility. Second, Hannig has developed efficient procedures for removing the large amount of heat still produced in the chamber despite the reduction in ionic strength. Cell viability is maintained throughout the separation procedure.

Zeiller and associates have made extensive studies of the electrophoretic separation of lymphoid cells. They find that the electrophoretic distribution of lymphocytes in both rats and mice is heterogeneous and characteristic of the organ from which the lymphocytes are taken [54-56]. Lymphocytes from spleen separate into two broad peaks that contain approximately equal numbers of cells. Lymphocytes from these peaks are designated as being from either the high-mobility region (HMR) or the low-mobility region (LMR). In contrast to spleen, the majority of lymphocytes in both bone marrow and thymus are found in the LMR. In rat spleen, cells capable of producing GVH disease are confined to the HMR [57]. Therefore, the LMR in spleen is presumed to be free of T cells. The distribution of B and T cells in mouse lymphoid tissue was investigated by transplantation of irradiated mice with various combinations of separated and unseparated cells along with sRBC, followed by assay for antibody-producing cells [56]. In thymus, active T cells were found only in the HMR, despite the fact that the bulk of thymocytes are in the LMR. In spleen, T cells are again confined to the HMR. B cells, however, are found in both regions. Bone marrow contains only B cells, which are found exclusively in the LMR. They conclude that there are two populations of B cells in mouse spleen and speculate that these populations correspond to different stages of B-cell differentiaton. Antibody-producing cells also separate into two populations, both in the LMR. The more slowly moving peak is composed of immature blast cells, and the faster is composed of mature plasma cells [58], clear evidence that cell surface change density can change with development.

The above results have in large part been confirmed by Nordling et al. [52], who investigated the electrophoretic distribution of mouse lymphoid tissue from thymus, bone marrow, lymph node, blood, and spleen. Again, thymocytes were predominately in the LMR, but pretreatment of the donors with hydrocortisone simultaneously increased both the number of thymocytes in the HMR and the response of unfractionated thymocytes to PHA. Bone marrow lymphocytes were all in the LMR. Spleen, lymph node, and blood all showed biphasic lymphocyte distributions; the proportions were consistent with all LMR cells being B cells and all HMR cells being T cells.

Spleen or lymph node cells from the peaks of the HMR or LMR regions were further tested. Results of tests with anti-θ serum (to detect T cells) and anti-mouse B lymphocyte antigen serum were consistent with HMR cells all being T cells and LMR cells all being B cells. HMR (but not LMR) spleen cells could produce GVH disease and cytotoxic lymphocytes, both of which are T-cell functions. When spleen cells from mice previously immunized with sheep erythrocytes were analyzed, antibody-producing cells were predominately in the LMR, whereas RFC were in both regions.

The work of Nordling et al. [52] is inconsistent with that of Zeiller et al.

[56] in one respect. Nordling et al. found no evidence for B cells in the HMR, whereas Zeiller et al. did find B cells in this region. More recent work by von Boehmer et al. [59] appears to resolve this discrepancy. They studied the detailed electrophoretic distribution profiles of cells in mouse spleen carrying the θ antigen (T-cell marker) or carrying a high surface density of immunoglobulin (B-cell marker). According to these workers, T cells are, indeed, primarily confined to the HMR, but the B-cell distribution, although more than half in the LMR, has a long shoulder that extends into the T-cell region and that comprises about 40% of the B-cell population. In addition, there was a small population of lymphocytes (less than 15% of the total) of intermediate mobility that carried neither marker. The HMR B cells appear to be primarily large cells and can be selectively eliminated by passage of the cell suspension through a glass bead column (see Sec. IV). Nordling et al. pretreated all of their samples in a manner which may well have selectively reduced large adherent lymphocytes.

von Boehmer et al. find that high-mobility B cells are naturally absent from thoracic duct lymph and that essentially 100% pure B and T cells can be obtained from the LMR and HMR, respectively. They also found, in agreement with Wioland et al. [51], that spleen cells from athymic (*nu/nu*) mice moved primarily in the LMR, consistent with the conclusion that these mice have no T cells.

IV. Adherence Separation

When a heterogeneous suspension of cells is placed on a glass or plastic surface, some cells will stick to the surface. The process can be made both more efficient and more rapid by increasing the area of the adsorbing surface, such as by passing the cell suspension through a column packed with small glass beads. When a lymphoid or myeloid cell suspension is analyzed, a substantial fraction of the lymphocytes pass through the column, while the phagocytic cells are retained on the column. Studies of Shortman et al. [60] suggest that this sort of column should be used with some caution. They distinguish among four different mechanisms by which cells are trapped on the column:

(1) Active Adherence. This mechanism requires that the cells be capable of metabolism. Thus, cells will undergo active adherence when a column is run at 37°C, but not when it is run at 4°C. Macrophages and granulocytes, but not lymphocytes, appear to adhere by this mechanism.

(2) Physical Adherence. This process does not require that the cells be capable of active metabolism. Thus, cells will adhere with nearly equal efficiency when the column is run at either 37° or 4°C. Neither macrophages nor granulocytes adhere by this mechanism, but a substantial fraction of lymphocytes do.

(3) Size Filtraton. This mechanism occurs only when bead diameters less than 100 μm are used. Some of the larger cells are trapped on the column.

(4) Nonspecific Stickiness. This process appears to remove all damaged cells.

Shortman et al. [61] found a rough correlation between the physical adherence properties and density of lymphocytes, in that adherent lymphocytes were generally light, and nonadherent lymphocytes were generally dense. B and T lymphocytes each contain subpopulations of both adherent and nonadherent cells. These subpopulations can differ in function; e.g., nonadherent T cells give a much larger PHA response than do adherent T cells [20]. AFC (derived from B cells) and cytotoxic lymphocytes (derived from T cells) are predominately low-density adherent cells. They speculate that lymphoid cells which will undergo physical adherence are lymphoid cells which are basically tissue fixed, whereas nonadherent lymphoid cells are primarily circulating cells.

Adherence separation has played an important role in unraveling the cells involved in the initiation of a humoral immune response to sRBC. Mosier [62] fractionated mouse spleen cells into adherent and nonadherent fractions by use of plastic dishes and showed that both populations were required to initiate an in vitro immune response. Subsequent studies have shown that the adherent population provides a cell whose function is radiation resistant [63], presumably a macrophage, whereas the nonadherent population appears to provide both B and T lymphocytes [64]. A radiation-resistant adherent cell is also required in the in vivo response, and this cell is probably identical to the one required in vitro, according to analytic cell separation experiments that used both density and sedimentation separation [65].

Several adherence procedures that depend more upon the biologic specificity of membrane receptors than on physical principles might be mentioned. Antigen-binding cells can be specifically depleted from a cell suspension by passage of the suspension through a column that contains antigen-conjugated gel beads [66,67]. These columns appear to retain cells of the B-cell lineage capable of binding with the antigen on the column. The usual technical problems associated with such columns are that there is considerable nonspecific sticking of cells to the column and that it tends to be difficult to recover the bound cells. A more promising procedure appears to be the use of antigen-derivatized nylon fibers, for which there appears to be antigen-specific binding of both B and T cells. Either or both can be almost completely recovered from the fibers [68].

V. Fluroescence-activated Cell Sorting

The objective is to separate lymphocytes on the basis of differences in cell surface components, such as θ antigen or membrane-bound immunoglobulin.

The membrane marker chosen is in some way specifically labeled with fluorescein. The technical problem is to find some way of specifically selecting out those cells so labeled. A system for achieving this goal has been developed by Bonner et al. [69]. The cell suspension that contains the fluorescein-conjugated cells is forced under pressure through a fine nozzle to form a narrow (approximately 50 μm in diameter) jet. The nozzle is so designed as to create a coaxial flow system in which the cells are restricted to lie within 6 μm of the axis. The jet is perturbed by a high-frequency oscillating crystal, which guarantees that it breaks up into small drops of a fixed size and that the break-up point is at a fixed point along the jet. Conditions are usually adjusted so that each drop contains no or one cell only, rarely more than one cell. A short distance upstream from the break-up point, a laser beam is focused on the jet. The laser beam excites fluorescence from any fluorescein-conjugated cell that passes through its focal point; the fluorescent light is detected by an appropriate detector. Whenever a sufficiently large fluorescence signal is detected, the whole jet is charged electrically with a short charging pulse, with timing such that the detected cell will be trapped in the droplet formed during the charging pulse. Droplets formed at other times will be uncharged. After droplet formation, the drops pass through an electrostatic field which causes the deflection of charged droplets into one container, while uncharged droplets continue undeflected and are collected in a second container.

In one study [70], this system was successfully used to separate specific B cells from other cells in mouse spleen. Spleen cells from mice previously immunized against keyhole limpet hemocyanin (KLH) were incubated with fluorescein-conjugated KLH, and fluorescent cells were separated from all other cells. Both the deflected (fluorescent) and undeflected cells were separately inactive on transfer with KLH into irradiated recipient mice. However, on recombination of the two fractions, or on addition of thymus cells to the deflected fraction, activity was regained. Superficially, one might conclude from this experiment that T cells do not have antigen-specific surface receptors. However, the fluorescein labeling conditions and the sensitivity of the instrument were such that a cell would be deflected only if it had more than 10^4 antigen molecules bound to its surface. Therefore, one concludes that if T cells have antigen-specific surface receptors, there must be fewer than 10^4 per cell. Similar results were obtained with human serum albumin (HSA) as the antigen and fluorescein-conjugated antibody against HSA as the label.

In a more recent version of the instrument, a second laser has been added, and the light scattered by cells into very small forward angles is monitored. It can be shown that the magnitude of this scatter signal is proportional to the size of the cell that produced it [71]. Thus, by appropriate analysis of the scatter and fluorescence signal, it is possible to deflect fluorescent cells of a specified size range. Nonviable lymphocytes tend to pick up fluorescent label nonspecifically. However, they produce a smaller scatter signal than do viable lymphocytes and can, therefore, be easily removed from the deflected beam.

The concept of detecting some property of a cell in a jet, charging the jet just before a droplet that contains the cell of interest breaks from the jet, and subsequently deflecting out that droplet is a very powerful one, in that many different properties of cells can be used as the basis for selection. The first system that successfully exploited this concept for cell separation was that of Fulwyler [72]. He incorporated a Coulter aperture in the nozzle of the jet, which gave him a measure of the volume of each cell as it passed through the nozzle. With this information, he could subsequently deflect cells of any desired volume from the jet.

VI. Conclusions

This chapter has dealt with three truly analytic separation procedures: density, sedimentation, and electrophoretic separation. Adherence separation and fluorescence-activated cell sorting are actually only semianalytic. A fourth analytic separation procedure, countercurrent cell separation [73], has not been dealt with, primarily because it has not yet been extensively applied to lymphoid cell populations. It probably yields separations similar (but not equivalent) to those obtained with electrophoresis. The above procedures are all complementary. Their serial application to the same cell population is a fruitful area which is only beginning to be exploited.

A set of numbers (ρ, s, μ) for a particular lymphocyte is certainly a more complete description of that cell than any morphologic description. It is also more detailed than is necessary to describe the biologic function of the lymphocyte at our present level of understanding: many more subpopulations are defined than can be accounted for in terms of known differences in biologic function. This is particularly true for subpopulations defined by ρ. The fond hope of investigators in the field is that each subpopulation represents a discrete step in development. The complete road map of lymphocyte differentiation is already available; we merely need to learn how to read it!

Acknowledgment

Some of the work described in this chapter was supported by the National Cancer Institute of Canada and the Medical Research Council of Canada (Grant MA-3017).

References

1. K. Shortman, Annu. Rev. Biophys. Bioeng. **1**, 93 (1972).
2. E. G. Olmsted, *Mammalian Cell Water,* Lea and Febiger, Philadelphia, 1966.
3. E. C. Anderson, D. F. Petersen, and R. A. Tobey, Biophys. J. **10**, 630 (1972).
4. H. R. MacDonald and R. G. Miller, Biophys. J. **10**, 834 (1970).
5. R. C. Leif and J. Vinograd, Proc. Nat. Acad. Sci. USA **51**, 520 (1964).
6. R. C. Leif, in *Automated Cell Identification and Cell Sorting* (G. L. Wied and G. F. Bahr, eds.), Academic Press, New York, 1970, p. 21.
7. K. Shortman, Aust. J. Exp. Biol. Med. Sci. **46**, 375 (1968).
8. N. Williams, N. Kraft, and K. Shortman, Immunology **22**, 885 (1972).
9. R. M. Gorczynski, R. G. Miller, and R. A. Phillips, Immunology **19**, 817 (1970).
10. K. A. Dicke, J. I. M. van Hooft, and D. W. van Bekkum, Transplantation **6**, 562 (1968).
11. D. J. Raidt, R. I. Mishell, and R. W. Dutton, J. Exp. Med. **128**, 681 (1968).
12. A. Böyum, Scand. J. Clin. Lab. Invest. **21** (Suppl. 97), (1968).
13. K. Shortman, J. Cell. Physiol. **77**, 319 (1971).
14. J. S. Haskill, D. G. Legge, and K. Shortman, J. Immunol. **102**, 703 (1969).
15. N. Kraft, K. Shortman, and J. Marchalonis, Immunology **20**, 919 (1971).
16. N. Kraft and K. Shortman, J. Cell. Biol. **52**, 438 (1972).
17. T. Takiguchi, W. H. Adler, and R. T. Smith, J. Exp. Med. **133**, 63 (1971).
18. K. Shortman, J.-C. Cerottini, and K. T. Brunner, Eur. J. Immunol. **2**, (1972).
19. S. Konda, Y. Nakao, and R. T. Smith, J. Exp. Med. **136**, 1461 (1972).
20. K. Shortman, W. J. Byrd, J.-C. Cerottini, and K. T. Brunner, Cell. Immunol. **6**, 25 (1973).
21. G. Janossy and M. F. Greaves, Clin. Exp. Immunol. **9**, 483 (1971).
22. R. M. Gorczynski, R. G. Miller, and R. A. Phillips, Immunology **20**, 693 (1971).
23. R. G. Miller and R. A. Phillips, J. Cell. Physiol. **73**, 191 (1969).
24. H. C. Mel, J. Theoret. Biol. **6**, 159, 181, 307 (1964).
25. E. A. Peterson and W. H. Evans, Nature (London) **214**, 824 (1967).
26. C. W. Boone, G. S. Harell, and H. E. Bond, J. Cell. Biol. **36**, 369 (1968).
27. T. G. Pretlow, II and C. W. Boone, Science **161**, 911 (1968).
28. T. G. Pretlow, II, C. W. Boone, R. I. Shrager, and G. H. Weiss, Anal. Biochem. **29**, 230 (1969).
29. T. G. Pretlow, II, Anal. Biochem. **41**, 248 (1971).
30. R. G. Miller, in *Techniques in Biophysics and Cell Biology* (R. Pain and B. Smith, eds.), Wiley, London, 1973, Vol. 1.
31. R. G. Miller and R. A. Phillips, Proc. Soc. Exp. Biol. Med. **135**, 63 (1970).

32. D. Osoba, J. Exp. Med. **132**, 368 (1970).
33. W. D. Armstrong and N. E. Kraft, J. Immunol. **110**, 157 (1973).
34. E. Diener, N. Kraft, and W. D. Armstrong, Cell. Immunol. **6**, 80 (1973).
35. R. A. Phillips and R. G. Miller, Cell Tissue Kinet. **3**, 263 (1970).
36. K. T. Brunner, A. A. Nordin, and J.-C. Cerottini, in *Second International Convocation of Immunologists,* Karger, Basel, 1971, p. 220.
37. H. R. MacDonald, R. A. Phillips, and R. G. Miller, J. Immunol. **111**, 575 (1973).
38. L. C. Andersson and P. Häyry, Cell. Immunol. **8**, 470 (1973).
39. K. Shortman, K. T. Brunner, and J.-C. Cerottini, J. Exp. Med. **135**, 1375 (1972).
40. G. E. Edwards, R. G. Miller, and R. A. Phillips, J. Immunol. **105**, 719 (1970).
41. B. E. Elliott and J. S. Haskill, Eur. J. Immunol. **3**, 68 (1973).
42. L. Lafleur, R. G. Miller, and R. A. Phillips, J. Exp. Med. **135**, 1363 (1972).
43. L. Lafleur, B. J. Underdown, R. G. Miller, and R. A. Phillips, Ser. Haematol. **V**(2), 50 (1972).
44. L. Lafleur, R. G. Miller, and R. A. Phillips, J. Exp. Med. **137**, 954 (1973).
45. R. G. Worton, E. A. McCulloch, and J. E. Till, J. Cell. Physiol. **74**, 171 (1969).
46. R. A. Phillips and R. G. Miller, J. Immunol. **105**, 1168 (1970).
47. H. Abu-Zahara, D. Amato, M. T. Aye, D. E. Bergsagel, A. M. Clarysse, D. H. Cowan, V. L. Fornasier, R. Hasselback, N. N. Iscove, E. A. McCulloch, H. Messner, R. G. Miller, R. A. Phillips, A. H. Ragab, W. D. Rider, and J. S. Senn, Ser. Haematol. **V**(2), 189 (1972).
47a. R. A. Phillips, unpublished observations.
48. H. A. Abramson, L. S. Moyer, and M. H. Gorin, *Electrophoresis of Proteins and the Chemistry of Cell Surfaces,* Reinhold, New York, 1942.
49. L. Weiss, In Vitro **5**, 48 (1970).
50. S. Nordling, L. C. Andersson, and P. Häyry, Science **178**, 1001 (1972).
51. M. Wioland, D. Sabolovic, and C. Burg, Nature [New Biol.] **237**, 274 (1972).
52. S. Nordling, L. C. Andersson, and P. Häyry, Eur. J. Immunol. **2**, 405 (1972).
53. K. Hannig, in *Methods in Microbiology* (J. R. Norris and D. W. Ribbons, eds.), Academic Press, London, 1971, Vol. 5B, pp. 513-548.
54. K. Zeiller and K. Hannig, Hoppe-Seyler's Z. Physiol. Chem. **352**, 1162 (1971).
55. K. Zeiller, H. G. Liebich, and K. Hannig, Eur. J. Immunol. **1**, 315 (1971).
56. K. Zeiller, E. Holzberg, G. Pascher, and K. Hannig, Hoppe-Seyler's Z. Physiol. Chem. **353**, 105 (1972).
57. K. Zeiller, K. Hannig, and G. Pascher, Hoppe-Seyler's Z. Physiol. Chem. **352**, 1168 (1971).
58. K. Zeiller, G. Pascher, and K. Hannig, Prep. Biochem. **2**, 21 (1972).
59. H. von Boehmer, K. Shortman, and G. J. V. Nossal, J. Cell. Physiol. **83**, 231 (1974).

60. K. Shortman, N. Williams, H. Jackson, P. Russell, P. Byrt, and E. Diener, J. Cell. Biol. **48**, 566 (1971).
61. K. Shortman, W. Byrd, N. Williams, K. T. Brunner, and J.-C. Cerottini, Aust. J. Exp. Biol. Med. Sci. **50**, 323 (1972).
62. D. E. Mosier, Science **158**, 1573 (1967).
63. J. Roseman, Science **165**, 1125 (1969).
64. D. E. Mosier, F. W. Fitch, D. A. Rowley, and A. J. S. Davies, Nature (London) **225**, 276 (1970).
65. R. M. Gorczynski, R. G. Miller, and R. A. Phillips, J. Exp. Med. **134**, 1201 (1971).
66. H. Wigzell and B. Andersson, J. Exp. Med. **129**, 23 (1969).
67. P. Truffa-Bachi and L. Wofsy, Proc. Nat. Acad. Sci. **66**, 685 (1970).
68. U. Rutishauser and G. M. Edelman, Proc. Nat. Acad. Sci. USA **69**, 3774 (1972).
69. W. A. Bonner, H. R. Hulett, R. G. Sweet, and L. A. Herzenberg, Rev. Sci. Instr. **43**, 404 (1972).
70. M. H. Julius, T. Masuda, and L. A. Herzenberg, Proc. Nat. Acad. Sci. USA **69**, 1934 (1972).
71. P. F. Mullaney and P. N. Dean, Biophys. J. **10**, 764 (1970).
72. M. J. Fulwyler, in *Automated Cell Identification and Cell Sorting* (G. L. Wied and G. F. Bahr, eds.), Academic Press, New York, 1970, pp. 97-109.
73. P. A. Albertsson, *Partition of Cell Particles and Macromolecules,* 2nd edit., Wiley, New York, 1972.

SECTION IV

Immune Functions of Lymphocytes

CHAPTER 6

Observations and Speculations on the Influence of T Cells in the Cellular Events of Induction of Antibody Formation and Tolerance In Vivo

Graham F. Mitchell*

The Basel Institute for Immunology
Basel, Switzerland

I. Introduction: Lymphocytes and Lymphoid Tissue

This chapter will describe recent experimental findings and several ideas on the cellular events and consequences of the encounter between antigen and antigen-reactive cells in vivo; the emphasis will be on studies that used mice as the

*Present address: Experimental Pathology Unit, The Walter and Eliza Hall Institute of Medical Research, Royal Melbourne Hospital, Victoria, Australia.

experimental animal. The lymphocyte is accepted, almost universally, as the only specific antigen-reactive cell, even though this statement is virtually meaningless, simply because of regular demonstrations of extreme heterogeneity in the lymphocyte population. As is common practice, the two major types of antigen-reactive lymphocyte, thymus-influenced (T) lymphocytes and precursors of antibody-secreting cells (B lymphocytes), will be referred to throughout as T cells and B cells [1]. After contact with antigen, both T and B cells are believed to be sensitive to various "signals": "*on signals,*" which result ultimately in populations of B cell-derived antibody-secreting cells, such as plasma cells, and memory cells, or T cell-derived sensitized lymphocytes (→ immune induction); "*off signals,*" which result in cell paralysis, "functional silence," and, perhaps ultimately, cell death (→ tolerance induction); and, for completeness, "*no signals,*" the case in which neither "on" nor "off signals" are generated. T cells modify the antibody-producing activity of the B-cell population, and popular belief is that a T cell-dependent "second signal" modifies, either directly or indirectly, the antigen-dependent "first signal" at the B-cell surface (see, e.g., Refs. 2-10).

Any consideration of the in vivo events of antibody production and tolerance must take into account the organization of lymphoid tissue. This is difficult, since we know nothing about the influence of anatomic location on the outcome of the interaction among T cells, B cells, ancillary cells, and antigen in the various peripheral or secondary lymphoid organs and tissues (i.e., spleen, lymph nodes, gut-associated lymphoid tissue, unorganized lymphoid aggregates, bloodstream, and lymphatics). Both T and B cells are contained in Gowans' "recirculating pool of lymphocytes" [11-13], and both can be recruited into, or out of, the lymphoid organs by antigen (J. Sprent, chapter 2). It seems that the general picture of lymphoid tissue architecture and organization has changed very little in the past few years (Fig. 1), except for the findings that germinal centers probably contain many T cells [14], that intralymphatic "backwaters" of accumulated lymphocytes and inflammatory cells in lymph nodes and spleen may be important in the response to antigen [15-17], and that there is now a problem of placing the spleen into the scheme of things (see Fig. 1).

The spleen has long been recognized as a hematopoietic organ in mice and a major site of antibody production. Because of the latter property, the spleen has been classified as a secondary lymphoid organ, along with the lymph nodes, as distinct from the primary lymphoid organs, such as the thymus and avian bursa of Fabricius [18]. Many recent studies, including those of Cantor and colleagues on $T_1 \rightarrow T_2$ cell differentiation [19-21] and Lafleur and colleagues on B-cell precursor (PB) → B-cell differentiation [22], indicate that the spleen may have several immunological functions which are lacking in lymph nodes. The spleen, as distinct from lymph nodes, is rich

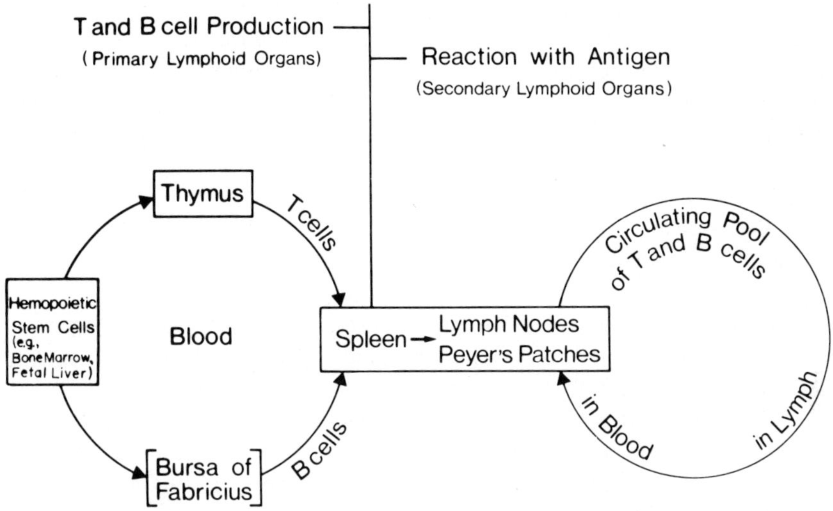

FIG. 1. Scheme of lymphoid tissue organization. The major unknown is still the site of B-cell production in mammals (i.e., the mammalian equivalent of the avian bursa of Fabricius). Likely candidates are the bone marrow and spleen, or conceivably the blood as it passes through some organ or tissue. The spleen appears to have several unique functions in the processing of T and B cells.

in T_1 cells and PB cells. Thus, the spleen may be an organ involved in the generation of B cells [23,24], an organ involved in the "processing" of early thymus migrants (T_1 cells) to potentially long-lived T_2 cells [25-27], an organ that contains "thymus-repopulating cells" within the population of hematopoietic cells [28], and an organ that contains B cells and T_2 cells since it is part of the recirculating pool. [The deficiency of PB cells in lymph nodes speaks against a bursa function for scattered lymphoid follicles in mammalian species. The recent findings that thymocytes from asplenic mice are defective (albeit marginally) in their "helper" function further complicates the picture [29,30].]

The induction of an antibody response in vivo involves more than an interaction between antigen and specifically reactive cells. Ancillary cells such as macrophages and granulocytes, phagocytose antigen and subpopulations or related cells (e.g., dendritic reticulum cells) may retain antigen at the cell surface for presentation to T and/or B cells [31,32]. Moreover, serum factors, such as antibody (±complement components), must also alter humoral immune responses by modifying the availability of antigen for T and/or B cells and its location in lymphoid organs. What is the function of antibody

(±complement)-dependent follicular localization of antigen (reviewed in Ref. 33)? Follicles and germinal centers remain the most enigmatic structures in secondary lymphoid organs, and it is not yet clear whether follicular localization of antigen serves to *sequester antigen within,* or *exclude it from,* relevant sites of immune induction.

II. T Cell-dependent and T Cell-independent Antibody Responses

The finding that T cell-depleted animals respond normally to some antigens but not to others has led to the division of antibody (B cell) responses into T-cell independent and T-cell dependent and the use of the corresponding terms to describe the antigens, "T cell-independent antigen" and "T cell-dependent antigen." In this discussion, the terms T cell-dependent B cell (D-B cell) and T cell-independent B cell (I-B cell) have been used as a means of differentiating between B cells which require the T-cell influence for the generation of "on signals" and those which do not have this requirement. (Playfair and Purves [23] have used the designiations B_2 and B_1 to describe these two B cell types.) If T cells increase total antibody production in the B-cell population as measured by a particular assay, this function of T cells is referred to as a "helper" function.

Various systems have been used to study T-cell dependence/independence of antibody production in vivo: (a) relatively long-term T cell-depleted animals, depletion being achieved by neonatal thymectomy, adult thymectomy followed by lethal irradiation and stem cell transplantation (e.g., "B mice"), injection of heterologous anti-T antisera, and congenital absence of the thymus [e.g., athymic, nude (*nu*/*nu*) mice]; (b) injection of irradiated mice with sources of B cells versus T plus B cells, the sources of B cells being anti-Thy-1 (θ) isoantisera-treated mixed T- and B-cell populations or fetal hematopoietic tissue, for example; the sources of T cells being thymocytes, cortisone-resistant thymocytes, or B cell-depleted mixed T- and B-cell populations; (c) the use of an antigen which addresses itself to B cells but for which there are few, if any, immunologically active T cells for genetic reasons; and (d) the use of animals in which T cells, but not B cells, have been rendered tolerant. Obviously, a significant deficiency of specifically reactive T cells must be demonstrated before an antibody response qualifies as a T cell-independent response (discussed in Ref. 8).

There are several general statements which can be made about T-cell dependence/independence.

a. Secondary responses are highly T-cell dependent, whereas many primary responses are not [34-38]. Only two observations are apparently contrary to this statement. Sinclair obtained normal secondary, but reduced primary, responses to sheep erythrocytes (sRBC) in neonatally thymectomized mice [39]. Primary *and secondary* responses to sRBC are certainly reduced in *nu/nu* mice [40]. Thus, in Sinclair's system, and in that of Svet-Moldavsky et al. [41], a small pool of reactive T cells, present after neonatal thymectomy, is probably being expanded such that increasing numbers of reactive T cells are available for "helper" functions at later time points after the primary injection of antigen [8,42].

The other apparent exception is the observation that in hapten-carrier antigen systems, the requirement for homologous carrier "help" does not apply to long-term primed animals [43-45]. That is, hapten-carrier 1-primed animals respond well to a hapten-carrier 2 complex injected many months after the initial antigen priming. With the assumption that carrier-reactive T cells are involved in these systems, as they are in mice [46,47], one interpretation of the finding is that primed B cells of high affinity have acquired the capacity of responding to antigen and no longer depend on T-cell "help." Several other interpretations can be made. A trivial one is that the longer animals are maintained in colonies the greater the probability of being exposed to either carrier 2 or an antigen with which it cross reacts. More seriously, in the one host system in which the observation has been made, high-affinity antihapten antibodies may be reducing the tolerogenicity of antigen for the cell combination *primed* antihapten B cells plus *virgin* anticarrier 2 reactive T cells [44] (Sec. III). [Experiments with the apparently non-T cell-stimulating antigens, DNP-lys-SIII and DNP-D-GL, suggest that primed anti-DNP B cells are markedly more sensitive to the tolerogenic effects of these antigens than are unprimed anti-DNP B cells [6,48,49].] Another interpretation is that a slow increase in the affinity of anticarrier 1-reactive T cells (cf. Ref. 50) has increased their cross reactivity to carrier 2. Or, related to this possibility, relatively "immunosilent" common new antigenic determinants (NAD) that result from haptenation of the two carrier proteins [51,52] may be relatively "immunodominant" at late time points after priming with hapten-carrier 1.

Evidence from other systems does not support the contention that B cells, at late time points after antigen contact, are less demanding on the T-cell influence for expression of their antibody-producing potential. That is, there is much evidence against the notion that a D-B cell-rich population can become an I-B cell-rich population with time after exposure to antigen. Thus, anti-Thy-1 (θ) isoantiserum treatment of primed spleen cells obliterates an adoptive secondary response for many months after priming the spleen cell donor [47,53-56]. Can D-B cells be encouraged to respond simply by increasing the antigen dose? Antibody titers or plaque-forming cell (PFC) numbers comparable to those in control mice have been obtained in some systems [57-63], but not in others [64,65], with large doses of antigen injected into T cell-deficient mice. Thus, either the division D-B cell/I-B cell is misleading and simply dependent on antigen dose, or one of the three following possibilities pertains. 1. The increased antigen dose increases the probability of recruiting residual T cells, thus inducing expression of D-B cells. (Since T cells are known to be primed by *small* doses of antigen, such as sRBC in vivo [53,66], one needs to postulate further that T-cell priming does not necessarily involve expression of "helper" functions.) 2. With increasing antigen dose, one is titrating for ancillary (e.g., mitogenic) substances which boost the response of B cells [67-72]. (The results on T-cell dependence of some adjuvants [65,73-75] restricts the number of ancillary substances that possibly mediate this effect. "Mitogen signals" may increase the amount of antibody produced by the progeny of triggered I-B cells or increase the *range* of B cells induced into antibody production.) 3. Increasing antigen dose converts a "no signal" to "on signals" in I-B cells of ultralow antigen-binding capacity (ABC), which are never recruited in the face of antibody production by D-B cells of higher ABC (see below). Such B cells could be expected to produce low combining-site affinity IgM antibodies (see below). Obviously, it becomes important to determine combining-site affinities, class distribution, and clonal heterogeneity of the additional antibody produced in T cell-deficient mice injected with high doses of antigen.

b. Most IgG antibody responses are highly T-cell dependent, whereas many IgM antibody responses are not [37,40,61,62,76-81]. This is a diluted statement derived from "IgG responses are more T cell dependent than IgM responses." Many different antigens are capable of eliciting near normal primary IgM responses in "B" mice or *nu/nu* mice. Examples are (T,G)-A–L [37], rabbit IgG fragments [76], ϕX174 bacteriophage [38], SIII [82,83], DNP-levan [84], PVP [85,86], and LPS [87]. *Subnormal* IgM responses have been demonstrated in the response of T cell-deficient mice to heterologous erythrocytes, even though IgG responses are reduced far more drastically (reviewed in Ref. 8). In the response to phage fd, the predominantly IgM response in genetic low-responder strains of mice (e.g., DBA/2) is not affected by T-cell deprivation. By contrast, the predominantly IgG response of high responders (e.g., DBA/1) is markedly reduced in T cell-deficient mice [58,88]. Carrier preimmunization [46,89-95] increases primary IgM antihapten antibody responses to hapten-carrier complexes in vivo [Refs. 93 and 94 (in rats and rabbits)] and in vitro [92,95], even though in other in vivo situations the principal effect is an accelerated maturation of the IgG antibody response [89,90].

Antigens, such as ϕX174 [38], DNP-dextran [96], and sRBC [97], elicit allotype-bearing IgG responses (of low avidity in the case of anti-ϕX174 antibodies) in at least some *nu/nu* mice. The responses are low titered and/or short-lived; yet, there is no doubt that early IgG antibodies are present after primary immunization. As discussed by Mi tchell [8], previous indications that T cell-deficient mice produce IgG antibodies suffered from the problems of substantial numbers of residual T cells in "B mice," because low doses of irradiation were used [61], or that the indirect PFC detected with antigen-coated sRBC (PVP in this case [85,86]) were not shown to be IgG-secreting cells rather than facilitated IgM-secreting cells [98]. $IgG_1(\gamma G_1)$ antibodies [61,62], and now homocytotropic (IgE?) antibodies [99], seem to be the highly T cell-dependent (sub) classes of antibody in the mouse.

c. High combining-site affinity antibodies are more T-cell dependent than are low-affinity antibodies [100,101]. This statement is compatible with statements *a* and *b* above but has not been widely confirmed. The intrinsic combining-site affinity of IgM antihapten antibodies is low [102-109], as is that of antibodies formed early in the immune response ([110,111] cf. Ref. 112). If primary IgM antibodies are relatively T cell independent, T cell-independent antibodies can be expected to be of low combining-site affinity, even though the "functional affinity," or avidity, may be high as a result of polyvalency in circulating IgM molecules. With respect to T-cell dependence/independence, there may well be a switch in emphasis from Ig C genes to V genes in the near future.

There are some indications that IgA may be similar to IgM (in being relatively T-cell independent and of low combining-site affinity [113]), whereas IgE may be similar to IgG (in being highly T-cell dependent and of high combining-site affinity). Thus, SIII elicits non-IgM antibodies in some strains of mice [114-116], which have been identified as IgA [115]. NIP-SIII elicits both IgM and IgA anti-NIP antibodies in long-term cultures of mouse spleen fragments [117]. No clear answer is available, however, on the question of T-cell dependence/independence of circulating IgA antibody production [42,118]. Homocytotropic (IgE?) antibody production is negligible in nude mice but may be very sensitive to the number of T cells used in reconstitution [99] (and, perhaps, therefore to the amount of IgG antibody [119]). Circulating IgE anti-DNP antibodies, like IgG anti-DNP antibodies, are highly susceptible to the inhibitory effects of high doses of DNP-D-GL [120].

d. Several antigens which induce T cell-independent antibody responses in vivo are highly persistent, polymeric, non-T-cell stimulating and in vitro are able to stimulate B cells nonspecifically and cleave C3, the third component of complement. Such antigens are SIII, PVP, and LPS. The synthetic polypeptides composed of D-amino acids [121,122], levan [123], DNP-levan [84], and NIP-mRBC [124] are also slowly metabolized, highly persistent, repeating determinant antigens which induce responses in "B mice" or acutely irradiated mice injected with bone marrow cells, responses which are not increased by added thymocytes. IgM antibodies predominate in the in vivo responses to these antigens. None of them seem to stimulate T cells.

(The clearly "T cell-independent antigens," such as SIII, PVP, and LPS, do not stimulate T cells after injection into irradiated mice [125-127]. Antigens for which there has been some doubt, but which are now known to be T-cell dependent in vivo [59,63,64,118], do stimulate T cells in the system of Gershon et al. [126,127] and induce IgG responses in vivo, e.g., *Brucella abortus*, POL, and KLH.)

Attempts to induce delayed hypersensitivity to SIII in guinea pigs [128] or in vitro activation of rabbit lymphocytes by SIII [129] have been unsuccessful. SIII does not elicit a secondary response in primed mice [82,130] nor does it act as a carrier for antigens, such as sRBC [131]. Immunologic memory to D-TGL is very difficult to demonstrate, quite unlike memory to L-TGL [132]. Following a suggestion by Möller [133], several groups have shown that antigens with repeating determinants, such as heavily substituted NIP-BSA [57] and DNP-POL [134], may induce T cell-independent IgM responses in vivo and in vitro.

Which property, then, if any, is related to T-cell independence: persistence, polymeric structure, inability to recruit T cells, B-cell mitogenicity [135], or ability to activate C3 [136,137]? The difference between D- and L-amino acid polypeptides [121,122] suggests an involvement of resistance to degradation (and therefore of in vivo persistence *if the antigen is of high molecular weight*). Does increasing the haptenic density on proteins reduce the susceptibility of such antigens to enzymatic degradation, which, in turn, increases the persistence of the antigen? Preliminary data indicate that this interpretation is correct. Heavily conjugated haptenated and labeled proteins, such as N*IP-FγG and DNP-BSA*, when injected in aqueous solution, are cleared rapidly from the blood, but, at the whole body level, counts persist long after counts have been lost from mice injected with lightly conjugated proteins [138]. Thus, at least a portion of the antigen of high epitope density may be resistant to degradation and behave as SIII and other highly persistent antigens. Are the properties of C3 activation and mitogenicity simply "assays" for polymeric structure? Are the antigen molecules to which antibody is produced really mitogenic or is this a property of contained bacterial endotoxins [67-72] or a function of the affinity of other contained moieties for mammalian cells in general? The doses used in vitro to test for mitogenicity are orders of magnitude higher than the optimal immunogenic doses in vivo. The hypothesis developed in a later section emphasizes the *tolerogenicity* of persistent antigens for D-B cells (of high ABC), a protective role of activated T cells for D-B cells, and the *dependence* of I-B cells (of low ABC) on antigenic persistence and polymeric structure to be triggered into low-affinity antibody production.

e. Haptens on non-T-cell stimulating antigens readily induce hapten-specific tolerance. Hapten-specific tolerance in mice has been obtained with TNP, DNP, and NIP determinants on non-T cell-stimulating antigens, such as autologous proteins [139-141], autologous (syngeneic) red cells [142,143], SIII [48,49,116], and D-GL [144]. Presumably, B cells with antihapten specificity are rendered tolerant. If this assumption is correct, it can be said that B-cell precursors of IgG-secreting cells (B^{γ} cells) or primed B cells (presumably of high ABC) are more susceptible to tolerance than are B-cell precursors of IgM-secreting cells (B^{μ} cells) or unprimed B cells (presumably of low ABC). *Nu/nu* mice injected with sRBC respond poorly to a subsequent injection of T cells plus sRBC [97]. Adoptive transfer experiments suggest that this system involves a combination of a (T-cell independent antibody-mediated block to the expression of B^{μ} cells [145] and a defect in the responsiveness of B^{γ} cells. There is thus a similarity between the consequences of injecting *athymic* mice with T cell-stimulating antigens, such as sRBC, and the consequences of injecting *intact* mice with non-T cell-stimulating antigens. The defect appears to be at the level of B^{γ} cells. No experimental system has totally ruled out a defect in nonspecific ancillary cells, which acquire specificity [146-148], as being the primary lesion in these putative B cell-tolerance systems. At first sight, the possibility seems remote, simply because the number of cells with nonspecificity (macrophages, other phagocytes, such as granulocytes, and reticulum cells) vastly exceeds that of cells with specificity, and the total population must be capable of overcoming and compensating for inhibitory influences with ease. The counter to this is that we do not know the proportion of ancillary cells with "initial nonspecificity" which are relevant to the expression of cells with specificity for antigen, i.e., T cells and B cells. It is conceivable that, in the apparent B^{γ}-cell tolerance in athymic mice injected with sRBC [97], a critical population of splenic ancillary cells is unable to interact with B cells (or T cells) in the response to the second dose of sRBC, which is injected together with T cells. However, the finding that sRBC-injected athymic mice will respond to TNP, but not to sRBC, when injected with T cells plus TNP-sRBC is difficult to explain on the basis of a defect in the capacity of ancillary cells to accommodate sRBC.

The concept of T-cell dependence/independence has come under attack usually from those who wish to elevate the T cell to the status of obligatory cell for B-cell triggering according to the tenets of "self-nonself discrimination" (see, e.g., Refs. 149 and 150). The principal observation on T-cell independence is simply that some antigens elicit comparable antibody responses (at some, if not all, time points after antigen injection) in intact mice and in mice with a severe deficiency of T cells or specifically reactive T cells. It is presumed that such "T cell-independent antigens" would elicit poor responses in the alternate experimental animal, the B cell-deficient chicken. The perfectly valid question, of course, is "how severe is the severe T cell deficiency?"

Those who propose the existence of T cell-independent responses, take comfort in the nude (*nu/nu*), putatively athymic, mouse! (It may well become important to determine in these athymic mice whether, with respect to the response under investigation, one is looking at the activity of an "exposed" but normal B-cell population or of a markedly compensated B-cell population.)

The normal individual contains antiself-B cells and circulating IgM antiself antibodies [151-156]. Thus, autoreactive I-B cells (of low ABC) may well be triggered by antigen, the resultant low combining-site affinity IgM antibodies being of little harm to the individual. The triggering of autoreactive D-B cells by antigen plus T cells is presumably to be avoided. The lesion of natural or acquired tolerance at the T- or B-cell level is unknown. T cells are defective in at least their "helper" functions in low- and high-zone [157-159] tolerant mice, whereas B cells are affected only in high-zone tolerance [160,161]. Are "functionally silent" cells masked by antigen, devoid of the original antigen receptors, internally blocked, or eliminated? With a hypothetical sequence, such as the following, there is likely to be more than one means of ensuring "functional silence": antigenic reactivity → receptor occupation → failure of surface shedding → "blindfolding" → potentially cytotoxic effects → repair → failure of repair mechanisms → cell death → replacement from precursor sources. [Perhaps it is necessary to retain, rather than eliminate, autoreactive *B cells.* A regulatory role of anti-idiotypic antibodies has been proposed by Jerne [162]. Autoreactive antibody receptors on the surface of a B cell may be required to stimulate anti-idiotypic antibodies (perhaps of a special class) which penetrate the thymus and inhibit the development and export of autoreactive *T cells.* This notion can be extended further. Anti-*non*self antibodies on B cells may promote production of anti-idiotypic antibodies which, again by feedback control in the thymus, limit the number of exported T cells with reactivity against that particular nonself determinant. In this way, the number of T cells reactive to *B cell-stimulating determinants* will be reduced: hence, "carrier-reactive" T cells and "hapten-reactive" B cells. This mechanism would also account for any lack of T cells reactive to B cell-stimulating antigens with restricted epitope heterogeneity, such as SIII, PVP, and LPS.]

III. A Hypothesis on T-B Cell Collaboration Which Ascribes to T Cells a Deblocking and Protective Function for B Cells of High Antigen-binding Capacity (ABC)

The following observations suggest that the consequence of the reaction between antigen and B^{γ} cell is B^{γ}-cell tolerance ("functional silence") and that reactive T cells *protect* such B^{γ} cells from tolerance by converting "off signals" to "on signals": (a) haptens on nonmetabolizable, apparently non-T cell-stimulating antigens inhibit IgG antihapten antibody responses to haptenated foreign proteins [48,144]; (b) an injection of sRBC in athymic *nu/nu* mice preferentially inhibits the IgG anti-sRBC antibody response to a subsequent injection of T cells plus sRBC [97]; and (c) antigens, such as (T, G)-A–L, when injected into (T, G)-A–L "nonresponders," inhibit IgG responses to a subsequent injection of the B-cell cross-reactive antigen, (H, G)-A–L, for which the same mice are "responders" [163]. [In the latter system, there is much indirect evidence which suggests that T cells in "nonresponders" are "functionally silent," i.e., absent, readily tolerized, or unable to collaborate with antigen-binding B cells (see below): hence, no IgG response [37].]

The main features of the "deblocking and protection" hypothesis are shown in Figs. 2 and 3 [8,48]. Virgin B cells of high ABC bind much antigen if the amount available to the cell is large. Aggregation of many antigen receptors at the cell surface leads to γC_H gene expression (Fig. 2). Receptor *redistribution* leads to the generation of "on signals" (Fig. 3), the dissociation of antigen plus receptor aggregates, and redistribution of receptors on B cells of high ABC being effected by digestion or removal of the antigen. "On signals" are generated by dissociation of antigen plus receptor microcaps rather than by a general shedding

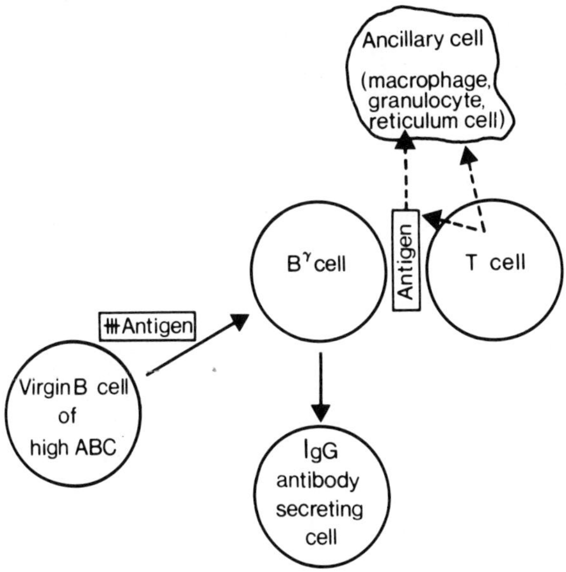

FIG. 2. Proposed scheme for the induction of antigen dose- and T cell-dependent high combining-site affinity IgG antibody production from virgin B cells.

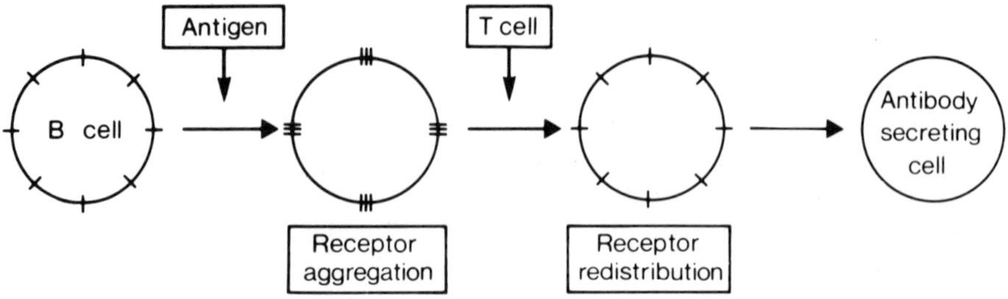

FIG. 3. Scheme of T cell-dependent generation of "on signals" (immune induction) in B cells (D-B cells).

of antigen plus receptor macrocaps [5,164-166]. T cells effect antigen digestion or removal at the B-cell surface either by T-cell dependent, locally active digestive enzymes [167] or via phagocytes which are attracted to, and activated in, the area by T cell-dependent "lymphokines" [168]. Thus, the "second signal" for antigen-binding B cells follows from a reduction in the amount of antigen in antigen plus receptor aggregates at the cell surface. Antigens which are nonmetabolizable will block B cells of high ABC but *stimulate* B cells of low ABC, since the relatively low energy of binding ensures that surface aggregates dissociate. In this way, "on signals" are generated in B cells of low ABC (I-B cells) quite independently of any T-cell influence. Metabolizable, T cell-stimulating antigens will block B cells of high ABC (D-B cells) if reactive T cells are not present. This "blockade" may be quite transient if the antigen is unstable or removed en masse. Several predictions follow.

1. Polymeric structure of antigen will increase efficiency of induction of both immunity and tolerance in B cells [148], the outcome being dependent upon the ABC of the B cell, T cell involvement, antigen dose, and antigen persistence.

2. All antigens will stimulate I-B cells (of low ABC), provided that the antigen is not monomeric (large doses of monomeric antigens which are free of aggregates and endotoxin and which do not aggregate in vivo may block B-cell receptor aggregation and, perhaps by altering receptor turnover, also lead to tolerance [156,169]).

3. Certain doses of antibody will block B cells of low ABC either because of competition for antigenic determinants [170] or because of stabilization of otherwise readily dissociated antigen plus receptor complexes at the cell surface [171].

4. Close physical association of activated T cell and antigen-binding D-B cells increases the efficiency of immune induction (the linked-recognition principle.

5. Production of high combining-site affinity antibodies (perhaps IgG and IgE versus IgM, in general) will be highly dependent on the presence of activated T cells.

6. Hyperactive T cells (or a hyperactive T cell plus phagocyte axis) may in some cases depress expression of B cells (e.g., some "suppressor" T-cell and "antigenic competition" effects) simply because of rapid elimination of the antigen.

7. If T cells also require digestion of antigen at the cell surface before "on signals" are generated, T cells may bind nonmetabolizable antigens, such as SIII, PVP, and LPS, but will not respond to such antigens.

8. In the primary response, where few T cells are present, many D-B cells will be temporarily blocked, I-B cells will be triggered into antibody production, and the appearance of low combining-site affinity (IgM) antibodies will precede that of high combining-site affinity (IgG) antibodies. (Immune induction in B^{γ} cells may be a relatively late event. Axelrad [172] has shown that hyperimmune anti-sRBC antibodies will block the primary IgG PFC response to sRBC when injected at Day 3 after sRBC injection. Moreover, DNP-lys-SIII given 3 days after homologous DNP-protein antigen is still able to block the adoptive secondary IgG anti-DNP response [48]).

9. Complexes of antigen plus cytophilic antibody of the type described by Feldmann and colleagues [148,173,174] will have several effects; e.g., affinity for phagocytes will decrease the availability of antigen and prevent tolerance in B cells of high ABC, while affinity for nonphagocytic ancillary cells will increase the availability of antigen for B cells of low ABC.

10. T cells that mediate antigen digestion functions will be "killer cells"; T cells that influence only phagocyte activities will not be "killer cells" in in vitro cytotoxic reactions [175].

There are two observations on hapten-carrier antigens in rabbits which do not appear to fit with predictions of the "deblocking and protection" hypothesis. First, rabbits primed with a hapten-carrier antigen respond by producing *high*-affinity antihapten antibody upon challenge with the hapten on a heterologous carrier, and, second, carrier preimmunization leads to relatively low-affinity antibody in response to hapten-homologous carrier challenge [111,129]. The observations have been made in one-host systems. Thus, for hapten-primed animals that respond to hapten-heterologous carrier challenge, preexisting antihapten antibody may be reducing the availability, and therefore the tolerogenicity, of the antigen [44]. Klinman and Doughty [176-178] have shown that in vitro challenge of primed cells with high doses of hapten-heterologous carrier leads to inhibition. Low-dose challenge results in expression of hapten-primed B cells; limited expression is apparent even in the absence of any T-cell influence. This dose of antigen is presumably not high enough to induce tolerance in primed B cells of high ABC, and therefore no T cells are required to protect from tolerance. Concerning the effect of carrier preimmunization, one needs to postulate that expression of unprimed B cells of low ABC (which must be in vast excess over B cells of high ABC) prevents the T cell-dependent high-affinity antibody from significantly raising the average affinity measured. Stimulation of an *unprimed* B-cell population must invariably lead to relatively low-affinity antibody; the antibody from triggered B cells of high ABC goes undetected unless a PFC assay is used [112].

The T cell-dependent locally-active digestive enzymes (e.g., proteases) could be from many different origins: T-cell surface enzymes activated after antigen binding, B cell-derived enzymes which are activated by T-cell products, or plasma-derived enzymes activated by T-cell products or T cell-dependent B-cell products. If such extracellular digestive enzymes are not involved and phagocytosis is the critical step in releasing a D-B cell from antigen "blockade," defective phagocytosis should facilitate "blockade" in D-B cells (and "clonal deletion" if "blockade" is a prelude to cell death) just as should a lack of reactive T cells. Studies by Passwell et al. [179] and Sabet et al. [180] indicate that reticuloendothelial (RES) malfunction markedly reduces the titer of high-affinity or IgG antibodies but not that of low-affinity or IgM antibodies. In this respect, the response of mice with a defective RES resembles that of T cell-deficient mice.

Obviously, IgM antibody production to some antigens is T-cell dependent [e.g., sRBC vs (T,G)-A–L], and, in some cases, carrier preimmunization increases primary IgM antihapten antibody responses. Can this observation be accounted for on the basis of the above hypothesis? There need be no parallelism between the amount of antigen (= no. of "antigen signals") required to induce a C_H gene switch in B cells and the amount of antigen required to inhibit (i.e., induce "T cell-independent tolerance"). Thus, a D-B cell of high ABC may switch to γ, but a D-B cell of intermediate ABC may not switch from μC_H gene expression. Both are able to bind enough antigen to be blocked, if not eliminated, in the absence of the T-cell deblocking and protective influence.

In the primary response to aqueous (T,G)-A–L, the number of antigen-reactive T cells recruited can be expected to be low; in the primary response to sRBC, the number of antigen-reactive T cells recruited can be expected to be high. Therefore, in the primary response to (T,G)-A–L, T cells play virtually no role in intact or T cell-deficient mice. By contrast, in the primary response to sRBC, substantial T-cell involvement releases D-B cells of intermediate ABC from "blockade" in intact but not in T cell-deficient mice. In both the sRBC and (T,G)-A–L systems, I-B cells of low ABC are triggered into antibody production independently of any T-cell involvement. In the case of SIII, for example, *only* I-B cells are triggered into antibody production in both intact and T cell-deficient mice. With appropriate T cell (plus phagocyte) stimulation, some anti-SIII D-B cells of intermediate ABC will be protected from tolerance induction because of more efficient phagocytosis and temporary sequestration of SIII in the induction period [131,181,182].

On the point of "linked-recognition," the experiments of Miller et al. [183] suggest that to effect "helper" functions in vivo, T cells must be activated. The efficiency of activated T cells in enhancing B-cell responses is increased by inducing the T-cell activation in the vicinity of antigen-binding B cells. This proximity requirement is best illustrated by the "carrier effect," in which much lower doses of the homologous hapten-carrier conjugate are required to stimulate carrier-primed T and hapten-primed B cells than of a mixture of the same hapten and carrier on separate molecules [6,46,184]. In the "allogeneic effect" in vivo, in which reactions that involve histoincompatible T and B cells markedly increase antibody production, the optimal conditions usually involve a reaction of T cells against histocompatibility antigens on the B cells which are presumably binding haptenic determinants ([6,185-187], cf. Ref. 188).

IV. B^{μ} and B^{γ} Cells

The terms B^{μ} and B^{γ} cell have been used as short hand for "B-cell precursor of IgM antibody-secreting cell" and "B-cell precursor of IgG antibody-secreting cell," respectively. As discussed above, many B^{μ} cells are I-B cells (i.e., I-B^{μ} cells), whereas most B^{γ} cells are D-B cells (i.e., D-B^{γ} cells). The designation B^{γ} is not meant to infer that these cells are expressing a γC_H gene at the time of contact with the test antigen. With the assumption that all virgin B cells are B^{μ} cells, B^{γ} cells reactive to a particular test antigen can be of two types: *preformed* and expressing a γC_H gene, or *inducible* and expressing a μC_H gene, at the time point under consideration. (With respect to the notation "virgin B cell," recent studies by Pernis and Rowe [189] suggest that, in the human at least, δ-chain expression may well accompany μ-chain expression in the maturation of B cells from their precursors.) Anti-μ chain sera are able to block IgG antibody responses and production of all subclasses of IgG immunoglobulin [190-193]. Yet, if the target cells for T cell-dependent allotype suppression in mice [194,195] are B cells (rather than early progeny of B cells), such B cells must express the γ chain at the cell surface. A positive identification of γ chains at the cell surface has been obtained in many studies (reviewed in Refs. 196 and 197).

In view of the finding that IgM and IgG antibodies often differ in intrinsic combining-site affinities for a particular determinant, virgin B^μ cells of high ABC must switch to B^γ cells, perhaps simply as a consequence of contact with relatively large amounts of antigen. Such B cells (D-B^γ cells) will then be highly dependent on the deblocking and protective T-cell influence for their further maturation to IgG antibody-secreting cells. By invoking antigen only as the pressure for switch, IgG antibodies, but not IgM antibodies, will invariably have a high combining-site affinity for the antigenic determinant *which effected the switch.* With respect to antigen A, a cross-reacting T cell-stimulating and/or readily metabolized antigen A′ may effect a switch in B^μ cells of high ABC, no tolerance induction, and the development of preformed B^γ cells capable of responding to antigen A. If the association constant of receptor site plus A is low (cf. receptor plus A′), this B^γ cell may well be "turned on" by antigen A independently of T cells. That is, the switched nonvirgin cell is an I-B^γ cell for antigen A but a D-B^γ cell for antigen A′. With this reasoning, a small amount of T-cell independent low-affinity IgG antibody production to a particular test antigen can be expected in athymic *nu/nu* mice previously exposed to cross-reacting antigens. The experiments of Chiller and Weigle [67], Roelants and Askonas [198], and Tao-Wiedmann [38] indicate that the induction of B-cell memory (e.g., expansion and/or switch and/or switch plus expansion) need not be T-cell dependent, provided that low amounts of antigen are used or late time points after antigen administration are examined. Moreover, studies on the inhibition of antigen-binding cells in "nonresponders" to (T,G)-A–L suggest that B^μ cells switch to B^γ cells independently of any T-cell influence [199]. As mentioned above, the *expression* of this memory status in B cells is greatly enhanced by reactive T cells.

Lafleur [200] has been able to partially enrich and deplete for B^γ cells by vigorously agitating splenic rosette-forming cells (RFC) against foreign red cells or haptenated red cells and separating the residual RFC by velocity sedimentation. RFC-rich fractions, when injected with T cells plus antigen into irradiated recipients, preferentially induce IgG PFC responses. Agitation presumably selects against cells of low ABC, but it is not yet known whether the residual RFC (of high ABC?) are expressing μ and/or γC_H genes.

Certain difficulties of interpretation are inherent in experiments that involve putative separations of B^μ and B^γ cells as tested by subsequent IgM versus IgG antibody production. Removal of B^γ cells from a mixed B-cell population will reduce the amounts of IgG antibody synthesized by residual cells on adoptive transfer. If this antibody normally has a marked negative influence on total IgM antibody production, the amount of IgM antibody produced by the depleted fraction of cells may well be high. However, until additional information is available on the number of IgM clones present in recipients of the depleted fraction, it is premature to assume that most B^{μ} cells have not been removed along with the B^{γ} cells. For example, a RFC fraction may contion 100% of the B^{γ} cells and 90% of the B^{μ} cells. The remaining 10% B^{μ} cells in the RFC-depleted fraction of cells may be capable of producing much IgM antibody in the absence of IgG antibodies. Conversely, the expression of the B^{μ} cells in the RFC fraction will be limited by the IgG antibodies produced by B^{γ} cells. Information of the type which can be obtained from isoelectric focusing techniques (modified for the detection of IgM) becomes essential in this type of experiment.

The outcome of the reaction among B^{μ} cells, B^{γ} cells, and antigen is highly dependent on the dose of antigen used and on the duration of contact with antigen. As discussed above, inhibition of B^{γ} cells is readily induced in vivo by high doses of metabolizable, T cell-stimulating antigens in athymic mice or by nonmetabolizable, apparently non-T cell-stimulating antigens in intact mice. Dose effects are quite pronounced: low doses of DNP-lys-SIII readily inhibit adoptive secondary IgG anti-DNP responses to DNP-MSH [48, 116], whereas much higher doses are required to block a primary IgG anti-DNP response to DNP-FγG [8,49]. Moreover, large doses of DNP-lys-SIII (milligram amounts) will also partially inhibit the primary IgM anti-DNP responses [201]. Low-affinity IgM antibody production is relatively resistant to tolerance induction [202-205]; such antibodies are derived from I-B cells.

Variable results have been obtained in experiments designed to test the effects of low or high epitope density on IgG versus IgM antibody production in vivo. It seems that antigen dose, antigen persistence, and epitope density all contribute to the class distribution of antibodies. *High* doses of *lightly* conjugated haptenated proteins [206,207] and cells ([143] cf. Ref. 207) preferentially induce IgG responses in mice, and polymeric structure is required to induce an IgM response [206]. Very low doses of sRBC induce *IgM* and not IgG antibody responses [208]. Are the B^{μ} cells which respond to *low*-dose sRBC (by producing IgM antibodies) of high ABC, and are they identical to those which switch to γG_H gene expression with *high* doses of antigen (e.g., Fig. 4)? Unfortunately, there is no experimental evidence which bears on this question.

V. Linkage of Ir Genes to Loci That Code for Cell Surface Antigens, Such as Histocompatibility and Ig Allotypic Antigens

The evidence is compelling that T cells are "functionally silent" in H-linked genetic low responsiveness to antigens, such as (T,G)-A–L, in mice. Specifically

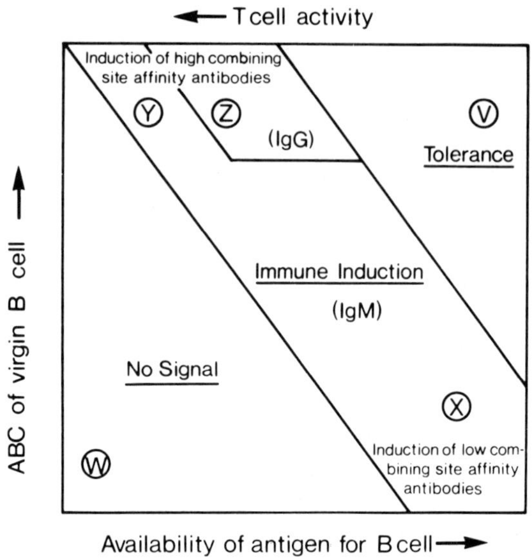

FIG. 4. An attempt to highlight the main features of the hypothesis developed in this chapter in diagram form (the slopes of lines and areas of compartments are meaningless). As extremes, tolerance is the consequence of an encounter between antigen and a virgin B cell of high ABC, provided the availability of antigen is high (point V), whereas no signals are generated in B cells of low ABC when the availability of antigen is low (point W). B cells of low ABC are induced into antibody production (IgM), provided the availability of antigen is high (point X). B cells of high ABC are switched from μ (point Y) to γG_H gene expression (and thus IgG antibody production) with certain amounts of antigen (point Z) and tolerized by excessive amounts of antigen (point V).

T cells reduce the availability of antigen for B cells and thereby deblock and prevent tolerance in B cells of high ABC. By the same token, hyperactive T cells (± phagocytes) will *prevent* expression of antibody formation in some B cells by reducing the availability of antigen. Production of high combining-site affinity antibodies will be highly T-cell dependent, quite unlike production of low combining-site affinity IgM antibodies. It must be emphasized that these considerations apply to virgin B cells. As discussed in the text, B cells with low ABC for an antigenic determinant A may have switched from μ to γ in response to a cross-reacting determinant A′ for which the cell has a high ABC. The production of *low*-affinity anti-A IgG antibody by this *primed* B cell may well be initiated independently of T cells, provided the availability of determinant A is high.

reactive T cells are either absent (but see Ref. 209), readily tolerized [126], or unable to interact with specifically reactive B cells [210-212]. It is proposed in the above hypothesis that B cells of high ABC (D-B^γ cells) contact antigen readily and are susceptible to inhibition by such antigen. Moreover, it is proposed that T cells react with cell surface-associated antigen, particularly with antigen on B cells of high ABC, where the antigen is arranged at the cell surface in aggregates or microcaps in the case of polymeric antigens. Conceivably, therefore, the recognition of B^γ cell-associated antigen by T cells may well be dependent on the H specificities in the local area of the B-cell receptor. The findings in an ingenious experiment by Katz et al. [212] can be interpreted in this way. Parental "GLT nonresponder" B cells primed to DNP are not able to interact with F_1 "GLT responder" T cells primed to GLT in a T-cell dependent, acute, adoptive anti-DNP antibody response to DNP-GLT.

Certain allotypic specificities at the cell surface may similarly present a "block to interaction" between hapten-reactive B^γ cells and carrier-reactive T cells. An association between Ig allotype and antibody production has been demonstrated in several systems; one is the response of mice to a decapeptide from TMVP [213]. Preliminary antigen-binding studies by Roelants [214] have thus far shown no differences in the number of splenic decapeptide-binding, Ig positive cells in *unprimed* low and high responders, a finding analogous to the observations on antigen-binding B cells in H-linked low and high responsiveness [199].

The prediction is that only high-affinity (IgG) antibody responses will be subject to regulation by B-cell surface-associated antigens. B^μ cells of low ABC, which do not require T cells for expression of low-grade IgM antibody production to (T,G)-A–L, for example [37], will not be influenced by the fickleness of T cells to react with antigen when bound to B cells. Ready dissociation of receptor plus antigen complexes ensures that such cells are induced into IgM antibody production. In fact, such cells may not bind antigen in sufficient amounts at any one time to ensure recruitment of reactive T cells. In "nonresponders," the B^γ cells that bind antigen will be blocked as a consequence of their failure to recruit T cells in their immediate neighborhood. If virgin B cells in mice are B^μ and are not expressing IgG allotypes, the allotype-linked genetic control may only apply to secondary immune responses, not to early primary IgM or *IgG* antibody production.

If, indeed, T cells of either "responder" or "nonresponder" genotype are incapable of interacting with antigen-binding "nonresponder" B^γ cells, the results in tetraparental mice and radiation chimeras require an explanation [215,216]. "Nonresponder" allotype antibody production to (T,G)-A–L is markedly increased in chimeras of "nonresponder" (of one Ig allotype) and "responder" cells (of another Ig allotype). Perhaps, in these apparently stable chimeras, there is sufficient residual anti-"nonresponder" histocompatibility antigen reactivity, or even *anti-"nonresponder" allotype* reactivity of "responder"-strain T cells, which enables antigen-binding "nonresponder" B^{γ} cells to be triggered. It would be interesting to know (and relevant to the question of IgG expression on B^{γ} cells) whether antiallotype-reactive T cells [194] of one *H-2* type would stimulate IgG anti-(T,G)-A–L antibody production in (T,G)-A–L "nonresponder" mice of the same *H-2* type but different Ig allotype.

VI. "Suppressor" T Cells

It is now readily accepted that activated T cells play a regulatory role in antibody production and do not invariably increase the total amount of antibody produced by B cells. Increased antibody responses in T cell-deficient mice and reduced titers after injection of excess T cells have been reported (reviewed in Refs. 126 and 217). These observations, together with those of others [218, 219] on the influence of T cells on homocytotropic (IgE?) versus IgG antibody synthesis, have led to the postulate that T cells may enhance ("helper" function) or inhibit ("suppressor" function) the expression of the various types of B cells reactive to a particular antigen. Much care is required in interpretation of "suppressor" T-cell effects if only one (sub) class of antibody or one type of antibody assay is being examined. "Helper" T-cell activities, by increasing one (sub) class of antibody, may *indirectly* suppress the expression of another (sub) class by means of feedback inhibition by antibody (e.g., IgG versus IgM and IgE).

As discussed by Droege [217] and Gershon [126], several different phenomena are likely to be involved in what are currently called "suppressor" T-cell effects. For example, Backer et al. [220] have reported that antilymphocyte serum (ALS) administration markedly increases the PFC response to SIII in some, but not all, strains of mice and in intact, but not athymic, *nu/nu* mice. We have found that CBA mice in the National Institute for Medical Research laboratories, Mill Hill, are poor responders to SIII, that C_3H are good responders, and that CBA, but not C_3H, mice contain high serum titers of "natural" anti-SIII antibody [116]. Therefore, in the system of Baker et al., it is possible that ALS, by acting on antibody-secreting cells and T cells, but not B cells, reduces levels of natural anti-SIII antibodies, which leads to an increased response to low doses of SIII. Reversal of the ALS effect by additional T cells would then reflect the high absorptive capacity of T cells for ALS and the resultant protection of "natural" anti-SIII antibody-secreting cells. Alternatively, ALS may activate phagocytes and thereby reduce the availability and tolerogenicity of SIII for B cells, which have a higher ABC than do I-B cells [131,181,182].

What, then, of the Kerbel and Eidinger [221] observation that mere adult thymectomy leads to a six- to eightfold increase in the response of mice to PVP, another persistent antigen? An unknown in this system is the effect of reinjected thymocytes, but one is pushed to explain this observation in terms other than "suppressor" T cells. Virtually nothing is known about the role of the thymus as a large reservoir of target lymphocytes for various regulators. Levels of serum substances with affinity for lymphocytes (e.g., hormones, autoantibodies) could be markedly increased for some time after thymectomy. Such substances in increased amounts may stimulate B cells responding to antigens, such as PVP and SIII. These substances may increase responses to persistent non-T cell-stimulating antigens, but not to metabolizable, T cell-stimulating antigens. Perhaps relevant to this point is the observation that in *primary* responses, the "allogeneic effect" increases the antibody response to non-T cell-stimulating and/or persisting antigens, but not the response to T cell-stimulating antigens [222,223].

In T cell-dependent allotype suppression [194,195], the "suppressor" T cell is presumably a normal T cell of the antigen-reactive type which responds to the paternal Ig allotype (when cell associated?) in the (SJL × BALB/c) F_1 mouse. Such a T cell never survives thymic processes of selection against "self" [224] when the paternal allotype is expressed and not masked by antibody early in life. [Jerne [162] and others [151] have speculated on the regulatory role of anti-Ig reactive T cells. If anti-*idiotype*-reactive T cells exist, such cells may well bind B-cell products (i.e., antibodies) and possibly acquire reactivity to specific antigen if the valence of the antibody is high (IgM) such that a net excess of combining sites is available for antigen binding [225]. In this way, some antigen-reactive T cells would have an identical antigen reactivity spectrum as some antigen-reactive B cells, simply because a B-cell product mediates recognition in both cells (c.f. the above speculation (Sec. II) on antiidiotypic antibody-mediated regulation of T cell reactivities).]

As part of the specific "suppressor" T-cell effect, it has been proposed that T cells are required for tolerance induction in B cells [126]. The experiments on which this proposal is based were performed with "B mice" given small numbers of T cells at the time of injection of large amounts of sRBC [226]. As mentioned previously, anti-sRBC B^{γ} cells in athymic *nu/nu* mice are highly susceptible to tolerance induction [97]; this observation is incompatible with that discussed above. A comparison of the two systems is difficult: in the Gershon and Kondo experiments [226], half of the mice were discarded at the time of testing for tolerance, hemagglutination titers were very low in all mice, and the majority of "sRBC-tolerant" mice responded poorly to an injection of T cells plus hRBC. Therefore, there seems to be no good evidence that T cells are required for tolerance induction in B cells, and the numerous studies cited above (and used as the basis of the hypothesis in Sec. III) speak strongly against the idea.

"Suppressor" T-cell effects can be readily explained by the above hypothesis, which ascribes to the T cell plus phagocyte axis the role of converting antigen-dependent "off signals" to "on signals" by antigen elimination. In some situations after priming with antigen, the T cell plus phagocyte combination may be excessively efficient at eliminating antigen, and fewer B cells receive any "on signals" at all. Both I-B cells and D-B cells could be affected by reduced amounts of available antigen. "Antigenic competition" may have a similar basis.

Parish [227] has demonstrated that partially modified flagellin antigens are potent inducers of cellular hypersensitivity but are tolerogens for antibody production. Since the sensitized T cells are present at the time of testing for tolerance, it would be interesting to know whether the hyperactivity of T cells (±phagocytes) actually caused the reduced expression of B cells. Information on antigen-binding T and B cells would be useful in this system. Hyperactive phagocytes have been implicated in an increasing number of inhibitory phenomena [181,182,228,229]. If the end result of an excess of activated T cells and hyperactive phagocytes is rapid antigen elimination, there is presumably not much left for the B cell to do and certainly no reason to produce antibody.

VII. Concluding Comments

This chapter has been concerned with the outcome of the encounter between B cells and antigen in vivo and the manner in which T cells modify the outcome. Emphasis has been placed on the availability of antigen for B cells of various binding capacities and the influence of T cells in regulating the availability of antigen for B cells (Fig. 4). By releasing B cells from antigen "blockade," T cells not only protect antigen-binding B cells from "of signals" (→tolerance) but also promote "on signals" (→immunity), perhaps via redistribution of released B-cell receptors.

Why this "deblocking and protection" hypothesis on the nature of the interaction between T and B cells rather than "antigen presentation" (see, e.g., Refs. 9 and 146-148) or "soluble differentiative or proliferative factor" (see, e.g., Ref. 6) hypotheses? There are difficulties with the two latter hypotheses. First, antigen presentation proposals infer that B cells not able to bind antigen are encouraged to do so by T cells or their products. Thus, T cells, either directly or indirectly, would increase production of low-affinity antibody production by the B-cell population. This is not the case in vivo [100,101]. Second, soluble factor proposals infer that the ever-present B cells with antiself reactivity will be encouraged to produce antibodies by factors secreted by nearby T cells responding to foreign antigens. This may be risky for a system that wishes to preserve self-tolerance [150].

The approach in this paper has been nothing but speculative, with an attempt to fit certain experimental data into a favored hypothesis on the early events in induction of antibody production and tolerance and the interactions among T cells, B cells, antigen, and ancillary cells and substances. Such an approach is naturally biased.

Acknowledgments

I wish to thank Dr. Niels Jerne and the members of The Basel Institute for Immunology for the opportunity of working in the excellent environment of the Institute, also my immediate colleagues Louis Lafleur, John Hamilton, and Russell Little for numerous discussions, Mrs. Kerstin Andersson for outstanding technical assistance in the experiments performed at this Institute and referred to in the paper, Mr. H. Stahlberger for the illustrations, and Penny Hamilton, Mary Watton, and Catherine Takacs for typing the manuscript.

References

1. I. M. Roitt, M. F. Greaves, G. Torrigiani, J. Brostoff, and J. H. L. Playfair, Lancet ii, 367 (1969).
2. H. N. Claman and D. E. Mosier, Progr. Allergy **16**, 40 (1972).
3. M. Cohn, Cell. Immunol. **5**, 1 (1972).
4. A. L. de Weck, Transplant. Rev. **10**, 3 (1972).
5. E. Diener and R. E. Langman, Progr. Allergy **18**, 6 (1975).
6. D. H. Katz and B. Benacerraf, Advan. Immunol. **15**, 1 (1972).
7. J. F. A. P. Miller, A. Basten, J. Sprent and C. Cheers, Cell. Immunol. **2**, 469 (1971).
8. G. F. Mitchell, in *Contemporary Topics in Immunobiology* (M. D. Cooper and N. L. Warner, eds.), Plenum Press, New York, 1973, Vol. 3, p. 97.
9. N. A. Mitchison, K. Rajewsky, and R. B. Taylor, in *Developmental Aspects of Antibody Formation* (J. Steřzl and I. Rihǎ, eds.), Academia, Prague, 1970, p. 547.
10. M. C. Raff, Nature (London) **242**, 19 (1973).
11. J. C. Howard, S. W. Hunt, and J. L. Gowans, J. Exp. Med. **135**, 200 (1972).

12. J. Sprent and J. F. A. P. Miller, Eur. J. Immunol. **2**, 384 (1972).
13. S. Strober and J. Dilley, J. Exp. Med. **137**, 1275 (1973).
14. G. Gutman and I. L. Weissman, Immunology **23**, 465 (1972).
15. B. Balfour, in *Proceedings of the International Conference on the Spleen,* Cluj, Romania, 1973.
16. K. Borum and M. H. Claesson, Acta Pathol. Microbiol. Scand. Sect. A **79**, 561 (1971).
17. R. H. Kelly, Nature (London) **227**, 510 (1970).
18. J. F. A. P. Miller and A. J. S. Davies, Annu. Rev. Med. **15**, 23 (1964).
19. H. Cantor, Cell. Immunol. **3**, 461 (1972).
20. H. Cantor, in *Cell Interactors: Third Lepetit Colloquium* (L. G. Silvestri, ed.), North-Holland, Amsterdam, 1972, p. 172.
21. M. C. Raff and H. Cantor, in *Progress in Immunology* (B. Amos, ed.), Academic Press, New York, 1971, p. 83.
22. L. Lafleur, R. G. Miller, and R. A. Phillips, J. Exp. Med. **137**, 954 (1973).
23. J. H. L. Playfair and E. C. Purves, Nature [New Biol.] **231**, 149 (1971).
24. K. Zeiller, E. Holzberg, G. Pascher, and K. Hannig, Hoppe-Seyler's Z. Physiol. Chem. **353**, 105 (1972).
25. J.-F. Bach and M. Dardenne, Cell. Immunol. **6**, 394 (1973).
26. J. F. A. P. Miller and G. F. Mitchell, in *Lymphatic Tissue and Germinal Centers in Immune Response* (L. Fiore-Donati and M. G. Hanna, Jr., eds.), Plenum Press, New York, 1969, p. 455.
27. L. Olsson and M. H. Claesson, Nature [New Biol.] **244**, 50 (1973).
28. D. Metcalf and M. A. S. Moore, Haemopoietic Cells, North-Holland, Amsterdam, 1971.
29. J. R. Battisto, F. Borek, and R. A. Bucsi, Cell. Immunol. **2**, 627 (1971).
30. R. A. Bucsi, F. Borek, and J. R. Battisto, J. Exp. Med. **136**, 761 (1972).
31. B. A. Askonas and G. E. Roelants, Eur. J. Immunol. **4**, 1 (1974).
32. D. H. Katz and E. R. Unanue, J. Exp. Med. **137**, 967 (1973).
33. G. J. V. Nossal and G. L. Ada, *Antigens, Lymphoid Cells and the Immune Response,* Academic Press, New York, 1971.
34. R. S. Basch, Int. Arch. Allergy Appl. Immunol. **30**, 105 (1966).
35. M. W. Hess and R. D. Stoner, Int. Arch. Allergy Appl. Immunol. **30**, 37 (1966).
36. E. Kolsch, A. J. S. Davies, and E. Leuchars, Eur. J. Immunol. **2**, 541 (1972).
37. G. F. Mitchell, F. C. Grumet, and H. O. McDevitt, J. Exp. Med. **135**, 126 (1972).
38. T. W. Tao-Wiedmann, Personal communication (1973).
39. N. R. St. C. Sinclair, Immunology **12**, 549 (1967).
40. E. M. Pantalouris and P. A. Flisch, Eur. J. Immunol. **2**, 236 (1972).
41. G. J. Svet-Moldavsky, S. N. Zinzar, and N. M. Spector, Nature (London) **202**, 353 (1964).
42. J. F. A. P. Miller and D. Osoba, Physiol. Rev. **47**, 437 (1967).

43. H. N. Eisen, J. R. Little, L. A. Steiner, E. S. Simms, and W. Gray, Israel J. Med. Sci. **5**, 338 (1969).
44. S. Kontiainen and O. Mäkelä, Immunology **20**, 101 (1971).
45. W. E. Paul, G. W. Siskind, B. Benacerraf, and Z. Ovary, J. Immunol. **99**, 760 (1967).
46. N. A. Mitchison, Eur. J. Immunol. **1**, 18 (1971).
47. M. C. Raff, Nature (London) **226**, 1257 (1970).
48. G. F. Mitchell, J. H. Humphrey, and A. R. Williamson, Eur. J. Immunol. **2**, 460 (1972).
49. G. F. Mitchell, J. H. Humphrey, and J. A. Hamilton, in *Proceedings of the International Conference on the Spleen,* Cluj, Romania, 1973.
50. E. Möller, W. W. Bullock, and O. Mäkelä, Eur. J. Immunol. **3**, 172 (1973).
51. B. Rubin, Eur. J. Immunol. **3**, 11 (1972).
52. B. Rubin, V. Schirrmacher, and H. Wigzell, in *Microenvironmental Aspects of Immunity* (B. D. Jankovic and K. Isakovic, eds.), Plenum Press, New York, 1973, Vol. 29, p. 133.
53. A. J. Cunningham and E. E. Sercarz, Eur. J. Immunol. **1**, 413 (1971).
54. G. F. Mitchell, E. L. Chan, M. S. Noble, I. L. Weissman, R. I. Mishell, and L. A. Herzenberg, J. Exp. Med. **135**, 165 (1972).
55. J. E. Niederhuber and E. Möller, Cell. Immunol. **6**, 407 (1973).
56. T. Takahashi, E. A. Carswell, and G. J. Thorbecke, J. Exp. Med. **132**, 1181 (1970).
57. J. Aird, Immunology **20**, 617 (1971).
58. E. Kolsch, E. Diller, G. Weber, and A. J. S. Davies, Eur. J. Immunol. **1**, 201 (1971).
59. G. F. Mitchell, R. I. Mishell, and L. A. Herzenberg, in *Progress in Immunology* (D. Amos, ed.), Academic Press, New York, 1971, p. 324.
60. N. R. St. C. Sinclair and E. V. Elliot, Immunology **15**, 325 (1968).
61. R. B. Taylor and H. H. Wortis, Nature (London) **220**, 927 (1968).
62. G. Torrigiani, J. Immunol. **108**, 161 (1972).
63. E. Unanue, J. Immunol. **105**, 1339 (1970).
64. B. A. Askonas, A. J. S. Davies, E. B. Jacobson, E. Leuchars, and G. E. Roelants, Immunology **23**, 791 (1972).
65. D. Dresser, Eur. J. Immunol. **2**, 50 (1972).
66. R. Falkoff and J. Kettman, J. Immunol. **108**, 54 (1972).
67. J. M. Chiller and W. O. Weigle, J. Exp. Med. **137**, 740 (1973).
68. I. Gery, J. Krüger, and S. Z. Spiesel, J. Immunol. **108**, 1088 (1972).
69. J. M. Jones and P. Kind, J. Immunol. **108**, 1453 (1972).
70. G. Möller, J. Andersson, and O. Sjöberg, Cell. Immunol. **4**, 416 (1972).
71. J. R. Schmidtke and F. J. Dixon, J. Exp. Med. **136**, 392 (1972).
72. J. W. Schrader, J. Exp. Med. **137**, 844 (1973).
73. A. Allison and A. J. S. Davies, Nature (London) **233**, 330 (1971).
74. P. Del Guercio, Nature [New Biol.] **238**, 213 (1972).
75. R. N. Taub and R. K. Gershon, J. Immunol. **108**, 377 (1972).
76. P. Hunter and A. J. Munro, Immunology **23**, 69 (1972).

77. K. Isaković, S. B. Smith, and B. H. Waksman, J. Exp. Med. **122**, 1103 (1965).
78. B. Kindred, Eur. J. Immunol. **1**, 59 (1971).
79. J. F. A. P. Miller, P. Dukor, G. Grant, N. R. St. C. Sinclair, and E. Sacquet, Clin. Exp. Immunol. **2**, 531 (1967).
80. N. R. St. C. Sinclair, Clin. Exp. Immunol. **2**, 701 (1967).
81. H. H. Wortis, Clin. Exp. Immunol. **8**, 305 (1971).
82. J. G. Howard, Transplant. Rev. **8**, 50 (1972).
83. J. K. Manning, N. D. Reed, and J. W. Jutila, J. Immunol. **108**, 1470 (1972).
84. P. Del Guercio and E. Leuchars, J. Immunol. **109**, 951 (1972).
85. B. Andersson, Doctoral Thesis, Tryckeri Balder, Stockholm, 1972.
86. B. Andersson and H. Blomgren, Cell. Immunol. **2**, 411 (1971).
87. G. Möller and G. Michael, Cell. Immunol. **2**, 309 (1971).
88. E. Kölsch, A. J. S. Davies, and E. Leuchars, Eur. J. Immunol. **2**, 541 (1972).
89. C. Cheers and J. F. A. P. Miller, J. Exp. Med. **136**, 1661 (1972).
90. M. Hurme, S. Kontiainen, I. J. T. Seppälä, O. Mäkelä, Eur. J. Immunol. **3**, 191 (1973).
91. D. H. Katz, W. E. Paul, E. A. Goidl, and B. Benacerraf, J. Exp. Med. **132**, 261 (1970).
92. J. Kettman and R. W. Dutton, Proc. Nat. Acad. Sci. USA **68**, 699 (1971).
93. S. Kontiainen, Eur. J. Immunol. **1**, 276 (1971).
94. V. Schirrmacher and K. Rajewsky, J. Exp. Med. **132**, 1019 (1970).
95. I. S. Trowbridge and H. R. Andersson, Eur. J. Immunol. **2**, 565 (1972).
96. J. Wrede, M. L. Gundelach, and E. Rüde, Personal communication.
97. G. F. Mitchell, L. A. Lafleur, and K. Andersson, Scand. J. Immunol. **3**, 39 (1974).
98. P. J. Baker and P. W. Stashak, J. Immunol. **103**, 1342 (1969).
99. G. Michael, Personal communication (1973).
100. R. K. Gershon and K. Kondo, Immunology **23**, 335 (1972).
101. R. K. Gershon and W. E. Paul, J. Immunol. **106**, 872 (1971).
102. M. M. Frank and J. H. Humphrey, J. Exp. Med. **127**, 967 (1968).
103. C. L. Hornick and F. Karusch, Immunochemistry **9**, 325 (1972).
104. O. Mäkelä, and A. M. Cross, Progr. Allergy **14**, 145 (1970).
105. O. Mäkelä, E. Ruoslahti, and I. J. T. Seppälä, Immunochemistry **7**, 917 (1970).
106. E. Merler, L. Karlin, and S. Matsumoto, J. Biol. Chem. **243**, 386 (1968).
107. H. Metzgar, Advan. Immunol. **12**, 52 (1970).
108. E. W. Voss, Jr. and H. N. Eisen, Fed. Proc. **27**, 684 (1968).
109. E. W. Voss, Jr. and M. M. Sigel, J. Immunol. **109**, 665 (1972).
110. G. W. Siskind, P. Dunn, and J. G. Walker, J. Exp. Med. **127**, 55 (1968).
111. L. A. Steiner and H. N. Eisen, J. Exp. Med. **126**, 1161 (1967).
112. L. Claflin and B. Merchant, J. Immunol. **110**, 252 (1973).
113. S. Fazekas de St. Groth and A. L. Notkins, in *Progress in Immunology*

(D. Amos, ed.), Academic Press, New York, 1971, p. 1215 (Workshop no. 15).
114. J. L. Fahey and J. H. Humphrey, Immunology **5**, 104 (1962).
115. R. Kearney and W. J. Halliday, Immunology **19**, 551 (1970).
116. G. F. Mitchell and J. H. Humphrey, in *Microenvironmental Aspects of Immunity* (B. D. Jankovic and K. Isakovic, eds.), Plenum Press, New York, 1973, Vol. 29, p. 125.
117. A. Ray, I. Nakamura, and O. Mäkelä, Unpublished results (1972).
118. P. Crewther and N. L. Warner, Aust. J. Exp. Biol. Med. Sci. **50**, 625 (1972).
119. T. Tada and K. Okumura, J. Immunol. **106**, 1002 (1971).
120. D. H. Katz, T. Hamaoka, and B. Benacerraf, Proc. Nat. Acad. Sci. USA, **70**, 2776 (1973).
121. M. Sela, Harvey Lect., **67**, 213 (1973).
122. M. Sela, E. Mozes, and G. M. Shearer, Proc. Nat. Acad. Sci. USA **69**, 2696 (1972).
123. J. J. Miranda, Immunology **23**, 829 (1972).
124. A. J. Munro, Personal communication (1972).
125. A. J. S. Davies, R. L. Carter, E. Leuchars, V. Wallis, and F. M. Dietrich, Immunology **19**, 945 (1970).
126. R. K. Gershon, in *Contemporary Topics in Immunobiology* (M. D. Cooper, and N. L. Warner, eds.), Plenum Press, New York, 1973, in press, Vol. 3.
127. J. Krüger and R. K. Gershon, J. Immunol. **108**, 581 (1972).
128. R. J. Gerety, R. W. Ferraresi, and S. Raffel, J. Exp. Med. **131**, 189 (1970).
129. W. E. Paul, G. W. Siskind, B. Benacerraf, and Z. Ovary, J. Immunol. **99**, 760 (1967).
130. W. J. Halliday, Bacteriol. Rev. **35**, 267 (1971).
131. P. Byfield, Cell. Immunol. **3**, 616 (1972).
132. C. A. Janeway, Jr. and M. Sela, Immunology **13**, 29 (1967).
133. G. Möller, Cell. Immunol. **1**, 573 (1970).
134. M. Feldmann and A. Basten, J. Exp. Med. **134**, 103 (1971).
135. A. Coutinho and G. Möller, Personal communication (1973).
136. P. Dukor, Personal communication (1973).
137. P. Dukor and K.-U. Hartmann, Cell. Immunol. in press (1976).
138. G. F. Mitchell, S. Kontiainen, J. A. Hamilton, and G. G. Klaus, Unpublished observations (1972).
139. D. T. Golan and Y. Borel, J. Exp. Med. **134**, 1046 (1971).
140. H. F. Havas, Immunology **17**, 819 (1969).
141. C. S. Walters, J. W. Moorhead, and H. N. Claman, J. Exp. Med. **136**, 546 (1972).
142. J. A. Hamilton and J. F. A. P. Miller, Eur. J. Immunol. **3**, 457 (1973).
143. D. Naor, S. Morecki, and G. F. Mitchell, Eur. J. Immunol., **4**, 311 (1974).
144. D. H. Katz, T. Hamaoka, and B. Benacerraf, J. Exp. Med. **136**, 1404 (1972).

145. F. C. Grumet, in *Genetic Control of Immune Responsiveness* (H. O. McDevitt and M. Landy, eds.), Academic Press, New York, 1972, p. 34.
146. P. J. Lachmann, Proc. Roy. Soc. London Ser. B **176**, 425 (1971).
147. M. J. Taussig and P. J. Lachmann, Immunology **22**, 185 (1972).
148. M. Feldmann and G. J. V. Nossal, Transplant. Rev. **13**, 3 (1972).
149. P. Bretscher, Transplant. Rev. **11**, 218 (1972).
150. M. Cohn, in *Genetic Control of Immune Responsiveness* (H. O. McDevitt, and M. Landy, eds.), Academic Press, New York, 1972, p. 367.
151. A. C. Allison, A. M. Denman, and R. D. Barnes, Lancet **ii**, 135 (1971).
152. L. E. Glynn and E. J. Holborrow, Autoimmunity and Disease, Oxford University Press, Oxford, 1965.
153. B. Halpern and G. Bourdon, C. R. Acad. Sci. Paris **273**, 2712 (1971).
154. G. M. Iverson and J. Lindenmann, Eur. J. Immunol. **2**, 195 (1972).
155. J. H. L. Playfair and S. Marshall-Clark, Nature [New Biol.] **243**, 214 (1973).
155a. M. Schlesinger, Progr. Allergy **16**, 214 (1972).
156. W. O. Weigle, Advan. Immunol. **16**, 61 (1973).
157. D. W. Dresser, Immunology **5**, 378 (1962).
158. N. A. Mitchison, Proc. Roy. Soc. London Ser. B **161**, 275 (1964).
159. G. R. Shellam and G. J. V. Nossal, Immunology **14**, 273 (1968).
160. N. A. Mitchison, in *Cell Interactions: Third Lepetit Colloquium* (L. G. Silvestri, ed.), North-Holland, Amsterdam, 1972, p. 112.
161. K. Rajewsky, C. Brenig, and I. Melchers, in *Cell Interactions: Third Lepetit Colloquium* (L. G. Silverstri, ed.), North-Holland, Amsterdam, 1972, p. 196.
162. N. K. Jerne, in *Proceedings of the Pasteur Memorial Symposium,* Pasteur Institute, Paris, 1973.
163. J. Ordal, F. C. Grumet, and H. O. McDevitt, Personal communication (1973).
164. E. Diener and V. H. Paetkau, Proc. Nat. Acad. Sci. USA, **69**, 2364 (1972).
165. M. C. Raff, M. Feldmann, and S. de Petris, J. Exp. Med. **137**, 1024 (1973).
166. G. Roelants, L. Forni, and B. Pernis, J. Exp. Med. **137**, 1060 (1973).
167. B. Levine, in *Genetic Control of Immune Responsiveness* (H. O. McDevitt and M. Landy, eds.), Academic Press, New York, 1972, p. 271.
168. Anonymous, Lancet **i**, 1490 (1973).
169. D. W. Dresser and N. A. Mitchison, Advan. Immunol. **8**, 129 (1968).
170. J. W. Uhr and G. Möller, Advan. Immunol. **8**, 81 (1968).
171. E. Diener and M. Feldmann, Transplant. Rev. **8**, 76 (1972).
172. M. Axelrad, J. Exp. Med. **133**, 857 (1971).
173. R. E. Cone, M. Feldmann, J. J. Marchalonis, and G. J. V. Nossal, Immunology, **26**, 49 (1974).
174. M. Feldmann, J. Exp. Med. **136**, 737 (1972).
175. K. T. Brunner and J. C. Cerottini, in *Progress in Immunology* (B. Amos, ed.), Academic Press, New York, 1971, p. 385.
176. N. R. Klinman, J. Exp. Med. **133**, 963 (1971).

177. R. A. Doughty and N. R. Klinman, J. Immunol. **111**, 1140 (1973).
178. N. R. Klinman and R. A. Doughty, J. Exp. Med. **138**, 473 (1973).
179. J. H. Passwell, M. W. Steward, and J. F. Soothill, Paper presented at the Meeting of the British Society for Immunology, Oxford, July 1973.
180. T. Sabet, C. Newlin, and H. Friedman, Immunology **16**, 433 (1969).
181. P. Byfield, G. H. Christie, and J. G. Howard, J. Immunol. **111**, 72 (1973).
182. J. G. Howard, G. H. Christie, and M. T. Scott, Cell. Immunol. **7**, 290 (1973).
183. J. F. A. P. Miller, A. Basten, N. L. Warner, J. C. S. Breitner, G. Rowland, J. Hamilton, H. Silver, and W. J. Martin, J. Exp. Med. **134**, 1266 (1971).
184. K. Rajewsky, V. Schirrmacher, S. Nase, and N. K. Jerne, J. Exp. Med. **129**, 1131 (1969).
185. H. W. Kreth and A. R. Williamson, Nature (London) **234**, 454 (1971).
186. J. C. Ordal and F. C. Grumet, J. Exp. Med. **136**, 1195 (1972).
187. K. Rajewsky, G. E. Roelants, and B. A. Askonas, Eur. J. Immunol. **2**, 592 (1972).
188. P. J. McCullagh, J. Exp. Med. **132**, 916 (1970).
189. B. Pernis and D. S. Rowe, Personal communication (1973).
190. H. G. Herrod and N. L. Warner, J. Immunol. **108**, 1712 (1972).
191. A. R. Lawton, R. Asofsky, M. B. Hylton, and M. D. Cooper, J. Exp. Med. **135**, 277 (1972).
192. D. D. Manning and J. W. Jutila, J. Exp. Med. **135**, 15 (1972).
193. C. W. Pierce, R. Asofsky, and S. M. Salliday, Fed. Proc. **32**, 41 (1973).
194. L. A. Herzenberg, E. L. Chan, M. M. Ravitch, R. J. Riblet, and L. A. Herzenberg, J. Exp. Med. **137**, 1311 (1973).
195. E. B. Jacobson, L. A. Herzenberg, R. Riblet, and L. A. Herzenberg, J. Exp. Med. **135**, 1163 (1972).
196. M. F. Greaves, J. J. T. Owen, and M. C. Raff, in *T and B Lymphocytes: Origins, Properties and Roles in Immune Responses,* Excerpta Medica, Amsterdam, 1973.
197. N. L. Warner, in *Contemporary Topics in Immunobiology* (M. G. Hanna, Jr., ed.), Plenum Press, New York, 1972, Vol. 1, p. 87.
198. G. E. Roelants and B. A. Askonas, Nature [New Biol.] **239**, 63 (1972).
199. G. J. Hämmerling, T. Masuda, and H. O. McDevitt, J. Exp. Med. **137**, 1180 (1973).
200. L. Lafleur, Personal communication (1973).
201. G. F. Mitchell and J. A. Hamilton, Unpublished observations (1973).
202. M. B. Rittenberg and W. W. Bullock, Immunochemistry **9**, 491 (1972).
203. G. A. Theis, I. Green, B. Benacerraf, and G. W. Siskind, J. Immunol. **102**, 513 (1969).
204. G. Weber and E. Kolsch, Eur. J. Immunol. **2**, 191 (1972).
205. T. P. Werblin and G. W. Siskind, Transplant. Rev. **8**, 104 (1972).
206. S. Kontiainen, Int. Arch. Allergy Appl. Immunol. **41**, 729 (1971).
207. O. Mäkelä, S. Koskimies, and A. J. Pasanen, in *Progress in Immunology* (D. Amos, ed.), Academic Press, New York, 1971, p. 653.

208. S. Abrahams, Ph.D. Thesis, University of Toronto, Ontario, Canada, 1973.
209. G. M. Shearer, E. Mozes, and M. Sela, J. Exp. Med. **135**, 1009 (1972).
210. B. Benacerraf and H. O. McDevitt, Science **175**, 273 (1972).
211. G. M. Shearer, in *Genetic Control of Immune Responsiveness* (H. O. McDevitt and M. Landy, eds.), Academic Press, New York, 1972, p. 35.
212. D. H. Katz, T. Hamaoka, M. E. Dorf, P. H. Maurer, and B. Benacerraf, J. Exp. Med. **138**, 734 (1973).
213. L. A. Herzenberg, E. Benjamini, S. Cherry, E. Leung, M. Noble, and G. F. Mitchell, in *Genetic Control of Immune Responsiveness* (H. O. McDevitt and M. Landy, eds.), Academic Press, New York, 1972, p. 1717.
214. G. E. Roelants, E. Benjamini, and G. F. Mitchell, Unpublished observations (1973).
215. B. W. Chesebro, G. F. Mitchell, F. C. Grumet, L. A. Herzenberg, H. O. McDevitt, and T. G. Wegmann, Eur. J. Immunol. **2**, 243 (1972).
216. K. Bechtol and H. O. McDevitt, Personal communication (1973).
217. W. Droege, in Curr. Titles Immunol. Transplant. Allergy **1**, 95 (1973).
218. T. Tada, K. Okumura, and M. Taniguchi, J. Immunol. **108**, 1535 (1972).
219. T. Kishimoto and K. Ishizaka, J. Immunol. **109**, 612 (1972).
220. P. J. Baker, N. D. Reed, P. W. Stashak, D. F. Amsbaugh, and B. Prescott, J. Exp. Med. **137**, 1431 (1973).
221. R. S. Kerbel and D. Eidinger, Eur. J. Immunol. **2**, 114 (1972).
222. D. P. Osborne, Jr., and D. H. Katz, J. Exp. Med. **137**, 991 (1973).
223. J. A. Hamilton and J. F. A. P. Miller, J. Exp. Med. **138**, 1009 (1973).
224. F. M. Burnet, *The Integrity of the Body,* Harvard University Press, Cambridge, Mass., 1962.
225. S. R. Webb and M. D. Cooper, J. Immunol. **111**, 275 (1973).
226. R. K. Gershon and K. Kondo, Immunology **18**, 723 (1970).
227. C. R. Parish, J. Exp. Med. **134**, 21 (1971).
228. E. H. Perkins, J. Immunol. **94**, 765 (1965).
229. O. Sjöberg, Clin. Exp. Immunol. **12**, 365 (1972).

CHAPTER 7

Cellular Immune Reactions

Robert A. Prendergast
Christopher S. Henney

The Johns Hopkins University
School of Medicine
Baltimore, Maryland

Chase's pioneer experiments which showed that cutaneous hypersensitivity to tuberculin could be transferred to normal recipients by lymphoid cells but not by immune serum [1] led directly to a classification of immune responses which is now universally accepted. Those immune reactions mediated directly by serum-borne immunoglobulins are considered humoral; other immune reactivity, such as Chase transferred, is collectively considered as cell mediated. This terminology is a loose one, because not only are the mediators of humoral immunity obviously cell derived but, as we shall describe, cellular immune reactions are also often patently dependent on humoral factors. The division of immune responses into two major subclasses, cell mediated and humoral, although perhaps misleading semantically, is, nevertheless, a useful one. Immunologists currently argue little about which phenomena they consider primarily to be cell mediated. Of these, perhaps the most important are the delayed hypersensitivity skin test reaction, graft-versus-host reactivities, and allograft rejection. In this chapter, we will consider each of these phenomena separately, reviewing briefly the historic developments in the area and summarizing some current ideas on the mechanistics of the reaction.

I. Delayed Hypersensitivity Skin Test Reactions

The classic features of a delayed hypersensitivity skin test reaction, an erythematous lesion of delayed onset characterized by an infiltration of mononuclear cells, have been known for decades. Jenner, in 1798, described a "reaction of immunity" in revaccinated persons as a "papular erythematous reaction in the skin, reaching its maximum 24-72 hours after vaccination." Dienes and Schonheit described the mononuclear cell infiltrate in the 1920s [2], and, incidentally, showed that the skin test reaction was not confined to antigens of bacterial sources (until that time, it had been common to refer to the reaction as "bacterial allergy"). It was not, however, until the classic work of Landsteiner and Chase that such reactions were considered independently from other immune phenomena. These investigators observed that transfer of living lymphoid cells from delayed-sensitized animals to normal hosts conferred to the recipient the ability to respond to injection of antigen in a manner indistinguishable from that of the primarily sensitized host [1,3]. These findings led directly to a series of studies on the specific cellular kinetics of this response. By use of radiolabeled cell populations from sensitized donor animals, it became possible to quantitate the donor cell infiltrate at skin test sites and to estimate the contribution of both donor and host cells in the resultant inflammatory reaction.

In several such studies, tritiated thymidine was used to label newly reactive and dividing cells in animals sensitized to a variety of antigens. When cells from these animals were transferred to normals, and the recipients challenged with antigen, only a very small proportion of the infiltrating mononuclear cells that responded to specific antigenic stimulus was found to be of donor origin [4-6]. Furthermore, in a series of experiments in which recipients were labeled prior to transfer, it was seen that the vast majority of the cells that comprised the inflammatory infiltrate were, in fact, of host origin, even though the host was immunologically naive prior to the cell transfer. These results were interpreted as showing that although a relatively small number of "knowledgeable" cells suffice to transfer and initiate the delayed response, the vast majority of the actual cells in the lesion were, in fact, immunologically uncommitted and had recently divided.

At about the same time, similar results were reported with use of allograft rejection as a measure of responsiveness [7]. In this study, allografts were exchanged at two locations between rabbits of different strains and a third allograft from yet another unrelated strain. By instillation of minute amounts of tritiated thymidine beneath the first pair of grafts, it was possible to label a *single* lymph node that responded to this graft. At the time of graft rejection, sections of both the homologous and indifferent test grafts were examined for the presence of labeled cells from this draining node. In no instance was there evidence that a *preponderant* number of cells from the labeled node were engaged in rejection of the graft from the homologous donor compared to the unrelated third-strain donor. These experiments, which obviated the necessity for cell transfer with its inherent possibility of cell damage or transfer of "immature" cells, nevertheless gave results similar to those of cell transfer experiments. The conclusions from these data are that a very small number of cells that recognize specific antigen are both necessary and sufficient to initiate subsequent inflammatory responses and that the vast majority of the cells that comprise the delayed hypersensitivity skin test response are immunologically uncommitted. Inherent in this observation, of course, is the implication that the migratory behavior of nonimmune cells is in some way influenced by the presence of immune cells.

These observations led to a series of in vitro experiments designed to follow the effect of antigen on immunologically competent cells. From these studies has come much of our current understanding of cellular immunity.

In the 1930s, Rich and Lewis [8] had noted that the migration of cells from splenic explants of guinea pigs immune to human tubercule bacilli could be prevented by preparations of old tuberculin. This protein had no effect on the migration of cells from nonimmune animals. These observations were extended by George and Vaughan [9] and by David and his colleagues [10] and led to the development of an in vitro model of the delayed hypersensitivity skin test reaction. This model centered on the fact that in the presence of homologous antigen, peritoneal exudate cells from sensitized guinea pigs demonstrated impairment of their normal migratory capacity from capillary tubes during short-term tissue culture. This reaction was demonstrated to be exquisitely specific and to parallel uniquely the state of delayed hypersensitivity as demonstrated in vivo. An important advance in our understanding of this model was contributed by Bloom and Bennett when they showed that peritoneal cells from which lymphocytes had been removed behaved as if they had come from normal (nonsensitized) animals and demonstrated normal migration in the presence of specific antigen [11]. The readdition of a very small percentage of the lymphoid cell population to the macrophages reestablished the effect seen in the whole cell peritoneal exudate. This observation firmly established that the lymphocyte was the primary antigen-responsive cell in this model. More importantly, perhaps, it demonstrated that a very small number of these cells can change the normal physiologic behavior of a large number of nonspecific cells (in this case, macrophages). It is this point that connects the in vitro studies with the cell transfer studies noted above and that permits us to explore the mechanism of "amplification," whereby small numbers of specifically reactive lymphocytes act on large numbers of immunologically nonspecific cells to effect a cellular immune response.

Since the lymphocyte has been shown to be the key cell in both the in vivo and in vitro studies, attention was turned to the possibility that "sensitized"* lymphocytes, in the presence of antigen, might release soluble effector substances. This premise was soon confirmed simultaneously, and independently, by Bloom and Bennett and by David [12,13]. They showed that after incubation of sensitized lymphocytes with antigen, the cell-free supernatant could itself inhibit the migration of normal peritoneal macrophages. This material was termed migration-inhibitory factor (MIF) by Bloom and was found to be a protein with a molecular weight of from 25,000 to 50,000 daltons as estimated by Sephadex gel chromatography and that migrates anodically in acrylamide gel electrophoresis to a position adjacent to that of albumin. It has subsequently been shown that MIF can be produced from normal lymphocytes after stimulation with the plant mitogen concanavalin A (con A). It now seems likely that MIF acts on the macrophage by combining with a membrane-associated glycoprotein [14]; furthermore, α-L-fucose abolishes the activity of MIF if present in the culture medium through the incubation period required for demonstrable macrophage migration [15].

Since the description of MIF, numerous other biologic activities have been found to be mediated by the supernatants of sensitized lymphocytes and specific antigen. Among these activities are a macrophage aggregating factor (MAF) [16], a skin-reactive factor [17], a blastogenic factor which causes normal small lymphocytes to transform and divide [18,19], a factor chemotactic for mononuclear macrophages [20], and a cytotoxic factor (lymphotoxin) [21].

It is obvious that many biologic activities can be mediated by supernatants of lymphoid cells exposed for relatively brief periods to specific antigen. Whether, in fact, each of thse biologic activities resides in a separate molecular moiety is still open to question. The primary problem in investigation of this aspect of the cellular immune response has been the difficulty of isolating and purifying sufficient material with a known biologic activity in one test system to use in another.

In summary, then, there is considerable evidence that several lymphocyte-derived soluble mediators can influence the behavior of blood mononuclear

---

*The term "sensitized" lymphocyte as used here applies to lymphocytes from immune animals.

cells. It appears that these mediators play an important role in the characteristic manifestations of the delayed hypersensitivity skin test reaction. At least schematically, we can assume that antigen administered subcutaneously interacts with "sensitized" lymphocytes during normal trafficking of these cells through the peripheral circulation. Such interactions lead to the production of soluble mediators which act both to prevent cells from leaving the site (MIF, MAF, and so on) and which encourage, chemotactically, the infiltration of mononuclear cells into the site. In both cases, the net result is the same—a mononuclear cell infiltrate principally of nonimmune cells at the site of antigen.

II. Cell-mediated Immunity Demonstrated by Graft-versus-Host Disease In Vivo and by the Mixed Lymphocyte Response In Vitro

One of the most interesting and best understood of cell-mediated immune phenomena is the graft-versus-host reaction (GVHR). GVHRs are an example of a purely cellular immune response in which neither antibody formation nor the complement system plays a role. The prerequisites for a GVHR are that the graft be composed of immunologically competent cells and that they recognize and respond to the genetically determined immunogens on recipient cells. In experiments that investigate the mechanism of GVHR, it is of importance that the donor cells not be rejected by the allogeneic recipient, and therefore most of these responses are performed in a "one-way" system where parental cells are given to an F_1 hybrid. Under these circumstances, the recipient will not recognize the parental cells as foreign, but parental cells perceive the alloantigen from the other parental strain present on F_1 cells. In practical terms, the original investigations of Simonsen [22] have drawn attention to the increase in spleen size of the F_1 recipient after administration of parental cells. Indeed, a sufficient number of donor cells reacting against host allogeneic tissue may result in severe wasting disease and death [23]. It is apparent, then, that the host may suffer from an immunologically specific response of immunocompetent donor cells. There are several mechanisms by which damage to host tissue may occur: for example, direct cytotoxic effects of the donor cells, leading to lysis of host cells [24] (reactivity of this type will be discussed in detail in Sec. III); release of nonspecific cytotoxins from donor cells after "triggering" by host alloantigen [21]; and the production of specific antibody by donor cells, leading to immune complex formation and complement-mediated immunopathology.

It has been pointed out by Elkins [25] that donor cells home to and remain within the lymphoid tissue of the host. These cells, then stimulated by host antigens, may eventually destroy host lymphoid tissue. The protection afforded the animal by its ability to respond to infectious agents is thus reduced, and the animal may ultimately die of an infectious process.

Recent data of Asofsky and colleagues [26,27] indicate that the lymphoid cells responsible for achieving GVHRs are thymus (T) -derived. Indeed, there is reason to suppose that GVHRs result from a synergistic interaction between two T-cell subpopulations, one a precursor and the second an effector cell. Thus, a combination of thymus cells and peripheral blood lymphocytes from parental animals has been found to act synergistically, both in causing splenomegaly and death of the F_1 recipient. For example, 10^7 thymus cells alone cause low mortality over a 30-day period, but 10^5 peripheral blood lymphocytes cause no mortality over the same period. When these two donor cell types were given together, mortality reached 80% at 32 days. The authors' conclusion that there are two subsets of T cells which act cooperatively in producing optimal GVHRs seems a compelling one, although the nature of the cooperation is, at present unknown.

An in vitro correlate of the GVHR is the mixed lymphocyte reaction (MLR). In this model, immunologically competent cells from two donors of disparate genetic background are mixed in culture. The response of each cell to cocultured alloantigen is measured either by visually quantifying the extent of the ensuing blast transformation or, more usually, by uptake of tritiated thymidine. It is possible under these in vitro conditions to duplicate the in vivo GVHR situation, since F_1 cells may be mixed with parental cells, so that recognition can only occur in one direction (parent against F_1). It is also possible to treat one set of lymphocytes with mitomycin C, which renders them incapable of division without affecting their ability to stimulate the untreated allogeneic cells. By fractionation of mouse spleen cells into T- and B-cell pools, Andersson et al. have shown [28] that the T cell alone responds to allogeneic stimulation in a one-way MLR.

We have just noted that the GVHR and its in vitro analog, the MLR, are exclusive properties of thymus-derived lymphoid cells. It is now fashionable to extrapolate from the specific to the general case and to equate the B and T subpopulations of lymphoid cells with respective functions: B cells, the precursors of antibody-forming cells, with humoral immunity; T cells with cell-mediated immune reactions. There is both a clinical and an experimental framework for making such division. Patients with congenital thymic hypoplasia (DiGeorge syndrome) and neonatally thymectomized birds and rodents exhibit deficient cell-mediated immune responses in the presence of a frequently normal humoral response; on the other hand, individuals with congenital hypogammaglobulinemia and birds bursectomized shortly after hatching show impaired humoral immunity without affecting their capacity to mount cell-mediated immune responses. Many observations suggest, however, that the division is too exclusive. As is described in detail elsewhere in this book, T cells are often required for optimal humoral responses, and very recent evidence suggests that lymphokines, such as MIF, can be produced by both B and T cells. Certainly, the T cell is centrally important in cellular immune phenomena, but it has become apparent that the collaboration of other cell types may be of importance.

One aspect of cellular immunity in which the T cell functions autonomously is T-cell-mediated cytolysis, an activity of importance in allograft rejection and, in some circumstances, a crucial feature in the control of neoplastic growth.

III. Cytolytic Activity of Thymus-derived Lymphocytes

The lytic activity of lymphoid cells was initially described by Govaerts some 15 years ago [29]. He demonstrated that thoracic duct cells from dogs which had rejected kidney allografts lysed donor kidney cells in vitro. This lytic phenomenon was soon shown to be a general one: lymphoid cells from immunized donors are capable of lysing cells that bear antigens against which the donor is sensitized. Recently, several distinct pathways by which cells can mediate immunologically specific cytolysis have been delineated [for review, see refs. 24, 30, 31]. In this chapter we will confine our attention to that activity mediated by T cells, principally because this cytotoxic mechanism alone has been shown to be of significance in vivo. Evidence for this statement is provided by the observation that cytolytically active T-cell populations (but not B-cell or macrophage populations) taken from immunized animals cause accelerated allograft rejection in syngeneic mice [32]. Similarly, immune T-cell populations have frequently been shown to cause tumor cell regression on transfer to syngeneic recipients [33]. It can thus be inferred that cytolytically active T cells are of importance in allograft rejection and are perhaps a feature of the host's immune surveillance against the development of neoplastic growth.

Although the mechanism of the T cell-mediated lytic process remains unknown, the recent development of several in vitro assay systems has yielded important information. Perhaps the best known of these systems is the one initially described by Brunner and his collaborators [34] and illustrated in Fig. 1. These investigators immunized C57BL/6 mice with a mouse mastocytoma cell line derived from DBA/2 mice, an antigenic challenge across major histocompatibility loci. About 10 to 12 days later, spleen cells from the immunized mice were taken as a source of lymphoid

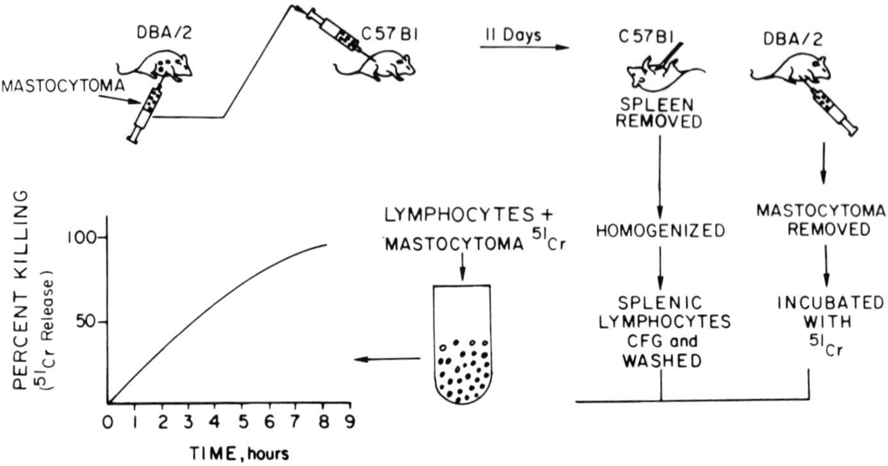

FIG. 1. Schematic representation of in vitro assay system for detection of T cell-mediated lysis. After Brunner et al. [34].

effector cells and were incubated with the DBA/2 mastocytoma cells. The lysis of the DBA/2 target cells was assayed by measuring the release of preincorporated ^{51}Cr. By use of this system, several requirements for the lytic process have been defined (see Table 1), and an overall scheme for the T cell-induced lytic process can be devised (Fig. 2).

Cytolysis is initiated by interactions between T lymphocytes and antigen-bearing cells. The interaction has to be an intimate one, because separation of the reactant partners by a semipermeable membrane or by a viscous medium (e.g., dextran or agarose) inhibits cytolysis. Furthermore, the association is an energy-requiring process and apparently requires membrane modulation to accommodate antigen into the T cell's antigen-binding site, because cytochalasin B (a known inhibitor of membrane modulatory activities) totally inhibits antigen-T-cell interactions and ablates cytolysis [35]. The effector lymphocyte must be viable to effect cytolysis. Lysis is independent of both antibody and the complement system [36].

It has been consistently observed that inhibitors of DNA synthesis have no effect on cytolysis. However, inhibitors of protein synthesis, while widely reported to suppress cytolysis [34, 38] apparently do so by compromising the viability of the effector cell rather than by impeding a specific metabolic pathway. In recent studies, prolonged inhibition of

TABLE 1

Requirements for T Cell-mediated Cytolysis[a]

Requirement	Comments
Viable T cell	X irradiation and metabolic inhibitors ablate cytolytic activity.
Intimate contact with target cell	No cytolysis when interacting cells separated in viscous medium or semipermeable membrane. Exquisite specificity of target cell destruction
Presence of divalent cations	Complete inhibition by EDTA. Mg^{2+} preferentially required for binding killer cells to target; Ca^{2+} required for cell lysis.
Intact cellular secretory organelles	By analogy, colchicine and drugs which augment lymphocyte cAMP levels inhibit cytolysis. These drugs interfere with cellular secretion in many systems.

[a]Adapted from Henney [37].

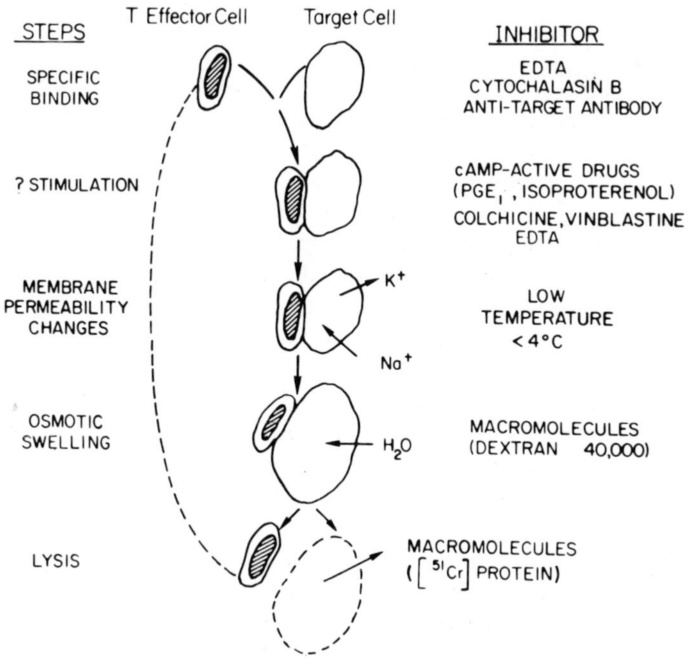

FIG. 2. Overview of stages in the T cell-mediated lytic cycle.

protein synthesis was without effect on the cytolytic activity of effector cells [39].

There is an interesting relationship between the cyclic-3′5′-adenosine monophosphate (cAMP) content of effector cell populations and their lytic efficiency [40]. Agents which augment intracellular cAMP, either by stimulating adenylate cyclase (e.g., isoproterenol, prostaglandins E_1 and E_2, and histamine) or by inhibiting the phosphodiesterase which catabolizes cAMP (e.g., theophylline), all inhibit cytolysis. This inhibitory effect is characterized by its reversibility—the inhibition of cytolysis proceeds only as long as the cAMP levels remain elevated—and by its specificity—propranolol reverses the inhibitory effect of isoproterenol but has no effect on inhibition due to prostaglandin E_1 or histamine. Prostaglandin $F_{2\alpha}$, which has no adenylate cyclase-stimulatory activity, does not inhibit cytolysis.

Inhibition of cytolysis by augmented cAMP levels is mediated by suppression of a lymphocyte function and not by conferring the target cells with a resistance to lysis. This conclusion is derived from studies with a relatively irreversible adenylate cyclase stimulator, cholera enterotoxin [41]. Toxin-treated effector cells show augmented cAMP levels and are incapable of effecting cytolysis. Toxin-treated target cells, on the other hand, show enhanced intracellular cAMP but are lysed to an extent and with an efficiency, comparable to that of unstimulated cells. The mechanistic level at which augmented cAMP levels suppress cytolysis remains puzzling [42].

Cytolysis is markedly, and irreversibly, inhibited by colchicine, an agent known to bind strongly to the dimeric subunits of microtubules and to prevent microtubular aggregation [43]. This binding has been shown to inhibit secretion in a wide variety of cell types [44].

Because cytolysis may be dependent on an intact cell secretory apparatus, it seems tempting to speculate that it involves secretion of a soluble, lytic factor. There are several problems with this hypothesis, however: T cell-mediated cytolysis is exquisitely specific, nonantigen-bearing (bystander) cells are not lysed, and cell-free supernatants derived from cultures in which all target cells have been killed are not, in themselves, lytic.

These findings are difficult to reconcile with a concept of lysis effected by a freely permeating lytic factor, analogous to Granger's lymphotoxin [21]. Recent studies make it appear even more unlikely that T cell-mediated cytolysis is dependent on either MIF or lymphotoxin production [39]. These studies showed that cytolytically active spleen cell suspensions incubated for 1 hr with 100 ng of cholera toxin and then washed extensively demonstrate no lytic activity. The same cell populations, however, produced, in the presence of homologous antigen, amounts of MIF and lymphotoxin comparable to the quantities produced by untreated lymphoid cells.

Not all activities of lytically active cells can be considered as being as beneficial to the host. There are well-documented instances of T cell-mediated destruction of host tissue. One example of this type, the graft-versus-host phenomenon, has already been described; others are often observed after viral infection. One of the best examples of this type has been observed after infection with lymphocytic choriomeningitis virus.

IV. Immunopathology Associated with Cell-mediated Immune Response: Lymphocytic Choriomeningitis Virus-induced Acute Central Nervous System Disease

Lymphocytic choriomeningitis (LCM) virus, when inoculated into the brains of normal adult mice, produces an acute inflammation of choroid plexus, ependyma, and leptomeninges, with a marked convulsive diathesis and death occurring 6 to 8 days after inoculation [45,46]. Animals subjected to immunosuppression by x-ray treatment or chemotherapy (e.g., with Cytoxan) before virus administration exhibit (or "carry") virus for their life-span but do not die or show virus-induced pathology [47].

In a series of investigations, Cole and his colleagues have demonstrated that adoptive immunization of such LCM virus "carrier" mice with LCM-immune spleen cells results in a lethal choriomeningitis essentially similar in pathologic manifestations to that demonstrated in normal mice inoculated with a lethal dose of LCM virus [48,49]. Further, they demonstrated that transfer of cells from nonimmune donors or immune serum was without effect [48]. LCM disease, however, can be produced by adoptive immunization of drug-induced carriers with viable immune lymphoid cells.

Investigation of the cells responsible for this immunopathogenic mechanism was undertaken. Spleen cell suspensions from adult mice immunized by intraperitoneal injection of LCM virus were treated with either normal or anti-θ serum to remove T cells. After incubation, cells were washed and inoculated into drug-induced "carrier" mice. Untreated immune cells transferred into LCM virus carrier mice resulted in death of these carriers. Treatment of these cells with normal rabbit serum plus complement did not alter this result. However, treatment of immune cells with anti-θ plus complement completely abrogated LCM disease and death in the drug-induced carrier [50]. A further observation from these experiments was unpredictable: although mice rendered LCM "carriers" by cyclophosphamide treatment died after adoptive immunization, neonatal LCM carrier mice (which do not require chemotherapy to manifest the carrier state) did not. It would appear, then, that the production of fatal choriomeningitis is determined in part by the distribution of viral antigen, and this distribution was markedly different in the neonatal and drug-induced carriers at the time of immune cell transfer. Where neonatal carriers have a high titer of circulating virus, drug-induced carriers have virus primarily in the central nervous system, at least early after intracerebral inoculation. It is likely, therefore, that adoptive immunization of the neonatal carrier results in exposure of specifically sensitized cells to virus outside the central nervous system, whereas adoptive immunization in the Cytoxan-induced carrier results in lymphocyte-virus interaction within the central nervous system [50].

Several recent reports have described techniques for demonstrating the cytolytic activity of LCM virus-specific T cells in vitro. In experiments published by Cole and his colleagues, BALB/c mice were made immune to LCM by three to four weekly intraperitoneal injections of LCM virus [51]. Spleen cells from these animals were then incubated with ^{51}Cr-labeled normal or LCM-infected L cells for 10 to 18 hr. These studies demonstrated that L cells acutely infected with LCM were readily lysed by specifically immune lymphocytes or by antibody in the presence of complement from virus-immune mice. In contrast, L cells chronically infected with LCM were relatively resistant to lysis by lymphocytes but were as susceptible to antibody-mediated lysis as were acutely infected cells. Immunofluorescent analysis of these L cells demonstrated that acutely infected L cells showed a relatively high proportion of the cells bearing LCM-specific antigenic determinants on their membranes. In contrast, chronically infected L cells demonstrated little, if any, LCM-specific antigen on their membranes. Both acutely and chronically infected cells showed an equivalent amount of virus-specific antigen within their cytoplasm.

It is reasonable to assume, then, that acutely infected target cells express a greater amount of virus-specific antigen at their surface and therefore are susceptible to lysis by cytolytically active T cells. Since cytolysis of infected cells, whether by antibody or mediated by T cells, must depend on the presence of antigens available at their surface for these specific agents, the distinction between acute and chronic infection of the target cells is presumably related to the distinction between antigen binding by T cells and by antibody.

More recent experiments by Volkert and his colleagues [52] demonstrate the kinetics of expansion of a T-cell population cytolytic for LCM-infected target cells. These experiments demonstrate that cytolytic cells are evident approximately 6 to 7 days after intraperitoneal immunization with LCM virus, reach a peak between Days 10 and 12, and rapidly decline, so that cytolytic cells are virtually absent 30 days after a primary immunization. Adoptive immunization with spleen cells at peak cytolytic activity 8 to 10 days after primary immunization does not result in significant LCM disease or death when transferred to drug-induced carriers. However, spleen cells taken

30 days after primary immunization, though demonstrating very little cytolytic activity in in vitro tests with infected L cells, are capable of inducing severe LCM disease and death in 100% of drug-induced carriers. It would appear, then, that cells taken late after immunization fulfill criteria for specific "memory" T cells and may, after exposure to antigen, be progenitors of effector T cells. Similarly, early immune cells would appear to have very little in the way of regenerative capacity for expansion to significant numbers of effector cells with resultant LCM disease on transfer. Both early and late immune cells are T cells, and the expression of their immunopathologic capacity and their cytolytic activity can be totally suppressed with anti-θ serum.

LCM virus-induced disease offers a virtually unique model system for investigation of cell-mediated immunopathology in vivo and in vitro. This virus, which is in itself harmless in situations where the immune response is suppressed or if the animal is exposed prior to the development of immunologic competence, is fatal when administered to a host with a normal complement of immunocompetent cells.

In addition to the cytolytic activity of T cells, there are other T-cell functions which can be regarded as "defensive" activities, in that they are of demonstrable benefit to the host in combating infection. Among the most interesting of these are the antibacterial activities first described by Mackaness [53].

V. Resistance to Infection by *Listeria monocytogenes*

The capacity to resist infection by some intracellular bacteria, such as *Listeria monocytogenes,* is cell mediated and requires the participation of both lymphoid cells and mononuclear phagocytes [53]. In the mouse, nonlethal infection gives rise to a population of specifically sensitized lymphocytes that are capable of passively transferring immunity [54]. The protection due to passive transfer of immune lymphocytes requires the accumulation of recipient phagocytic cells at sites of *Listeria* infection, since it is the macrophage whch is the ultimate effector cell that rids the host of bacteria [55]. Mackaness and his colleagues demonstrated that, after "activation" by the sensitized lymphocyte in the presence of *Listeria* antigen, the macrophage acts nonspecifically and also protects against infection with unrelated bacterial pathogens. The mechanism of activation of macrophages by lymphocytes is not completely understood, but it is probable that the sensitized lymphocyte releases a macrophage-activating factor after contact with specific antigen [56]. The host response to *Listeria,* then, is clearly a form of cell-mediated immunity and can be transferred only by viable lymphocytes and cannot be transferred by antibody.

In a recent study, it was shown that the transfer of immunity to *Listeria* was dependent on the inclusion in the sensitized lymphocyte population of T cells, since treatment of immune spleen cells with anti-θ serum abrogated the ability of this cell population to confer adoptive immunity on recipients [57].

The T cells responsible for the transfer of anti-*Listeria* immunity are apparently a rapidly dividing population. North has shown that after an intravenous immunizing infection with *Listeria,* there arises in the spleen a population of committed lymphocytes which can adoptively immunize normal recipients against a lethal challenge infection [58]. These cells are first produced in the spleen between 48 and 96 hr after immunizing infection and are maximal by Day 6. The cells are apparently short-lived in the environment of the spleen, and their presence can no longer be detected 20 days after immunizing infection. Following a 15-hr pulse of an antimitotic drug, vinblastine, 6 days after an immunizing infection, the ability to protect normal recipients against infection was completely ablated. These cells, therefore, are a rapidly dividing population following antigen stimulus.

In an attempt to activate macrophages in a nonspecific fashion during *Listeria* infection, we had recourse to a protein of invertebrate origin isolated from the coelomocyte (mononuclear phagocyte) of the sea star *Asterias forbesi.* This material demonstrates many of the effects of lymphokines as tested in mammalian systems. Thus, sea star factor (SSF) has the properties of migration inhibitory factor, delayed skin reactivity, mononuclear chemotaxis, and macrophage activation, all of which mimic activities demonstrable in the supernatants of sensitized T cells after incubation with specific antigen [59-61]. Another effect of SSF is its ability to suppress the primary but not the secondary response in development of cytolytic T cells following alloantigenic challenge in vivo or in vitro [60,62]. This latter effect of SSF was indeed the case in the response of mice to challenge with *Listeria.*

Mice became highly susceptible to infection with a normally sublethal dose of *Listeria* if treated with SSF from 96 hr before to 48 hr after intravenous inoculation of the organism. It was also shown that immunization of mice could be abrogated if the normally immunogenic quantity of *Listeria* was accompanied by SSF. On the other hand, treatment of suitably immunized mice with SSF did not alter their protected state. Further, treatment of immune spleen cells with high concentrations of SSF in vitro did not impair their ability to protect normal recipients from challenge with a lethal dose of *Listeria* [63]. In summary, the results of these experiments suggest that a primary immune response to *Listeria* could be impaired to a highly significant degree with low concentrations of SSF, but a secondary response was not under this constraint. Taken together with the data on the effect of SSR on the primary and secondary generation of cytolytic T cells in vitro, these experiments may indicate a qualitative as well as a quantitative difference between naive and "memory" T cells in their response to antigen.

VI. Thymus-derived Lymphocytes and Cellular Immune Reactions

The T-cell mediators of anti-*Listeria* immunity resemble the effector T cells that respond to allograft sensitization in terms of their kinetics of development. The appearance of cytotoxic T cells after immunization of mice with alloantigen-bearing tumor cells, as has already been pointed out, is evident 4 days after immunization and peaks at approximately Days 10 to 12. Thereafter, there is a rapid decline with little or no activity demonstrable by Day 30. The same time course has also been shown for effector T cells responsive to LCM antigen in animals immunized with this virus by intraperitoneal injection [52]. It would appear, then, that the effector cell in allograft immunity, the cells that respond to LCM antigen with demonstrable cytolysis of LCM-bearing target cells, and the lymphocytes responsible for transfer of anti-*Listeria* immunity belong to populations of thymus-derived lymphocytes characterized by rapid division, short half-life, and rapid recirculation. Are they, indeed, the same cells? Recent evidence suggests that they may not be, because cytotoxicity and mediator production can be experimentally dissociated. Thus, Henney et al. have shown [39] that although the activity of cytolytically active T-cell populations can be totally abolished by drugs which augment lymphocyte cAMP levels, the drugs had no effect on the capacity of the same cell populations to produce either of two mediators, MIF and lymphotoxin. This was true of antigen-induced lymphokine production from guinea pig lymph node cells and mitogen (con A) -induced mouse lymphotoxin. Similar dissociation of cytolytic activity from mediator production has been seen with the vinca alkaloids colchicine, Colcemid, and vinblastine. These drugs all suppress cytolysis but have no effect on either MIF or lymphotoxin production.

These findings do not, of course, imply that soluble mediators lack other important biologic functions in connection with delayed-type hypersensitivity reactions or in tumor or allograft rejection. Furthermore, although a dissociation between cytolytic activity and mediator production under the conditions employed was clear, it cannot be argued on the basis of these experiments that these two functions are necessarily performed by independent populations of T cells. This may, indeed, be likely; yet, the alternative possibility that mediator production and cytolytic activity are functions of the same cell line at different stages of maturation cannot, at this time, be excluded.

In this chapter we have described several reactions generally considered as cellular immune phenomena. As is apparent in all cases, thymus-derived lymphocytes play a major role, and, in some cases, they are the only cells required for the activity to be manifest. We have also attempted to stress that the exhibition of these T cell-controlled events is in almost all cases mediated by soluble factors produced by the immune lymphocyte on contact with homologous antigen. There is evidence that at least some of the mediators are synthesized de novo after antigen "triggering."

These concepts of cellular immune reactions are now widely (perhaps universally) accepted. Yet, they are really strikingly new: the first soluble mediator was described in 1966; the demonstration that cytolytic activity was a T cell-mediated event was reported in 1970. There are, of course, still many unknowns.

A central issue is the nature of the antigen-receptor site on the immune T cells, the receptor which imparts antigen specificity to the reactions we have described. This will be discussed in chapters 9 and 10 of this book.

Another intriguing question centers on the control of antigen-driven clonal proliferation. Antigenic stimulation clearly leads to the differentiation and proliferation of cells of both the B- and T-lymphocyte series. What halts the clonal proliferation of these cells? For the B cell, it seems reasonable that cell division ceases because the end cell of the expansion, the plasma cell, lacks sufficient surface immunoglobulin, the antigen receptor, and therefore may no longer be subject to antigen "drive." The end cell thus limits the proliferative capacity of the B-cell clone. The same mechanism clearly cannot control T cell expansion, because the end cell of this series, the "sensitized" (or effector) T cell, does possess an antigen receptor, as shown, for example, by demonstrations that it binds specifically to allogeneic cells that bear antigens against which the effector cell is directed [64]. These effector T cells should, therefore, be continually under antigenic influence to proliferate; why do they stop? This important question is, as yet, unresolved, but the following recent observations may provide some hint.

Several exogenous hormones are capable of negatively modulating lymphocyte T-cell function by augmenting intracellular cAMP levels. The inhibition of T cell-mediated cytolysis by prostaglandin E_1 and by histamine are good examples. This suppression of T-cell function is thought to be mediated via specific hormone receptor sites closely linked to membrane-associated adenylate cyclase. Not all effector T cell preparations are inhibitable by histamine, however, and thus, operationally, such cells do not possess histamine receptor units [65]. Most interestingly, Plaut et al. have recently shown that there is a linear correlation between time after antigenic stimulation and the

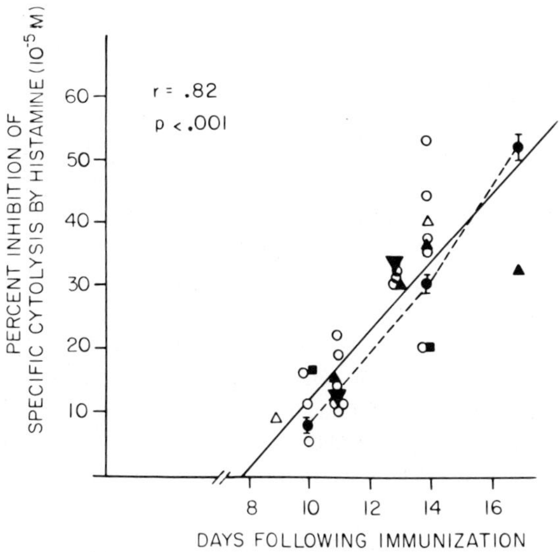

FIG. 3. Adult C57BL/6 mice were immunized intraperitoneally with 10^7 DBA/2 mastocytoma cells. The cytolytic activity of spleen cell suspensions was assessed at various times thereafter, and the inhibition of cytolysis by 10^{-5} M histamine was measured on each occasion. Data from 30 experiments are shown together with the linear regression line for all of the data. The open circles represent experiments where animals were tested at one time; in these cases, lymphoid pools from three to 10 animals were used. The other symbols represent experiments where different animals from simultaneously immunized groups were sequentially followed; in these cases, pools of three to five animals were used. In the group of animals represented by the filled circles, the mean percentage of inhibition of cytolysis due to 10^{-5} M histamine together with the standard error of the mean of triplicate assays are shown for 10, 14, and 17 days after immunization. [From Plaut et al. [66]. By permission of *Nature (London).*]

susceptibility of the lytically active cells to histamine inhibition in vitro [66]. The lytically active cells formed 10 to 12 days after immunization with alloantigen were unaffected by exogenous histamine, and thus lack histamine receptors. The activity of cells harvested 18 days after antigen, however, is markedly suppressed by the drug. Between Days 10 and 18, there is a linear relationship between inhibition and time (Fig. 3). Furthermore, the display of histamine receptors on effector cells is associated with a decline in the number of such cells in the animal. Plaut has demonstrated that this is true of several antigens in several mouse strains and is true for other hormone receptors, e.g., epinephrine.

Thus, the lytically active effector T cell is not a totally differentiated cell but begins to display hormone receptors after its acquisition of antigen receptor. The temporal relationship between the genesis of histamine receptors and the decline in effector cell proliferation suggests that these two events are interrelated. The hypothesis, then, is that the acquisition and display of hormone receptors by the "aging" effector T cell allows this cell to be modulated by hormones present in its environment. It is suggested that such modulation may serve to control T-cell expansion even in the face of antigen "drive."

The last decade has seen major changes in our concepts of cellular immune phenomena, perhaps primarily the realization that all of the reactions involve a subpopulation of lymphoid cells that bear a unique set of antigens and a characteristic developmental and circulatory pattern. To date, these thymus-derived lymphocytes have been shown to perform four major immunologic functions: "helper" activity in antibody formation, production of soluble mediators, regulation of immune responses (for example, the function of "suppressor" T cells), and cell-mediated cytotoxicity. It is not yet possible to determine whether the helper and suppressor activities of T cells are mediated by subpopulations different from those responsible for mediator production and direct cytolysis or whether a single T-cell line exhibits different capabilities during different stages of its differentiation or maturation. Such issues will clearly dictate the direction of investigations in the near future.

Acknowledgments

The references used in this chapter have been chosen rather arbitrarily and are offered merely as a guide to a huge literature.

The experimental work from these laboratories reported in the text was supported by Grants A1 06927 (R.A.P.) and A1 10280 (C.S.H.) from the National Institute of Allergy and Infectious Diseases and by a grant to Dr. Henney from the National Science Foundation. Dr. Prendergast is the recipient of a Research to Prevent Blindness, Inc. Professorship; Dr. Henney is the recipient of a Research Career Development Award from the National Institute of Allergy and Infectious Diseases.

This is communication 139 from the O'Neill Memorial Laboratories.

Note Added in Proof

In the two years since this chapter was written, there has been considerable advance in our understanding of some aspects of cellular immunology. For example, the question of T-cell subpopulations posed in the final paragraph of this chapter has been partially resolved. The demonstration by Cantor and Boyse of distinctive (Ly) antigens on the lymphoid cell surface during differentiation enabled those investigators to show that helper and killer T cells belong to two different subpopulations with distinctive precursors [67, 68]. The relationship between the suppressor and killer cells is less clear since they display the same Ly antigens.

The precise mechanism of T cell-mediated cytolysis remains unknown, but it now seems unlikely that a soluble factor is involved in target-cell lysis [31,69,70]. In fact, recent observations seem to implicate cell-surface-associated enzyme systems in the lytic process [71]. Ferluga and Allison have demonstrated that isolated plasma cell membranes from regional lymph node cells of mice skin-sensitized to oxazalone were lytic for P815 target cells, in a manner directly proportional to the plasma cell membrane concentration [72].

The T cell-mediated destruction of virally-infected target cells has received much attention following Zinkernagel and Doherty's fascinating observation that effector and target cell must be syngeneic at the H-2 locus for lysis of the virally-infected target to occur [73-75]. Whether this is an *absolute* requirement is still not completely settled.

References

1. M. W. Chase, Proc. Soc. Exp. Biol. Med. **59**, 34 (1945).
2. L. Dienes and E. W. Schonheit, Proc. Soc. Exp. Biol. Med. **24**, 32 (1926).
3. K. Landsteiner and M. W. Chase, Proc. Soc. Exp. Biol. Med. **49**, 688 (1942).
4. R. T. McCluskey, B. Benacerraf, and J. W. McCluskey, J. Immunol. **90**, 466 (1963).
5. S. Cohen, R. T. McCluskey, and B. Benacerraf, J. Immunol. **98**, 269 (1967).
6. J. S. Najarian and J. D. Feldman, J. Exp. Med. **114**, 779 (1961).
7. R. A. Prendergast, J. Exp. Med. **119**, 377 (1964).
8. A. R. Rich and M. R. Lewis, Bull. Johns Hopkins Hosp. **50**, 115 (1932).
9. M. George and J. H. Vaughan, Proc. Soc. Exp. Biol. Med. **111**, 514 (1962).
10. J. R. David, H. J. Lawrence, and L. Thomas, J. Immunol. **93**, 264 (1964).
11. B. R. Bloom and B. Bennett, Fed. Proc. **27**, 3 (1968).
12. B. R. Bloom and B. Bennett, Science **153**, 80 (1966).
13. J. R. David, Proc. Nat. Acad. Sci. USA **56**, 72 (1966).
14. H. G. Remold and J. R. David, J. Immunol. **107**, 1090 (1971).

15. H. G. Remold, J. Exp. Med. **138**, 1065 (1973).
16. L. Samsak, S. Dray, and S. P. Gotoff, J. Immunol. **104**, 296 (1970).
17. B. Bennett and B. R. Bloom, Proc. Nat. Acad. Sci. USA **59**, 756 (1968).
18. D. C. Dumonde, R. A. Wolstencroft, G. S. Panayi, M. Matthew, J. Morley, and W. T. Howson, Nature **224**, 38 (1969).
19. F. T. Valentine and H. S. Lawrence, Science **165**, 1014 (1969).
20. P. Ward, H. G. Remold, and J. R. David, Science **163**, 1079 (1969).
21. G. A. Granger and W. P. Kolb, J. Immunol. **101**, 111 (1968).
22. M. Simonsen, Progr. Allergy **6**, 349 (1962).
23. G. W. Santos and A. H. Owens, Nature (London) **210**, 139 (1966).
24. P. Perlmann and G. Holm, Advan. Immunol. **11**, 117 (1969).
25. W. L. Elkins, Progr. Allergy **15**, 78 (1971).
26. R. Asofsky, R. Tigelaar, and H. Cantor, in *Progress in Immunology* (B. Amos, ed.), Academic Press, Inc., New York, 1971, p. 369.
27. H. Cantor and R. Asofsky, J. Exp. Med. **131**, 235 (1970).
28. L. C. Andersson, S. Nordling, and P. Hayry, J. Exp. Med. **138**, 324 (1973).
29. A. Govaerts, J. Immunol. **85**, 516 (1960).
30. J.-C. Cerottini, A. A. Nordin, and K. T. Brunner, Nature (London) **228**, 1308 (1970).
31. C. S. Henney, in *Mechanisms of Tumor Immunity* (I. Green and B. Benacerraf, eds.), John Wiley, New York, in press (1976).
32. J. Sprent and J. F. A. P. Miller, Nature (New Biol.) **234**, 195 (1971).
33. B. T. Rouse and H. Wagner, J. Immunol. **109**, 1282 (1972).
34. K. T. Brunner, J. Mauel, J.-C. Cerottini, and B. Chapuis, Immunology **14**, 181 (1968).
35. C. S. Henney and J. E. Bubbers, J. Immunol. **111**, 85 (1973).
36. C. S. Henney and M. M. Mayer, Cell. Immunol. **2**, 702 (1971).
37. C. S. Henney, Transplant. Rev. **17**, 37 (1973).
38. R. M. Thorn and C. S. Henney, J. Immunol. **116**, 146 (1976).
39. C. S. Henney, J. Gaffney, and B. R. Bloom, J. Exp. Med. **140**, 837 (1974).
40. C. S. Henney, H. R. Bourne, and L. M. Lichtenstein, J. Immunol. **108**, 526 (1972).
41. L. M. Lichtenstein, C. S. Henney, H. R. Bourne, and W. B. Greenough, J. Clin. Invest. **52**, 691 (1973).
42. H. R. Bourne, L. M. Lichtenstein, K. L. Melmon, C. S. Henney, Y. Weinstein, and G. M. Shearer, Science **184**, 19 (1974).
43. M. Plaut, L. M. Lichtenstein, and C. S. Henney, J. Immunol. **110**, 771 (1973).
44. E. Becker and P. Henson, Advan. Immunol. **17**, 94 (1973).
45. C. Armstrong and R. D. Lillie, Publ. Health Rep. **49**, 1019 (1934).
46. J. Hotchin, Cold Spring Harbor Symp. Quant. Biol. **27**, 479 (1962).
47. J. Hotchin and H. Weigard, J. Immunol. **87**, 675 (1961).
48. D. H. Gilden, G. A. Cole, A. A. Monjay, and N. Nathanson, J. Exp. Med. **135**, 860 (1972).

49. D. H. Gilden, G. A. Cole, and N. Nathanson, J. Exp. Med. **135**, 874 (1972).
50. G. A. Cole, N. Nathanson, and R. A. Prendergast, Nature (London) **238**, 335 (1972).
51. G. A. Cole, R. A. Prendergast, C. S. Henney, in *Lymphocytic Choriomeningitis Virus and Other Arenaviruses* (F. Lehmann-Grube, ed.), Springer-Verlag, Berlin, 1973, p. 61.
52. M. Volkert, O. Marker, and K. Bro-Jorgenson, J. Exp. Med. **139**, 1329 (1974).
53. G. B. Mackaness, Sem. Hematol. **7**, 172 (1970).
54. G. B. Mackaness, J. Exp. Med. **129**, 973 (1969).
55. S. P. Tripathy and G. B. Mackaness, J. Exp. Med. **130**, 17 (1969).
56. C. F. Nathan, M. Karnovsky, and J. R. David, J. Exp. Med. **133**, 1356 (1971).
57. F. C. Lane and E. R. Unanue, J. Exp. Med. **135**, 1104 (1972).
58. R. V. North, J. Exp. Med. **138**, 342 (1973).
59. R. A. Prendergast and M. Suzuki, Nature (London) **227**, 277 (1970).
60. R. A. Prendergast, G. A. Cole, and C. S. Henney, Ann. N. Y. Acad. Sci. **234**, 7 (1974).
61. R. A. Prendergast and S. H. Liu, Scan. J. Immunol., in press (1976).
62. C. L. Reinisch, N. A. Gleiner, and R. A. Prendergast, submitted for publication.
63. D. O. Willenborg and R. A. Prendergast, J. Exp. Med. **139**, 820 (1974).
64. M. Feldmann, I. R. Cohen, and H. Werkle, Transplant. Rev. **12**, 57 (1972).
65. M. Plaut, L. M. Lichtenstein, and C. S. Henney, J. Immunol. **111**, 389 (1973).
66. M. Plaut, L. M. Lichtenstein, and C. S. Henney, Nature (London) **244**, 284 (1973).
67. H. Cantor and E. A. Boyse, J. Exp. Med. **141**, 1376 (1975).
68. H. Cantor and E. A. Boyse, J. Exp. Med. **141**, 1390 (1975).
69. C. S. Henney, J. Reticuloendothelial Soc. **17**, 231 (1975).
70. M. Gately, M. M. Mayer, and C. S. Henney, Cell. Immunol., in press (1976).
71. L. D. Frye and G. J. Friou, Nature (London) **258**, 333 (1975).
72. J. Ferluga and A. C. Allison, Nature (London) **255**, 708 (1975).
73. R. M. Zinkernagel and P. C. Doherty, Nature (London) **248**, 701 (1974).
74. P. C. Doherty and R. M. Zinkernagel, Transplant. Rev. **19**, 89 (1974).
75. P. C. Doherty and R. M. Zinkernagel, J. Exp. Med. **141**, 502 (1975).

CHAPTER 8

Cell Interactions in the Immune Response In Vitro

Marc Feldmann

I.C.R.F. Tumour Immunology Unit
Department of Zoology
University College London
London, England

I. Introduction

Biology has entered the molecular era. In a tentative way, so has immunology. We are now interested in knowning, in molecular terms, the details of the problems of cellular immunology which have been outlined in the last decade or so. Since molecular biology can be performed in the test tube, but not in intact animals, tissue culture approaches to cellular immunology have thrived, as they have in other fields of biology. The advantages of in vitro techniques are immediately apparent: it is possible to control the cells (type and number) that participate in immume responses; antigen concentrations may be varied at will; and the total response may be measured, as there is no net cell migration.

Access to the system is available at all times. Furthermore, it is possible to isolate and characterize the products which lymphocytes make. By varying the geometry of culture systems, the importance of cell-to-cell contact or of chemical mediators in cell interaction may be studied.

Yet there *are* disadvantages to the tissue culture approach. At best, in vitro techniques tell us about the cell biology of lymphoid cells and some aspects of the physiology of artificial cell mixtures. They cannot approach questions that involve the physiology of the entire immune system.

One important drawback is the loss of tissue organization. The architecture of the lymph node, for example, has progressively evolved over millions of years from the primitive jugular body of the amphibians [1] to the multifollicular lymph nodes of eutherian mammals, and thus lymphoid architecture must presumably serve some useful purpose. However, the common culture systems used in immunology employ single-cell suspensions. By teasing a spleen or lymph node into a suspension, the complex tissue organization is irrevocably destroyed. In an analogous way, the recirculation of lymphocytes from lymphoid organs through the blood and lymph must also be ignored in tissue culture studies.

Despite these potential drawbacks, the immune system in vitro behaves in many ways like the same cells in vivo. Nearly all of the immunologic phenomena which occur in intact animals may be reproduced, at least in part, in vitro. Both primary and secondary cell-mediated and humoral responses occur [2-5]. Antibody production of IgM, IgG, and IgA classes has been described [6,7]. High- and low-zone tolerance, in either T or B cells, has been described [8,9], as has antigenic competition [10-12] and T-cell suppression [13-15]. Furthermore, the Ly antigen phenotype of helper, suppressor, and killer T cells induced in vitro and in vivo is the same. For these reasons, and because different culture systems yield very similar results [16], confidence in the conclusions based on in vitro technology is increasing.

This chapter will survey some of the various forms of cell cooperation which have been studied in vitro. Of the four broad categories, emphasis will be placed on the one about which most is known, namely, cooperation between T and B cells. Of necessity, a chapter of this size can only consider a minute proportion of such an expanding field as cell collaboration.

II. Interaction Between T and B Lymphocytes

Due to the pioneering work of Claman, Miller, Davies, Mitchison, Taylor, Rajewsky, and their colleagues in the late 1960s, it is known that interactions between two populations of lymphocytes (T and B) are of major importance in the generation of many, but not all, antibody responses. More recently, however, it has become apparent that T cells do not invariably stimulate B cells. T cells may sometimes lead to the reverse, namely, to the suppression of antibody production [17]. Both of these phenomena are interlinked and will be discussed in this chapter.

A. Positive Interaction Between T and B Cells: "Cell Cooperation"

Based on studies performed in irradiated mice, Mitchison and colleagues [18] proposed a detailed mechanism of cell cooperation, which is illustrated in Fig. 1. Their experiments with hapten-protein conjugates had indicated that "linked regonition," namely, the simultaneous recognition of "haptenic determinants by B cells, and "carrier" determinants by T cells, was essential for optimal cell

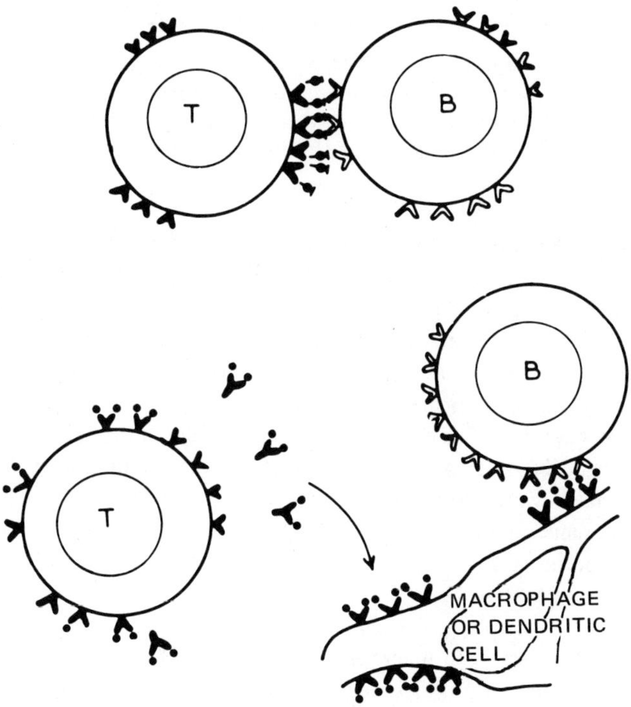

FIG. 1. Mechanisms of cell cooperation that involve linkage of T- and B-lymphocyte receptors. Upper diagram represents direct contact of lymphocytes, with antigens as the glue. Lower diagram demonstrates IgT, completed with antigen which binds to macrophages or dendritic cells. B cells are immunized on the lattice of determinants thus formed. (From [141]. By permission of *Transplantation Proceedings.*)

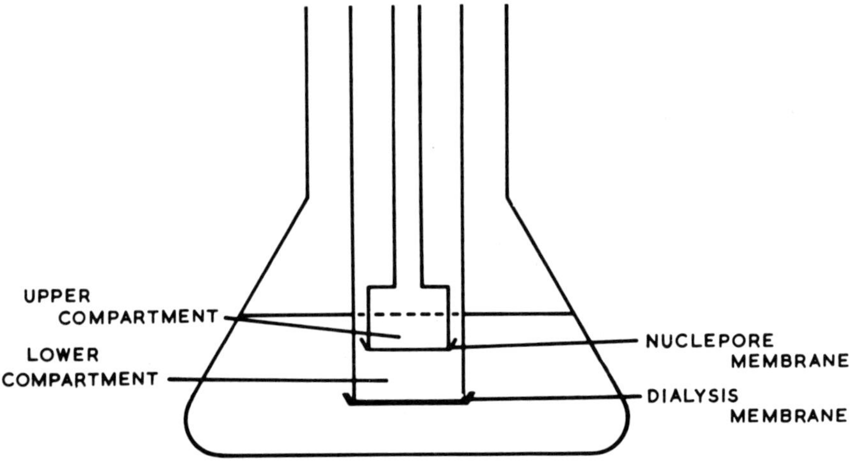

FIG. 2. Double-chapter culture formed by concentric glass tubes, suspended in a reservoir of medium. T cells were placed in the upper compartment, and B cell-containing populations were placed in the lower compartment. (From Feldmann and Basten [142]. By permission of the *Journal of Experimental Medicine.*)

cooperation. Two possible forms of linked recognition are shown in Fig. 1. One involves a direct contact between T and B lymphocytes, whereas the other is indirect, involving a third-party cell, represented as a macrophage or dendritic cell. Although experiments in vivo could not discriminate between these two possibilities, this discrimination was possible in vitro by the use of tissue cultures with two compartments, as illustrated in Fig. 2. With this system, populations that contained T cells were cultured in one compartment, separated by a cell-impermeable nucleopore membrane from the population of B cells in the other chamber. Since cooperation occurred just as efficiently in the presence as in the absence of the membrane, direct cell contact between T and B cells was not essential (Fig. 3). This conclusion has been extensively confirmed (e.g., Refs. 19-24).

Current concepts of T-B cell cooperation may be summarized as follows: cooperation involves both macrophages and T and B cells [25]; factors are important in cooperation. Two categories have been described: specific factors, with specificity for a given antigen, and nonspecific factors.

1. Antigen-specific Factors in Cell Cooperation

Various groups of workers have reported the presence of antigen-specific factors (SF) derived from populations of cells which mediate cell cooperation.

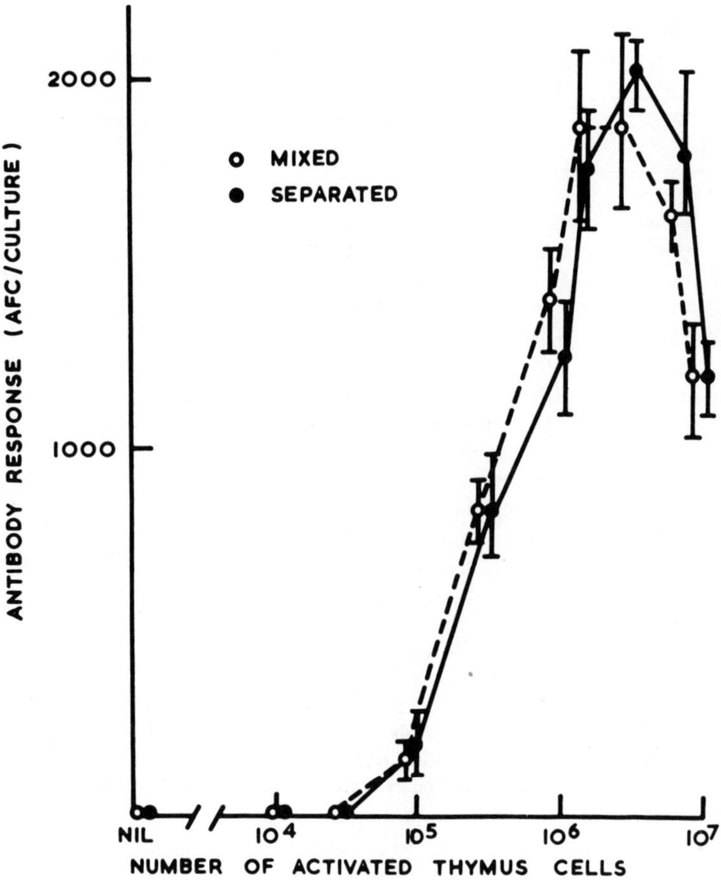

FIG. 3. Cooperation between T and B cells was as efficient when they were mixed or separated by a 1-μm nucleopore membrane. ATC_{KLH} were cultured with DNP Fla-primed spleen cells and 1 μg/ml DNP KLH. Anti-DNP response was assessed 4 days later.

a. Antigen-specific Migration-inhibitory Factor. This cooperative factor with activity (MIF) was reported by Lachmann and Amos [26]. Its chemical nature has yet to be characterized. It seems to be of low molecular weight (≃ 50,000).

b. IgT Antigen. Complexes of antigen and T cell-released antibody (IgT) were described as mediators of cell cooperation by Feldmann, Basten, and colleagues. Subsequent work by Rieber and Riethmuller [24,27] and by Tada and colleagues [28] have confirmed the presence of specific Ig-cooperative factors.

TABLE 1

Serologic Identification of Specific Cooperative Factor in T-cell Supernatants[a]

Cells	Immunogen (ml)		ATI-DNP Response (AFC/culture ± SE)
Normal spleen	NIL		20 ± 15
Normal spleen	DNP POL		715 ± 110
Normal spleen	S/N[b] ATC_{KLH} + DNP KLH	0.5	110 ± 55
Normal spleen	S/N[b] ATC_{KLH} + DNP KLH	0.1	310 ± 60
Normal spleen	S/N[b] ATC_{KLH} + DNP KLH	0.01	355 ± 190
Normal spleen	S/N[b] ATC_{KLH} + DNP KLH	0.001	85 ± 60
Normal spleen	S/N abs Sepharose-anti-Ig[c]	0.5	30 ± 25
Normal spleen	S/N abs Sepharose-anti-Ig[c]	0.1	50 ± 35
Normal spleen	S/N abs Sepharose-anti-Ig[c]	0.01	25 ± 15
Normal spleen	S/N abs Sepharose-NRG[d]	0.5	135 ± 70
Normal spleen	S/N abs Sepharose-NRG[d]	0.1	420 ± 115
Normal spleen	S/N abs Sepharose-NRG[d]	0.01	360 ± 110
Normal spleen	S/N abs Sepharose-anti-μ[e]	0.5	20 ± 75
Normal spleen	S/N abs Sepharose-anti-μ[e]	0.1	30 ± 25
Normal spleen	S/N abs Sepharose-anti-μ[e]	0.01	55 ± 40

[a]Spleen cells (1.5×10^7) were incubated for 4 days with immunogen as above; three cultures per group. Data from Feldmann and Greaves [139].
[b]S/N, supernatant.
[c]Sepharose-anti-Ig, polyvalent rabbit anti-Ig coupled to Sepharose.
[d]Sepharose-NRG, normal rabbit globulin coupled to Sepharose.
[e]Sepharose-anti-μ purified anti-μ antibodies (a gift of Drs. A. Lawton and M. Cooper) coupled to Sepharose.

c. *Other Specific Factors.* These factors have been reported by Yu and Gordon [21] and by Taussig and Munro [29].

Other workers, while not directly demonstrating the presence of specific cooperative factors, have not been able to reconstitute antibody responses fully in the absence of specific T cells (e.g., Refs. 30,31), thereby indirectly demonstrating specific T-cell function.

Taussig and Munro have reported the presence of an Ia antigen-containing specific T-cell factor of a molecular weight of approximately 50,000 [29]. No Ig determinants have been found in these factor preparations, which were reported to be highly unstable, so the possibility remains that Ia and Ig T-cell factors reported may be fragments of the same molecule.

Experiments performed in double-chamber flasks indicated that adherent cells were required in the B-cell compartment for cooperation to occur [25], which suggests that macrophages may be a necessary intermediate in specific cooperation [20]. This interpretation was confirmed by experiments in which macrophages were incubated with supernatants from ATC in the presence of antigen. The washed macrophages were capable of immunizing pure populations of B cells, either primed or unprimed [20]. These results substantiated, in broad outline, the concept shown in the lower half of Fig. 1.

Although it has been demonstrated that macrophage-bound complexes of antigen and IgT represent the moiety which actually immunizes B cells, the details of this last step remain to be fully established. It is not clear why IgT-bound antigen is a much more potent stimulator of B cells than is macrophage-bound antigen in the *absence* of IgT. Two possibilities, not mutually exclusive, stand out. First, the pattern of antigen distribution on the macrophage surface may be of importance, e.g., it may resemble that found on the surface of a thymus-independent antigen. Second, macrophages may, in response to IgT binding, release factors which facilitate the triggering of B cells.

Recent experiments have suggested that *both* mechanisms may operate. Evidence that suggests that the pattern of antigenic determinants present on the surface of a macrophage is critical to its immunogenicity was obtained in experiments performed with two populations of specific cooperative factors [33]. Basically, it was found that macrophages incubated with one specific factir (I) at 4°C could not bind a second specific factor (II) in an immunogenic way, as shown in Tables 2 and 3. If one macrophage population was incubated simultaneously at 4°C with two specific factors, the capacity to immunize B cells was abolished for *both* antigens (Tables 2 and 3). Two possible mechanisms for the abolition of immunogenicity may be considered. First, *total* binding of any one IgT population may be insufficient. Most of the receptors for IgT may have been saturated. While this mechanism may operate if one supernatant is added first, it does not seem likely if both T-cell supernatants are added simultaneously. The other alternative is that the *manner* of binding of IgT molecules is altered; i.e., the correct "lattice" of repeating determinants may not form if both sets of IgT bind randomly to any one macrophage. The results in Table 4 indicate that macrophages which had bound one population of IgT (and effectively absorbed most of it) could still bind a second population; these results strongly support the second alternative.

In view of recent demonstrations that mammalian membranes may be envisaged as fluid mosaics, with surface structures capable of redistribution [34], is it reasonable to think of patches or lattices of antigen *existing* on the surface of a macrophage long enough to be immunogenic? I think it is, for two reasons. First, although it has been demonstrated that many surface structures *can be* redistributed, there is no evidence that, in the absence of a

TABLE 2

Antigenic Competition with Helper Cell Products[a]

Macrophages Incubated with	Antibody Response DNP	$F_{\gamma}G$
I. ATC_{KLH} + DNP KLH	720	0
II. $ATC_{F_{\gamma}G}$ + $F_{\gamma}G$	0	470
III. I & II Separately	495	310
Together	55	75
Together + I	395	50

[a]Macrophages (10^6) were incubated for 2 hr at 4°C with supernatants I or II, obtained from 2×10^6 ATC. The macrophages were washed, and 10^5 or 3×10^5 were cultured with 1.5×10^7 DNP POL-primed spleen cells for 4 days. Data from Feldmann and Schrader [140].

TABLE 3

Ig Nature of Helper and Competitive Material from ATC[a]

Macrophages Incubated with Supernatants from	Antibody Response DNP	$F\gamma G$
I. $ATC_{F\gamma G + F\gamma G}$	0	445
II. ATC_{KLH} and DNP KLH	720	0
III. I and subsequently II	80	400
IV. I and II simultaneously	65	55
V. 1 incubated anti-Ig beads	0	0
VI. V and then II	375	0

[a]Macrophages (10^6) were incubated for 2 hr at 4°C with supernatants I or II, obtained from 2×10^6 ATC. The macrophages were washed, and 10^5 or 3×10^5 were cultured with 1.5 $\times 10^7$ DNP POL-primed spleen cells for 4 days. Data from Feldmann and Schrader [140].

cross-linking stimulus, these structures ever become aggregated, or "capped." Furthermore, some surface structure (e.g., θ antigen [35,36]) do not readily become redistributed, even in the presence of antibody. Thus, the interaction of IgT with its receptor need not imply that the spacing of receptors for IgT, if it is indeed critical, would be altered. Alternatively, IgT antigen complex may induce the formation of aggregates which may be immunogenic entities.

The results above implicate the exact *manner* of antigen binding to macrophages via IgT as a factor in the mechanism of B-cell triggering. They do not, however, exclude an additional more active participation of macrophages in B-cell triggering. Waldmann and Munro [37] found that populations

TABLE 4

Activity of Macrophage-absorbed Supernatants

Stimulus (ml)	Antibody Response (AFC/culture)		
	Original[b]	abs A[c]	abs B[d]
Supernatant 1.0	325	65	83
Supernatant 10^{-1}	610	30	25
Supernatant 10^{-2}	305	25	30
Supernatant 10^{-3}	115	20	35
Supernatant 10^{-4}	30	35	20
	DNP		FγG
No antigen	30		0
DNP POL[e]	1,195		10
Macrophage A[f]	40		10
Macrophage B[g]	20		450

[a] Antibody response of DNP POL-primed cells after 4 days in culture.
[b] Original supernatant (1 ml from 10^6 ATC) from ATC_{KLH} and DNP KLH.
[c] One milliliter of original supernatant absorbed with 10^6 peritoneal exudate cells.
[d] One milliliter of original supernatant absorbed with 10^6 peritoneal exudate cells which had previously been absorbed with supernatant from $ATC_{F\gamma G}$ + FγG.
[e] One-tenth gram per milliliter of DNP POL.
[f] 10^5 peritoneal exudate cells/culture.
[g] 10^5 peritoneal exudate cells which had been incubated with supernatant from $ACT_{F\gamma G}$ + FγG.

of activated T cells from the spleen of irradiated mice produced more nonspecific factor (in the presence of antigen) if additional macrophages were added. None was produced if macrophages were removed. Schrader demonstrated that supernatants of activated macrophages augmented the response to FγG [38]. These results suggest, but by no means prove, that macrophages may make factors which influence B-cell triggering in cell cooperation. Other evidence, though still preliminary, on the capacity of macrophage products to influence B-cell triggering has come from a study of the effect of purified IgT (from a thymus lymphoma, the θ-positive EL4 or WEHI22 tumors) on the immune response to thymus-dependent and thymus-independent antigens. It was found that whereas EL4Ig, even at low concentrations, suppressed the IgM AFC response to a thymus-dependent antigen, TNP KLH, it augmented the IgG response to the same antigen [38a].

2. *Nonantigen-specific Factors (NSF)*

Various workers have reported that supernatants from various sources may nonspecifically augment immune responses in vitro. These factors have been obtained, in the absence of antigen, from thymocytes or spleen cell cultures [22,39] and also from antigen-stimulated cultures of spleen [30] or activated T cells [30].

The most effective supernatants have come from cultures stimulated with histocompatible cells ("allogeneic" supernatants or mixed lymphocyte reaction (MLR) supernatants, e.g., Refs. 19,22,40,41).

The production of these factors *depends* on T cells, as shown by the effect of anti-θ and complement [22] or by the effect of thymectomy [19]. Whether these factors are synthesized by T cells, or by macrophages, in response to T cells has not yet been clarified. The experiments of Sjöberg [42] and Waldmann and Munro [37], while perhaps favoring a macrophage origin, do not definitely establish it. In contrast, the cell separation studies of Schimpl and Wecker [43] have suggested a T-cell origin for NSF. In view of the sensitivity of tissue cultures to nonspecific stimuli, it is entirely possible that *both* activated T cells *and* activated macrophages synthesize a type of NSF.

Different functional types of nonspecific factors have been reported. Schimpl and Wecker have reported two; a T cell-amplifying factor was derived from normal spleen. It augmented the response to sheep red blood cells (sRBC) in vitro of spleen cells from ATxBM mice but *not* those from "nude" mice. In contrast, they described a T cell-replacing factor (TRF) which restores the sRBC response of spleen cells from nude mice [22]. Whether these agents are really distinct, or whether the "TRF" represents a higher concentration of the former, is yet not clear.

Gorczynski et al. [30,40,44] reported that a factor from ATC, stimulated to sRBC or alloantigens, augmented the response of certain B-cell populations to sRBC. The latter was active at lower concentrations than the former. By preparing an antiserum to the allogeneic factor, the serologic similarity of the "allogeneic" and "syngeneic" factors was demonstrated [44]. In their experiments, no responses to sRBC were obtained in the absence of a small number of specific helper cells [45], providing further evidence for the synergy of NSF and specific influences. An example of the need for the synergistic effect of NSF-specific cells is shown in Fig. 4.

The mechanism of action of "nonspecific factors," once they have been formed, is directly on B cells, as demonstrated by the use of a macrophage-independent antigen, DNP POL [19]. NSFs augment response to *both* thymus-dependent or thymus-independent antigens in vitro [19] and in vivo [46]. Whether NSF may stimulate B cells to respond to a totally T-dependent antigen in the total absence of specific T cells or specific factor is not known. Responses to sRBC in cultures of nude mouse spleen may be restored to normal levels by NSF (e.g., Ref. 22). In contrast, the response to sRBC of other B-cell sources could not be restored by Gorczynski et al. [45] in the absnece of a

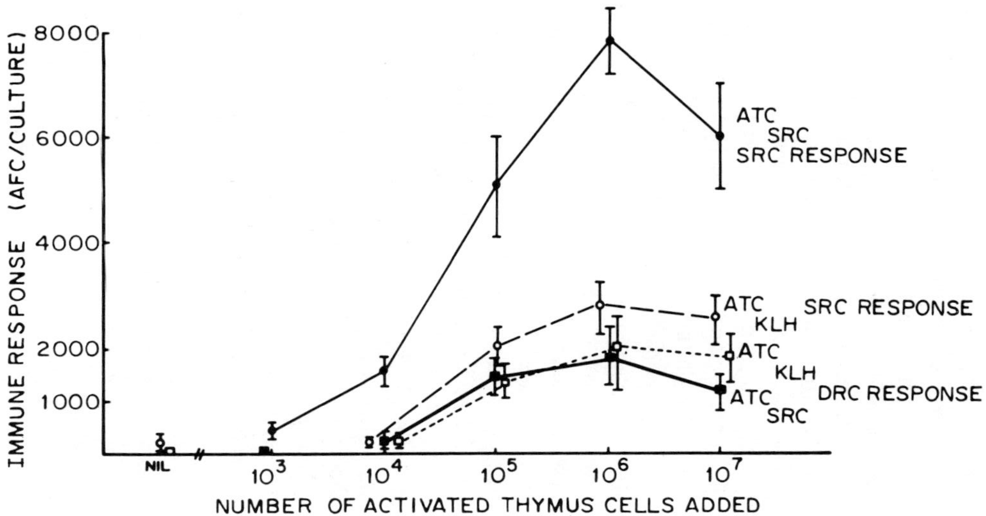

FIG. 4. Synergy of specific and nonspecific factors. Comparison of the effects of allogeneic CBA T cells on the responses of *nu/nu* spleen with sRBC and dRBC. (●) Response to SRC in the presence of ATC_{SRC}, (○) response to SRC in presence of ATC_{KLH}, (□) response to DRC in presence of ATC_{KLH}, response to DRC in presence of ATC_{SRC}. (From Feldmann and Basten [19]. By permission of the *Journal of Experimental Medicine.*)

small number of specific T cells. For example, B cells purified from the marrow could not respond to NSF alone, at any concentration. Spleen cells from nude mice which responded to sRBC did not respond to DNP FγG or DNP KLH in the prsence of NSF [19]. These observations are difficult to interpret. It is known that sRBCs have a thymus-independent component [47, 48] and that spleen cells from nude mice proliferate better than do other sources of B cells [49]. Furthermore, the very small percentage of θ-positive cells [50] (? functional T cells) in nude mouse spleen may be sufficient to affect the response to sRBC, but not to other antigens, which classically are more T dependent than are sRBC, e.g., FγG [51]. Whereas NSF did not permit a response of spleen cells from nude mice to a thymus-dependent hapten-protein, DNP FγG, responses to thymus-independent DNP POL are markedly augmented [19]. NSF augmented responses to red cells and to DNP POL antigens, to which the nudes respond, even without NSF, although with differing degrees of vigor, but NSF did not stimulate responses to DNP FγG or DNP KLH, to which there was no background response [19,52]. It was suggested that NSF amplified existing responses and that it did not facilitate antigen-specific triggering, which was a function of specific factor (or thymus-independent antigen). These considerations are supported by the fact that NSF worked just as efficiently if added 2 days after the initiation of culture as it did at the beginning [22]. More recent work by Schimpl and associates [53] has indicated that NSF acted chiefly to influence differentiation of cells which had already proliferated into AFC. NSFs have also been reported to augment IgG production in vitro [54,55].

At present, biochemical studies of NSF are difficult to summarize. Schimpl et al. [53] reported that their NSF was susceptible to proteolytic enzymes. Chromatography revealed a broad peak with a median molecular weight of 50,000. Other workers have reported several stimulating peaks of various molecular weights [57]. In contrast, Gorczynski et al. found a broad peak with a molecular weight $\simeq$ 150,000 [30].

Thus, T-B cooperation involves three cells and at least two classes of molecular factors. It seems reasonable to assume that the factors which may be demonstrated in vitro do, in fact, function in vivo, since Rieber and Riethmuller [24] have injected "specific complexes" (antigen and IgT) into ATxBM mice, which produced very good responses, and Tada's IgT experiments were performed in vivo. The allogeneic effect in vivo [58] suggests that NSFs are active in vivo.

Despite our expanding knowledge, there are still many aspects of cell cooperation which are not understood. The first of these aspects is the role of complement in the antibody response. Pepys [59] reported that the injection of cobra venom factor (CVF), at doses which virtually eliminated circulating C3, suppressed the response to thymus-dependent antigen sRBC but not to a thymus-independent antigen, such as pneumococcal polysaccharide SIII.

The timing of injection of CVF was critical; C3 depletion was necessary during the initial 2 to 3 days after antigen to cause suppression. Later suppression was uneventful, which suggested that C3 was involved in the triggering of responses to thymus-dependent antigens. Dukor and Hartmann [60] have suggested that C3b, bound to B cells, may be a "second isgnal" for B-cell activation. To support their theory, Dukor and colleagues have obtained results which indicate that many thymus-independent antigens may, at high concentrations, activate C3 by a bypass mechanism [61] and that B-cell activation of lymph node cells by mitogens was diminished in the presence of zymosan-treated serum [62]. All of these results are not, in my view, compatible with a single role of C3 on the antibody response. It could be argued that Pepys' [59] initial results with CVF may have been due to other effects of CVF, apart from C3 depletion. For example, CVF is highly immunogenic, so that the inhibition of the sRBC response could have been due to antigenic competition, which only affects T-dependent antigens. Nevertheless, more recent results have confirmed that lack of C3 suppresses cooperative responses. Anti-C3 antiserum suppresses the response to sRBC but not to pneumococcal polysaccharide SIII in mice [62a].

In vitro, purified anti-C3 antibodies inhibit the response to the thymus-dependent antigen TNP KLH but not that to thymus-independent DNP POL, as illustrated in Table 5. These experiments do not demonstrate any requirement for C3 in the response to DNP POL. However, they cannot exclude its participation, because it could be argued that much smaller amounts may be sufficient with a polymeric antigen. Some evidence that suggests that there may be an effect of C3 directly on B cells also has been obtained by using cultured spleen cells from mice at various times after priming. Preliminary experiments [62b] indicate that much more anti-C3 is needed to block responses soon after priming. This difference does not correlate with the magnitudes of the total response which can be elicited at various times after priming.

The regulation of the Ig classes produced in a cooperative response is another aspect which is not clearly understood at present. Various workers have suggested that IgG antibody production is more dependent on T cells than is that of IgM [63]. States where T cells are limiting depress the IgG response more than that of IgM, e.g., partial tolerance [64] and thymectomy [65]. The reasons for the greater T-cell dependence of IgG antibody production are *not* yet known. Several theoretical possibilities may be suggested:

1. IgG precursor cells need *more* of the same T-cell products for their stimulation;
2. IgG precursors need different factor(s) to be stimulated as well as, or instead of, those required by IgM;

TABLE 5

Effect of Anti-C3 on Antibody Response In Vitro[a]

Cells	Antibody (μ/ml)		Antigen	Anti-DNP Response (AFC/Culture ± SE)
KLH primed[b]	NIL		NIL	30 ± 20
KLH primed[b]	NIL		TNP KLH[c]	860 ± 110
KLH primed[b]	anti-C3[d]	10 μ/ml	TNP KLH[c]	110 ± 70
KLH primed[b]	anti-C3[d]	1 μ	TNP KLH[c]	95 ± 30
KLH primed[b]	anti-C3[d]	0.1 μ	TNP KLH[c]	210 ± 45
KLH primed[b]	anti-C3[d]	0.01 μ	TNP KLH[c]	480 ± 115
KLH primed[b]	sheep IgG_1[e]	10 μ/ml	TNP KLH[c]	680 ± 160
KLH primed[b]	sheep IgG_1[e]	1 μ	TNP KLH[c]	910 ± 215
KLH primed[b]	anti-C3	10 μ/ml	DNP POL[f]	560 ± 165
KLH primed[b]	anti-C3	1 μ	DNP POL[f]	710 ± 205
KLH primed[b]	sheep IgG_1	10 μ/ml	DNP POL[f]	605 ± 105

[a]Data from Feldmann and Pepys [62b].
[b]Spleen cells from mice, primed three times with KLH adsorbed on bentonite last time 8 weeks prior to culture. Responses at 4 days shown.
[c]0.1 μg/ml TNP KLH.
[d]Purified sheep anti-C3 antibody of $1gG_1$ class.
[e]Sheep IgG_1 devoid of anti-C3 activity.
[f]1 μg/ml DNP POL.

3. IgG response occurs later, and there is only sufficient T-cell effect in the presence of normal numbers of T cells.

While the early work on specific cooperation in vitro was chiefly concerned with the production of IgM antibody, since relatively little IgG antibody was made, more recent attempts to study IgG responses have been more successful. By use of spleen cells from mice primed three times with TNP KLH, Bullock and Rittenberg have regularly obtained IgG production in vitro [66,67]. Thus, experiments were performed with mice primed in this way to compare the production of IgM and IgG in double-chamber flasks in vitro. As shown in Fig. 5, IgG production requires the presence of significantly more ATC than does IgM production. This experiment confirms the in vivo work that indicates that more T-cell function is required for IgG production. It does not, however, establish that more *specific* factor is needed. These experiments could equally be interpreted as demonstrating that more NSF is needed, for IgG production, as described by Schimpl et al. [54,55]. The NSF acting in this system could be made either by ATC or by macrophages as a consequence of the binding of SF [37]. As mentioned above, it has been reported that higher concentrations of

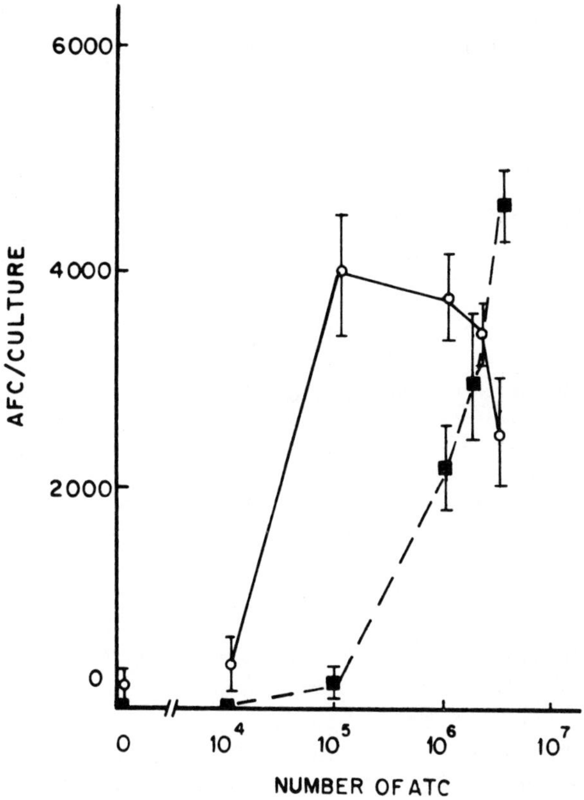

FIG. 5. Comparison of the number of ATC required for the induction of IgM and IgG responses in vitro. (○) IgM anti-DNP response; (■) IgG anti-DNP response. Data from Feldmann et al. [85].

NSF are needed to trigger an IgG response to sRBC than an IgM response [54]. Similar results have been obtained with DNP POL, as illustrated in Table 6. The experiments of Cheers and Miller [68], who reported an increased IgG anti-NNP response to NNP sRBC after carrier red blood cell priming, are also interpretable in terms of a T cell-dependent factor which influences Ig class selection.

Whether IgG synthesis and secretion require a qualitatively *different* stimulus from that of IgM is not known. It is known that IgG synthesis needs both types of T-dependent cooperative factors, specific and nonspecific (see above). Whether the material in the allogeneic supernatants or in supernatants of *Corynebacterium parvum*-treated macrophages which increases IgG production is the same as that which increases IgM, or whether it is a different

TABLE 6

Augmentation of IgG Responses by MLR Supernatants

Cells	Stimulus (μg/ml)	Anti-DNP Response (AFC/culture)	
		IgM	IgG
DNP POL primed[a]	DNP POL 1	2,480	310
DNP POL primed[a]	DNP POL 10^{-1}	1,680	720
DNP POL primed[a]	DNP POL 10^{-2}	1,270	1,040
DNP POL primed[a]	DNP POL 10^{-3}	340	550
DNP POL primed[a]	DNP POL 1 + MLR S/N[b]	5,680	550
DNP POL primed[a]	DNP POL 10^{-1}	2,970	1,350
DNP POL primed[a]	DNP POL 10^{-2}	1,560	2,780
DNP POL primed[a]	DNP POL 10^{-3}	650	2,590
DNP POL primed[a]	DNP POL 10^{-4}	410	1,920

[a]Spleen cells from mice primed with 20 μg DNP POL 6 weeks previously.
[b]Supernatant from CBA × BALB/c culture.

molecule, will not be known until these factors are purified. However, the simplest explanation which fits the available data is that there is a distinct T-dependent (possibly macrophage produced) molecule which is required for B cells in large numbers to develop into IgG AFC.

The development of higher-affinity antibody-producing cells with time after immunization has been documented with many antigens in different species [69]. This selection toward affinity depends markedly on antigen dose and on time after injection (reviewed by Siskind and Benacerraf [69]). Traditional concepts attribute this phenomenon to the selective pressure of limiting residual antigen. As the antigen concentration falls, only cells with higher-affinity receptors bind sufficient antigen to become triggered. Current concepts of collaboration fit well with this view. For example, as antigen concentration declines, the amount of IgT-antigen complexes, the immunogenic form of antigen for B cells, also becomes limiting. Only B cells with sufficient numbers of high-affinity receptors may bind long enough to these smaller complexes of macrophage-bound antigen to become triggered. It has been reported that the production of high-affinity antibody depends on the presence of T cells in near normal numbers [70,71], whereas in their absence, only low-affinity antibody is produced. In my opinion, this observation has been used in a misleading manner, to argue against the importance of antigen presentation mechanisms of cell collaboration in vivo (e.g., Mitchell, Chapter 6 of this volume). There is increasing evidence of the role of T cells in antigen persistence [72-75], and thus in T-deficient animals, there would be much less antigen remaining at late stages after immunization, perhaps insufficient to trigger even high-affinity B cells. In agreement with this interpretation is the well-known fact that the highest-affinity antibody does not develop in intact animals if the dose of antigen is too low or if the adjuvant is omitted [69]. Siskind and Benacerraf [69] developed a probability argument to explain this observation. With insufficient antigen, too little would reach the rare high-affinity cells, and thus the *average* affinity of serum antibody is lower. Studies which measure the binding of antibody released by single AFC have clarified these concepts of antigen-driven selection in the maturation of affinity. For example, Claflin et al. [75,76] have reported that very early AFC include a small proportion of cells of the highest affinity ever detectable in that species. These experiments emphasize the need for selection of precursor cells and their prolonged proliferation driven by persisting antigen to eventually become the dominant species. Since T cells make factors which promote B-cell proliferation (vide supra), this is another way in which T cells influence the selection toward higher-affinity cells, which make better use of the residual antigen. Furthermore, if more NSF is needed to facilitate the differentiation of B cells into IgG AFC, the latter, which release high-affinity antibody, would only appear in the presence of sufficient numbers of T cells. It can also be argued that the selective influence of limiting residual antigen would also affect Ig class selection that favors IgG precursor cells, with receptors of higher affinity than the IgM precursor cells which seem to have receptors of a uniform low affinity (e.g., Refs. 77-79).

Schlossman and Williamson [80] have reported that guinea pigs immunized with DNP oligolysines, e.g., α-DNP lys_{10}, produce antibody of restricted heterogeneity, compared with the antibody produced against, for example, DNP KLH. Why do some antigens trigger fewer B-cell clones? Again, this observation is compatible with the two-factor concept of cell collaboration developed above. It is known that the size of the combining site of antibody molecules is such that it will fit about three or four amino acid molecules [81]. Thus, the specificity of B-cell receptors is not only for DNP, which is merely the immunodominant tip of the hapten, but also for DNP and its neighboring amino acids. With a synthetic antigen, such as α-DNP lys_{10}, there is thus only one "DNP" determinant, whereas there would be many in DNP KLH, since the amino acids adjacent to the DNP would vary in DNP KLH. For this reason, a smaller number of clones would have high binding affinity for "DNP" in α-DNP lys_{10} than "DNP" in DNP KLH. Thus, the restricted heterogeneity would depend on the same factors as does affinity regulation described above.

Another question of interest with respect to concepts is the role of immune response (Ir) genes in the T-B-cell collaboration that controls the immune response. Several types of genetic control have been reported. Many antibody responses are genetically linked to the major histocompatibility loci.

The genes that control these responses in the mouse have been termed Ir-1. These genes appear to control T-cell functions [82]. Other genes, Ir-3, control the function of antibody-forming cell precursors [83]. The view is held by some that Ir-1 genes code for T-cell surface receptors for antigen [82]. Although this view is compatible with some results, it is by no means the only hypothesis consistent with the known facts of Ir gene action and ignores much other evidence on the chemical nature of T-cell receptors. Other hypotheses of Ir gene function have been discussed elsewhere [84].

Although there is compelling evidence from various groups of the existence of specific cooperative factors, and three identifications of these factors as Ig-like [20,24,28], there are still many unanswered questions about "IgT," the T-cell component of the specific cooperative factor. The first questions concerns the cell type that actually synthesizes IgT. While there is much evidence that the cell which releases IgT is a T cell [85], and that only metabolically active T cells do so [86], there is as yet no conclusive evidence that IgT is not adsorbed from the serum onto the surface of a subpopulation of T cells [87]. This possibility is given some credence by the fact that some activated T cells have a receptor for the Fc of immunoglobulin [88]. However, the B-cell origin of IgT would not explain the marked cytophilia of IgT for macrophages [89], which is greater than that reported for any serum Ig class or for B-cell surface Ig [89]. It could still be argued that Ig of non-T cell origin could acquire, during its stay on the T-cell membrane, a "receptor" for the macrophage surface. Other circumstantial evidence for a T-cell origin of IgT is the occurrence of Ig+,θ+ thymomas, reported by Harris et al. [90], Boylston [91] and Pernis et al. [92]. Furthermore, Roelants et al. have elegantly shown that there are T antigen-binding cells for squid hemocyanin (MSH) by use of a radioactive label for antigen and a fluorochrome for the θ marker. They have shown that anti-Ig can induce capping of the antigen, with loss of receptors [93] and, more recently, that if the cells are left at 37°C for 6 hr, the receptors regenerate, can be recapped, and so on [94]. If this experiment is performed in the absence of B cells, once the original receptors have capped off, they can only be reacquired by synthesis by T cells. Preliminary experiments suggest that this is indeed the case [94a].

Another point of ignorance about IgT is its exact Ig class. Although SF reacts with "*specific*" anti-μ antibody, prepared and generously donated by several authorities in the field (Drs. N. L. Warner, R. M. E. Parkhouse, A. Lawton, and R. Asofsky), and with no other specific antiheavy-chain antisera, it is still possible, since it has yet to be isolated in a pure form, that it only shares a few determinants with IgM, or cross reacts weakly. It could be the product of one ancestral gene expressed in the common ancestor of T and B cells, which evolved in a somewhat different way from the B-cell μ gene.

Another point of ignorance about SF is whether it is comprised of only

IgT and antigen. For example, it could be argued that the binding of IgT antigen to the macrophage may be mediated by other factors. Conceivable candidates include Ia antigens, Ir gene products, C3, or perhaps even CIg.

B. Negative Interaction Between T and B Cells: T-cell Suppression

The now imposing evidence for the existence of suppressor T cells has been recently reviewed by Gershon and Kondo [95] and will therefore not be dealt with here. Suffice it to say that there is evidence for both *specific* T-cell suppression in tolerance induction [96-99] and for the regulation of the antibody response [100] and *nonspecific* T-cell suppression [95]. The augmented response to thymus-independent antigens found in T cell-depleted mice (thymectomized "nude" or ALS treated) may also be interpreted in terms of specific T-cell suppressor effects [101,102].

Experiments performed in vivo have not clarified the mechanism of specific T-cell suppression. In vitro specific T-cell suppression was first noted in experiments where ATC were cultured in double-chamber flasks separated from adherence column-purified lymphocytes. It was found that the lymphocytes were not only not immunized but were also refractory to challenge with the macrophage-independent antigen DNP POL, i.e., were tolerant. These findings led to the demonstration that ATC supernatants contain suppressive activity under certain conditions: if adherent cells are removed [100], in the presence of antimacrophage serum [103], and if high concentrations of supernatants are used [103].

The properties of the suppressive material in the ATC supernatant have been examined and are summarized in Table 7, which shows the effects of different ATC supernatants on adherent cell-depleted spleen (purified lymphocytes). After 6 hr, the cells were washed and challenged with TNP KLH and peritoneal exudate cell. These results indicate three resemblances between the specific cooperative factor and the specific suppressor: carrier specificity, adsorption by macrophages (absorption of "suppressor" renders the macrophages immunogenic), and adsorption by anti-Ig-coated Sepharose beads.

The above experiments describe a specific T cell-mediated suppression of the B-cell response. Analogous experiments have been performed on the suppression of T cells. It was found that T cells suppress other T cells more readily than they suppress B cells [103].

The existence of specific suppressor cells in vitro has been confirmed by Waldmann and Munro [104] in a slightly different system. They found that high doses of TNP KLH induced B-cell tolerance in TNP KLH-primed spleen only if KLH-reactive T cells were present. However, they have not yet reported attempts to identify the nature of the specific suppressor in their

TABLE 7

Immunoglobulin Nature of Specific T-Cell Suppressor

Cells	Supernatant	Challenge	Response[a] (AFC/culture)	
			IgM	IgG
TNP KLH-primed spleen	NIL	TNP KLH + PE[b]	2,200	1,560
TNP KLH-primed spleen	NIL	NIL	250	0
TNP KLH-primed spleen	S/N $ATC_{F\gamma G}$ + DNP FγG[c]	TNP KLH + PE	2,610	1,210
TNP KLH-primed spleen	S/N abs Sepharose-anti-Ig[d]	TNP KLH + PE	2,650	1,290
TNP KLH-primed spleen	S/N abs Sepharose-anti-NRG[e]	TNP KLH + PE	2,510	1,105
TNP KLH-primed lymphocytes	NIL	TNP KLH	150	0
TNP KLH-primed lymphocytes	NIL	TNP KLH + PE	1,330	640
TNP KLH-primed lymphocytes	NIL	NIL	10	0
TNP KLH-primed lymphocytes	S/N $ACT_{F\gamma G}$ + DNP FγG[c]	TNP KLH + PE	250	0
TNP KLH-primed lymphocytes	S/N abs Sepharose-anti-Ig[3d]	TNP KLH + PE	1,670	810
TNP KLH-primed lymphocytes	S/N abs Sepharose-anti-NRG[4e]	TNP KLH + PE	310	0

[a]Response at Day 6 was measured.
[b]10^5 peritoneal exudate cells per culture.
[c]Supernatant from $ATC_{F\gamma G}$ + DNP FγG (0.1 μg/ml).
[d]Same supernatant absorbed with Sepharose conjugated with anti-Ig antibody.
[e]Same supernatant absorbed with Sepharose conjugated with normal rabbit globulin.

system. Tada and colleagues have reported that extracts of thymocyte membranes from rats injected with *Ascaris* contain a carrier-specific suppressive activity for the IgE response. Their initial attempts to characterize the suppressor have indicated a difference between it and a specific factor which induces a response [28,105]. The "stimulator" was Ig in nature, but the suppressor was of lower molecular weight and was not adsorbed to anti-Ig columns, but was adsorbed into anti-Ia columns [143]. More recent studies have indicated that suppressor T cells and helper T cells are different [144], but it seems unlikely.

Various nonspecific forms of T-cell suppression have also been described, such as the diverse entities lumped together under the term "antigenic competition." Other examples have been described, such as during desensitization [106] and in the DNA synthetic response to alloantigens (summarized by Gershon and Kondo [95]).

Currently, it is not known whether all forms of nonspecific suppression are due to a single mechanism. The best studied example of nonantigenic specific suppression is antigenic competition. This phenomenon has been the subject of three exhaustive reviews, by Taussig [107], Liacopoulos and Ben Efraim [108], and Pross and Eidinger [109] and therefore will not be the subject of analysis here. In a model of antigenic competition initiated in vivo but expressed in vitro, Schrader and Feldmann [12] found that the suppressive effect could be overcome either by the addition of small numbers of anti-θ-treated peritoneal exudate cells or by trypsinization of the cell suspension. These experiments indicated that this model of antigenic competition was explained by a reversible block at the macrophage surface. This conclusion is reminiscent of the suppression of subsequent responsiveness to a second ATC supernatant, which may be induced by the addition of ATC supernatants, as described in Tables 2, 3, and 4. The concept that antigenic competition of this type is due to a temporary reversible block of macrophage cooperative capacity has also been suggested by other authors [110-112]. However, although the bulk of the data on competition between different molecules fit into this scheme, it seems unlikely that all forms of antigenic competition are due to this mechanism. Competition between two determinants on the same molecule, "intramolecular competition," is not compatible and is probably due to differences in the frequency of antibody-forming cell precursors [107]. Direct evidence for the existence of a nonspecific suppressor, believed by some to be the mediator of antigenic competition [95], has yet to be published. However, it seems likely that the suppressive effects of mitogen-stimulated cells, reported by Dutton [15] and Rich and Pierce [14], are probably due to nonspecific inhibitors.

III. Collaboration Between Subpopulations of T Cells

The work of Asofsky, Cantor, and Tigelaar has demonstrated synergy between populations of T cells. They found that mixtures of blood leukocytes (or lymph node cells) and thymocytes gave significantly greater graft-versus-host reactions than expected by summing the reactivity of the components measured separately (reviewed in Ref. 113). Studies with anti-θ serum established that both populations were T cells [113] and thus that this form of synergy was distinct from that which occurs between T and B cells.

Also, the phenomenon of synergy between populations of T cells in vitro has recently been described in several laboratories, by Wagner et al. [114], Tigelaar and Feldmann [115], and Hayry and Andersson [116], in both the cytotoxic and proliferative responses to allogeneic cells. The circumstances of the collaboration closely resemble those found in the GVHR in vivo: blood or lymph node (LN) cells interact with thymocytes. As in vivo, the T nature of the cooperating cells was established by the use of anti-θ serum [117]. Optimal cooperation (superaddition) *occurs in the presence* of relatively low numbers of LN cells. A relative excess of lymph node cells results in a suboptimal response from the thymocytes [115], which suggests the existence of T-dependent suppressor mechanisms in this response, as in the T-B cooperative response. The mechanism of T-T cooperation has not yet been delineated. For example, it is not known whether there is any specificity in the interaction, or whether factors are involved. The details of the specificity of the interacting cells are also not known. It is tempting to speculate that one cell may react to the so-called lymphocyte-defined (LD) antigens, which are important in the MLR, and that the other may react to serologically defined (SD) antigens, which are important in the cytotoxic response, in agreement with the elegant work of Eijsvoogel and Bach and their colleagues [118,119]. The function of macrophages in the T-T interaction in the response to cellular alloantigens is not known (see below). Cooperation between subpopulations of T cells in vitro has been discussed more extensively in a recent review by Wagner and Nossal [120], and also by Hayry and Andersson [116] and Tigelaar and Feldmann [115]. More recently, evidence has been obtained for T-T interaction, in the induction of helper cells [145] and in the induction of suppressor cells [146]. In both these examples, and in the generation of killer cells [114-116], the precursors are in the long-lived T_2 cell pool.

IV. Macrophage-lymphocyte Interaction

Macrophages are involved in the stimulation of both cell-mediated and humoral immune responses. Macrophages participate in the triggering of both T and B cells. Since we do not know whether effects reported for T cells also apply for B cells, and vice versa, these questions are discussed separately.

A. Interaction of Macrophages and B Cells

Since macrophages which have bound specific cooperative factor are instrumental in immunizing B lymphocytes, much of this topic has already been discussed under the heading of T-B cooperation. Macrophages also interact with B cells in other ways. For example, there are suggestions that B cells release factors which may facilitate the activation of B cells. These factors have been reported by Hoffmann and Dutton [121], Shortman and Palmer [122], and by Schrader [38]. These activities are probably similar to the "potentiating factor" in the MLR reported by Bach et al. [123].

The use of different assays for these factors has made it difficult to compare these results or predict whether these various activities are due to the same or to diverse factors. For example, Hoffmann and Dutton [121] looked at the capacity of macrophage supernatants to restore the response to sRBC macrophage-depleted spleen cells, as did Shortman and Palmer [122], while Schrader examined the capacity of macrophage supernatants to augment the response of athymic (nude) mouse spleen cells to respond to deaggregated FγG in vitro. Schrader interpreted his results as indicating that macrophages which had been stimulated, either in vivo or in vitro, produce a factor which can alter the reactivity of B cells to antigen. The results obtained with sRBC are even more difficult to interpret. For the sRBC results, it is conceivable that macrophage supernatants contained factors which digested sRBC, producing antigenic fragments of reduced size [122]. Since these "soluble sRBC antigens" can be both macrophage and thymus independent [122,124], the sRBC results need not imply any direct effects of these macrophage supernatants on B cells. Other evidence for an effect of macrophage supernatants on B cells comes from a study of the effects of *C. parvum*-treated macrophages in the antibody response in vitro. These macrophages augment IgG antibody production, even with unprimed B cells [68a].

Evidence for a suppressor function of macrophage products on antibody responses was obtained by Sjöberg [42] during a study of the effect of GVH responses in vitro. He found that removal of macrophages by carbonyl iron treatment abolished the suppressive effect, whereas anti-θ serum treatment did not. The suppressive effects were noted both with sRBC, a thymus-dependent antigen, and with the thymus-independent lipopolysaccharide (LPS). If LPS triggers B cells directly, as POL does [125], the suppressive effect reported must have been directly on B cells.

B. Interaction of Macrophages and T Lymphocytes

Macrophage-lymphocyte interaction is just as important in T-cell responses as it is in the antibody response. For example, macrophages have been implicated in the MLR [126], in cytotoxic responses [127], in blastogenic responses to antigen [128], in the induction of delayed hypersensitivity reactions, and in the augmentation of T-cell responses to mitogens [129].

Though the importance of these interactions is well established, the exact mechanism of interaction is not known, and the interpretations offered are highly speculative. One role of macrophages in T-cell responses in vitro, whose importance seems clear but is hard to quantitate precisely, is their effect on cell survival, which is often higher in their presence than in their absence. It is possible that this effect influences *all* the in vitro macrophage-T cell interactions. Other mechanisms which may be of importance include the digestion of antigen, since it has been reported that small antigen molecules favor the inducation of delayed hypersensitivity rather than antibody production [130].

Antigen bound to the surface of macrophages stimulates T cells efficiently. Mitchison [131] and Unanue and Askonas [132] found that macrophage-bound antigen, while only inducing weak primary responses, primed for very high anamnestic responses. Seeger and Oppenheim [133] have extended these findings to demonstrate that macrophage-bound antigen also efficiently induced delayed hypersensitivity. These results also have been obtained in vitro by Rosenthal and colleagues [134]. The reasons for the efficiency of macrophage antigen, but *not* lymphocyte, thymocyte, or hepatoma cell-bound antigen, is not clear [135]. Is it the spatial arrangements, or does the macrophage make factors which are important for triggering? By analogy with the results obtained by Gery et al. [129] in the T-cell response to mitogens, it seems possible that macrophage factors may be of importance. It is impossible, of course, to exclude a role of antigen presentation in the heightened immunogenicity of macrophage-bound antigen for T cells in vivo. This question can be resolved by the use of a totally in vitro system for the induction of helper cells [135].

A mechanism of macrophage-T lymphocyte interaction has been documented by Gery et al. [129, 136]. These workers studied the effect of supernatants from macrophages on the response of T cells to mitogens, phytohemagglutinin (PHA), or concanavalin A (con A). The production of the active factory by macrophages, which they termed lymphocyte-activating factor (LAF), was accelerated by the presence of lipopolysaccharide or other mitogens. The enhancement by other mitogens (PHA, con A) depends on the presence of T cells, i.e., was indirect. Factors active for mouse T cells were obtained from syngeneic, allogeneic, and xenogeneic (human, rabbit) macrophages [136]. These factors synergized with both light and dense peripheral T cells or thymocytes. It is not known at present whether LAF has any effect on the response of T cells to antigens.

Macrophage-T cell interaction is important in the inducation of helper cells. This interaction is greatly restricted; and the macrophages and T cells must be identical at the I-A subregion of the H-2 complex [147]. The interaction is mediated by a macrophage factor, having a molecular weight of approximately 55,000, which is a complex of Ia antigen and immunogen (broken down). It sends to a receptor on a T_1 cell [148]. Apart from this factor, there are others, acting on T_2 cells as well.

V. Conclusions

The overwhelming importance of cell cooperation of various types in the immune system is now only too apparent. While some aspects of the regulation of these responses have been discussed, the most important one has been conspicuously ignored, namely, the regulation of self-nonreactivity [137,138]. This phenomenon would take another chapter to discuss.

Acknowledgment

This study was supported by a C. J. Martin Fellowship from the National Health and Medical Research Council, Canberra, Australia. This chapter was written in 1973.

References

1. E. Diener and G. J. V. Mossal, Immunology **10**, 535 (1966).
2. R. I. Mishell and R. W. Dutton, J. Exp. Med. **126**, 423 (1967).
3. J. Marbook, Lancet **ii**, 1281 (1967).
4. E. Diener and W. D. Armstrong, Lancet **ii**, 1281 (1967).
5. H. Wagner and M. Feldmann, Cell. Immunol. **3**, 405 (1972).
6. C. W. Pierce, B. M. Johnson, H. E. Gershon, and R. Asofsky, J. Exp. Med. **134**, 395 (1971).
7. M. Hurme and O. Mäkelä, in *Proceedings of the 8th Leucocyte Culture Conference, Uppsala* (K. Lindahl-Kiessling and D. Osoba, eds.), Academic Press, New York, p.203, 1973.
8. M. Feldmann and G. J. V. Nossal, Transplant. Rev. **13**, 3 (1972).
9. E. Diener and M. Feldmann, Transplant. Rev. **8**, 76 (1972).
10. H. Pross, T. Novak, and D. Eidinger, Cell. Immunol. **2**, 445 (1971).
11. O. Sjöberg and S. Britton, Eur. J. Immunol. **2**, 282 (1972).
12. J. W. Schrader and M. Feldmann, Eur. J. Immunol. **3**, 771 (1973).
13. M. Feldmann, Nature [New Biol.] **242**, 82 (1973).
14. R. R. Rich and C. W. Pierce, J. Exp. Med. **137**, 205 (1973).
15. R. W. Dutton, J. Exp. Med. **136**, 1445 (1972).
16. M. B. Rittenberg and M. Feldmann, unpublished data (1972).
17. R. K. Gershon, Curr. Topics Microbiol. Immunol. **3**, 1 (1973).
18. N. A. Mitchison, K. Rajewsky, and R. B. Taylor, in *Developmental Aspects of Antibody Formation and Structure* (J. Šterzl and I. Říha, eds.), Academia Publishing House, Czechoslovak Academy of Science, Prague, Vol. 2, p. 547, 1970.
19. M. Feldmann and A. Basten, J. Exp. Med. **136**, 722 (1972).
20. M. Feldmann, J. Exp. Med. **136**, 737 (1972).
21. H. Yu and J. Gordon, Nature [New Biol.] **244**, 20 (1973).
22. A. Schimpl and E. Wecker, Nature [New Biol.] **237**, 15 (1972).
23. J. M. Fidler and E. Golub, Personal communication (1973).

24. E P. Rieber and G. Riethmuller, Z. Immunol. Forsch. **147**, 262 (1974).
25. M. Feldmann, J. Exp. Med. **135**, 1049 (1972).
26. P. J. Lachmann and H. E. Amos, in *Immunopathology, VIth International Symposium* (P. A. Miescher, ed.), Grune and Stratton, New York, Vol. 6, pp. 65-72, 1970.
27. E. P. Rieber and G. Riethmuller, Z. Immunol. Forsch. **147**, 276 (1974).
28. M. Taniguchi and T. Tada, J. Immunol. **113**, 1757 (1973).
29. M. J. Taussig and A. J. Munro, Fed. Proc. **35**, 206 (1976).
30. R. M. Gorczynski, R. M. Miller, and R. A. Phillips, J. Immunol. **110**, 968 (1973).
31. J. J. Mond, T. Takahashi, and G. J. Thorbecke, J. Exp. Med. **136**, 715 (1972).
32. M. Feldmann, R. E. Cone, and J. J. Marchalonis, Cell. Immunol. **9**, 1 (1973).
33. M. Feldmann and J. W. Schrader, Cell. Immunol. **14**, 235 (1973).
34. S. J. Singer and G. L. Nicolson, Science **175**, 720 (1972).
35. R. B. Taylor, W. P. H. Duffus, M. C. Raff, and S. de Petris, Nature [New Biol.] **233**, 225 (1971).
36. R. F. Ashman and M. C. Raff, J. Exp. Med. **137**, 69 (1973).
37. H. Waldmann and A. Munro, Nature (London) **243**, 256 (1974).
38. J. W. Schrader, J. Exp. Med. submitted for publication (1973).
38a. M. Feldmann, A. W. Boylston, and N. Hogg, Eur. J. Immunol. **5**, 429 (1976).
39. G. Doria, G. Agarossi, and S. di Pietro, J. Immunol. **108**, 547 (1972).
40. R. M. Gorczynski, R. G. Miller, and R. A. Phillips, J. Immunol. **108**, 547 (1972).
41. J. A. Hirst and R. W. Dutton, Cell. Immunol. **1**, 190 (1970).
42. O. Sjöberg, Clin. Exp. Immunol. **12**, 365 (1972).
43. A. Schimpl and E. Wecker, Personal communication (1973).
44. R. M. Gorczynski, R. Miller, and R. A. Phillips, Transplant. Proc. **5**, 607 (1973).
45. R. M. Gorczynski, R. Miller, and R. A. Phillips, J. Immunol. **111**, 900 (1973).
46. D. P. Osborne, Jr. and D. H. Katz, J. Exp. Med. **137**, 991 (1973).
47. J. H. L. Playfair and E. C. Purves, Nature [New Biol.] **231**, 149 (1971).
48. J. S. Haskill, J. Marbrook, and B. E. Elliott, Nature [New Biol.] **233**, 237 (1971).
49. H. Wagner, J. Immunol. **109**, 630 (1972).
50. M. C. Raff, Nature (London) **246**, 350 (1973).
51. J. F. A. P. Miller and N. L. Warner, Int. Arch. Allergy Appl. Immunol. **40**, 59 (1971).
52. H. Waldmann and A. Munro, Immunology **27**, 53 (1974).
53. B. A. Askonas, A. Schimpl, and E. Wecker, Eur. J. Immunol. **4**, 164 (1974).
54. A. Schimpl and E. Wecker, J. Exp. Med. **137**, 547 (1973).
55. M. Feldmann, Unpublished data (1973).
56. J. W. Schrader, Personal communication (1973).
57. J. D. Watson, J. Immunol. **111**, 1301 (1973).
58. D. H. Katz, Transplant. Rev. **12**, 141 (1972).
59. M. B. Pepys, Nature [New Biol.] **237**, 157 (1972).
60. P. Dukor and K. Hartmann, Cell. Immunol. **7**, 349 (1973).

61. P. Dukor, G. Schuman, R. H. Gisler, M. Dierich, W. Konig, U. Hadding, and D. Bitter-Sauerman, J. Exp. Med. **139**, 337 (1974).
62. G. Schuman, R. H. Gesler, M. Dierich, U. Hadding, D. Bitter-Sauerman, and P. Dukor, in *Proceedings of the 8th Leucocyte Culture Conference, Uppsala* (K. Lindahl-Kiessling and D. Osoba, eds.), Academic Press, New York, 1973.
62a. M. Feldmann and M. B. Pepys, Nature (London) **249**, 159 (1974).
63. N. R. St C. Sinclair, Immunology **12**, 549 (1967).
64. R. B. Taylor and H. H. Wortis, Nature (London) **220**, 927 (1968).
65. G. F. Mitchell, J. H. Humphrey, and A. R. Williamson, Eur. J. Immunol. **2**, 460 (1972).
66. W. W. Bullock and M. B. Rittenberg, Immunochemistry **7**, 310 (1970).
67. W. W. Bullock and M. B. Rittenberg, J. Exp. Med. **132**, 926 (1970).
68. C. Cheers and J. F. A. P. Miller, J. Exp. Med. **136**, 1661 (1972).
69. G. W. Siskind and B. Benacerraf, Advan. Immunol. **10**, 1 (1969).
70. R. K. Gershon and W. E. Paul, J. Immunol. **106**, 872 (1971).
71. R. K. Gershon and K. Kondo, Immunology **23**, 335 (1972).
72. J. Mitchell, J. Pye, M. C. Holmes, and G. J. V. Nossal, Aust. J. Exp. Biol. Med. Sci. **50**, 637 (1972).
73. S. Kontiainen and N. A. Mitchison, Immunology **28**, 523 (1975).
74. S. Kontiainen, Immunology **28**, 534 (1975).
75. L. Claflin, B. Merchant, and J. Inman, J. Immunol. **110**, 241 (1973).
76. L. Claflin and B. Merchant, J. Immunol. **110**, 252 (1973).
77. J. D. Wilson and M. Feldmann, Nature [New Biol.] **237**, 3 (1972).
78. R. Huchet and M. Feldmann, Eur. J. Immunol. **3**, 49 (1973).
79. E. Möller and O. Mäkelä, in *Proceedings of the 3rd Lepetit Colloquium*, North-Holland, Amsterdam, p. 214, 1972.
80. S. F. Schlossman and A. Williamson in *Genetic Control of Immune Responsiveness* (H. O. McDevitt and M. Landy, eds.), Academic Press, New York, p. 54, 1972.
81. I. Schechter, B. Schechter, and M. Sela, Biochim. Biophys. Acta **127**, 438 (1966).
82. H. O. McDevitt and M. Landy (eds.), *Genetic Control of Immune Responsiveness,* Academic Press, New York, 1972.
83. G. M. Shearer, E. Mozes, and M. Sela, J. Exp. Med. **135**, 1009 (1972).
84. M. Feldmann, Transplant. Proc. **5**, 111 (1973).
85. M. Feldmann, J. Sprent, and L. Hudson, Unpublished data (1973).
86. M. Feldmann and A. Basten, Eur. J. Immunol. **2**, 213 (1972).
87. J. H. Playfair, Presentation at BSI meeting, April 1973.
88. T. O. Yoshida and B. Andersson, Scand. J. Immunol. **1**, 401 (1972).
89. R. F. Cone, M. Feldmann, J. J. Marchalonis, and G. J. V. Nossal, Immunology, **26**, 49 (1974).
90. A. W. Harris, A. D. Bankhurst, S. Mason, and N. L. Warner, J. Immunol. **110**, 431 (1973).
91. A. W. Boylston, Immunology **24**, 851 (1973).
92. B. Pernis, P. Krammer, and L. Forni, Personal communication (1973).
93. G. Roelants, L. Forni, and B. Pernis, J. Exp. Med. **137**, 1060 (1973).

94. G. Roelants, A. Ryden, N. Hogg, and F. Loor, Nature (London) **247**, 106 (1973).
94a. G. Roelants, L. Form, and B. Pernis, J. Exp. Med. **137**, 1060 (1973).
95. R. K. Gershon and K. Kondo, Immunology **21**, 903 (1971).
96. M. Cooper, G. L. Ada, and R. E. Langman, Cell. Immunol. **4**, 289 (1972).
97. A. Basten, J. F. A. P. Miller, J. Sprent, and C. Cheers, J. Exp. Med. **140**, 199 (1974).
98. J. M. Phillips, F. Quagliata, and D. D. Benzinger, J. Immunol. **111**, 1712 (1973).
99. R. Huchet and M. Feldmann, Eur. J. Immunol. **3**, 49 (1973).
100. M. Feldmann, Eur. J. Immunol. **4**, 660 (1974).
101. P. J. Baker, R. F. Barth, P. W. Stashak, and D. F. Amsbaugh, J. Immunol. **104**, 1313 (1970).
102. P. J. Baker, N. D. Reed, P. W. Stashak, D. F. Amsbaugh, and B. Prescott, J. Exp. Med. **137**, 1431 (1973).
103. M. Feldmann, Eur. J. Immunol. **4**, 667 (1974).
104. H. Waldmann and A. Munro, Eur. J. Immunol. **4**, 410 (1974).
105. T. Tada, K. Okumura, and M. Taniguchi, J. Immunol. **108**, 1535 (1972).
106. J. M. Dwyer and F. S. Kantor, J. Exp. Med. **137**, 32 (1973).
107. M. J. Taussig, Curr. Topics Microbiol. Immunol. **60**, 125 (1973).
108. P. Liacopoulos and S. Ben Efraim, Progr. Allergy, **21**, 72 (1975).
109. H. Pross and D. Eidinger, Advan. Immunol. **18**, 1 (1974).
110. N. I. Brody and G. W. Siskind, Immunology **22**, 185 (1972).
111. N. I. Brody and G. W. Siskind, Immunology **22**, 75 (1972).
112. J. M. Rhodes and S. O. Larsen, Immunology **23**, 817 (1972).
113. R. E. Tigelaar and R. Asofsky, J. Exp. Med. **137**, 239 (1973).
114. H. Wagner, M. Rollinghof, and M. Feldmann, in *Proceedings of the 8th Leucocyte Culture Conference, Uppsala* (K. Lindahl-Kiessling and D. Osoba, eds.) Academic Press, New York, p. 111, 1973.
115. R. Tigelaar and M. Feldmann, Transplant. Proc. **5**, 1711 (1973).
116. P. Hayry and L. C. Andersson, Transplant. Proc. **5**, 1697 (1973).
117. H. Wagner, J. Exp. Med. **138**, 1379 (1973).
118. V. P. Eijsvogel, R. du Bois, C. J. M. Melief, W. P. Zeylemaker, L. Raat-Koning and L. de Groot-Kooy, Transplant. Proc. **5**, 415 (1973).
119. F. H. Bach, M. L. Bach, P. M. Sondel, and G. Sundharadas, Transplant. Rev. **12**, 30 (1972); F. H. Bach, Transplant. Proc. **5**, 23 (1973).
120. H. Wagner, M. Rollinghof, and G. J. V. Nossal, Transplant. Rev. **17**, 3 (1973).
121. M. Hoffmann and R. W. Dutton, Science **172**, 1047 (1971).
122. K. Shortman and J. Palmer, Cell. Immunol. **2**, 399 (1971).
123. F. H. Bach, B. J. Alter, S. Solliday, D. C. Zoschke, and M. Janis, Cell. Immunol. **1**, 219 (1970).
124. W. Byrd, M. Feldmann, and J. Palmer, Immunology **27**, 331 (1974).
125. M. Feldmann, Eur. J. Immunol. **2**, 130 (1972).
126. E. M. Hersh and J. E. Harris, J. Immunol. **100**, 1184 (1968).
127. H. Wagner, M. Feldmann, W. Boyle, and J. W. Schrader, J. Exp. Med. **136**, 331 (1972).
128. R. C. Seeger and J. J. Oppenheim, J. Exp. Med. **132**, 44 (1970).

129. I. Gery, R. K. Gershon, and B. H. Waksman, J. Exp. Med. **136**, 128 (1972).
130. J. L. Turk, *Delayed Hypersensitivity*, North-Holland, Amsterdam, 1967.
131. N. A. Mitchison, Immunology **16**, 1 (1969).
132. E. R. Unanue and B. A. Askonas, Immunology **15**, 287 (1968).
133. R. C. Seeger and J. J. Oppenheim, J. Immunol. **109**, 244 (1972).
134. D. L. Rosenstreich, J. T. Blake, and A. S. Rosenthal, J. Exp. Med. **134**, 1170 (1971).
135. S. Kontiainen and M. Feldman, Nature (London) **245**, 285 (1973).
136. I. Gery and B. H. Waksman, J. Exp. Med. **136**, 143 (1972).
137. M. Cohn, in *Genetic Control of Immune Responsiveness* (H. O. McDeivtt and M. Landy, eds.), Academic Press, New York, p. 367, 1972.
138. P. Bretscher, Transplant. Rev. **11**, 217 (1972).
139. M. Feldmann and M. F. Greaves, unpublished data (1973).
140. M. Feldmann and J. W. Schrader, Cell Immunol. **14**, 235 (1973).
141. Transplant. Proc. **5**, 43 (1973).
142. M. Feldmann and A. Basten, J. Exp. Med. **136**, 49 (1972).
143. T. Tada, in *Proceedings of the 9th Leucocyte Culture Conference* (A. S. Rosenthal, ed.), p. 771, 1975.
144. M. Feldmann, P. Beverly, M. Dunkley, and S. Kontiainen, Nature (London) **258**, 614 (1975).
145. M. Feldmann, D. Kilburn and J. Levy, Nature (London) **256**, 741 (1975).
146. M. Feldmann and S. Kontiainen, Eur. J. Immunol. **6**, 302 (1976).
147. P. Erb and M. Feldmann, J. Exp. Med. **142**, 460 (1975).
148. P. Erb, M. Feldmann, and N. Hogg, Eur. J. Immunol. **6**, 365 (1976).

CHAPTER 9

Genetic Factors in the Immune Response: The Immune Response Genes

James W. Goding

Cellular Immunology Unit
The Walter and Eliza Hall Institute of Medical Research
Royal Melbourne Hospital
Victoria, Australia

I. Introduction

The current explosion of knowledge in immunogenetics, as witnessed by the almost simultaneous appearance of two new journals devoted entirely to the subject, stems largely from the belief that in this field may lie the solution to many central problems in immunology. The elucidation of the structure of DNA [1] and the realization that there was, in general, a "one-way" flow of information from DNA to protein had enormous impact on immunology and was a major factor that led to the acceptance of "selectionist" theories of antibody formation [2]. Similarly, the influence of germ line genes on immune responsiveness might be seen in terms of protein structure, perhaps in some cases at the level of the amino acid sequences of secreted antibody and/or lymphocyte receptors for antigen [3]. If all antibody/receptor diversity were in the germ line [4], the interpretation of such "immune response gene" phenomena would be simplified, but at present this question is still very much under debate [5-7].

In this chapter, the principal known sites of genetic influence on the immune response will be surveyed, and then the role of the "immune response" (Ir) genes linked to the major histocompatibility complex (MHC) will be discussed in detail. The MHC consists of a group of closely linked (and possibly *functionally related*) [8] genes that control a variety of immunologic phenomena, including rejection of transplanted organs [9], susceptibility or resistance to viral [42], neoplastic [10], and autoimmune [11] disease, complement levels [12], and specific immune responses to a variety of antigens. There is a considerable body of evidence to suggest that these Ir genes control antigen recognition at the level of the thymus-derived lymphocyte (T cell), and it has been proposed [13] that they represent the structural genes for a nonimmunoglobulin T-cell receptor for antigen. In view of the continuing controversy over the nature of the T-cell receptor, this elegant and provocative hypothesis is currently being vigorously investigated.

This chapter will not attempt to cover in detail immunoglobulin genetics or the nature of the "generator of diversity" (GOD). Several excellent reviews of these topics have recently appeared [5-7,14]. It might be noted that the current interest in the MHC-linked Ir genes has been spurred on by a series of unexpected findings. The initial discovery of immune response genes to poly-L-lysine (PLL) and (T,G)-A-L* were unexpected [15,16], as was the subsequent demonstration of linkage of the Ir-1 locus to the MHC in the mouse [17,18]. The strong evidence for the functional expression of Ir-1 in T cells was met with an equally surprising finding of a new *B-cell* antigen controlled by a gene closely linked to, or possibly identical with, this gene [19,20]. These findings may represent a warning to approach the future with an open mind.

The genetics of the immune response have been frequently reviewed [3,13,21-26].

II. Survey of Mechanisms

In a system as complex as that involved in immune responsiveness, which depends on antigen processing and degradation, molecular recognition, gene activation, synthesis of macromolecules, and many other functions, there are many sites where genetics factors could operate. It should perhaps be pointed out that although many examples of genetic control of the immune response are known, the precise mechanism of action is known for only a few of them. Figure 1 is a much simplified plan of the immune system which illustrates a few points where genetic factors might act.

An obvious possible mechanism for genetic control of immune responsiveness is self-tolerance [27]. An individual would be expected to be unable to make an immune response against "self"-components, and therefore should be tolerant to antigenic determinants which are closely related to self. Most self-components are probably "thymus-dependent" antigens, and a case can be made for the idea that self-tolerance is largely, if not entirely, a T-cell function [28-30]. Therefore, such a model might well be expressed exclusively in T cells.

An F_1 heterozygote between a responder and a nonresponder to a given antigen would be expected to be a *nonresponder* in this model, since the individual concerned would express the relevant self-component. Such limited control cannot explain much of the available data, since in many situations where genetic control has been demonstrated, *response* is dominant. However,

---

*A synthetic branched polypeptide, which consists of a poly-L-lysine backbone, side chains of poly-D,L-alanine, and the amino terminal tips of tyrosine and glutamic acid in a randomly mixed sequence (Fig. 2, p. 325).

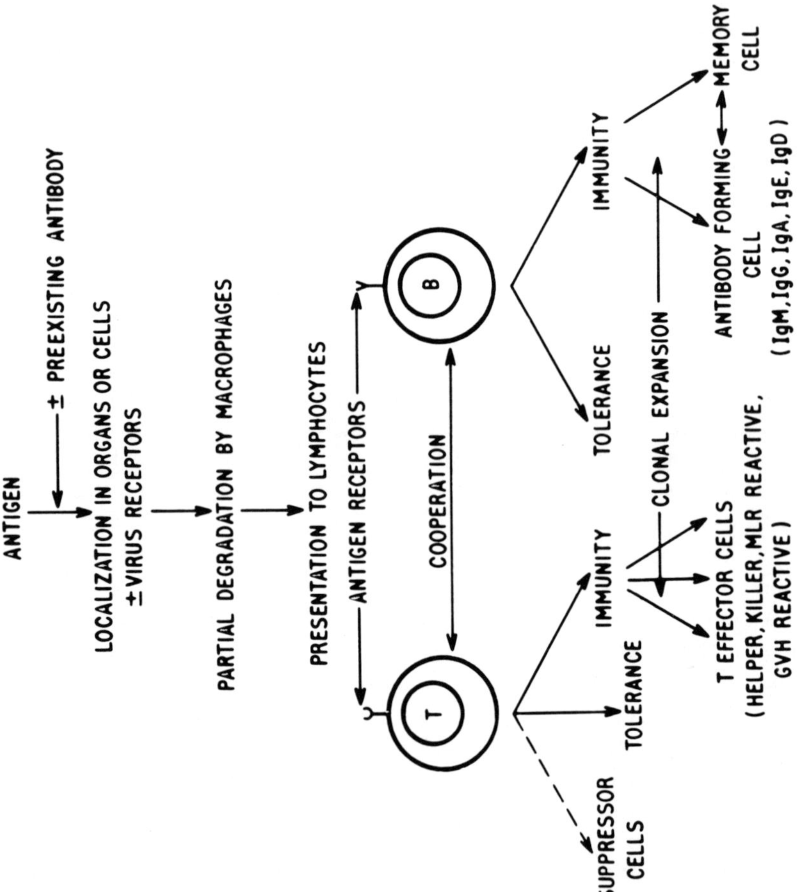

FIG. 1. Simplified plan of the immune response.

situations can be devised where a "self-tolerance" model may produce dominant responsiveness.

For example, consider the hypothetical case where an animal A makes an antibody with a particular variable region structure (idiotype) against animal B [31]. If this antibody is purified and reinjected into A, no anti-idiotypic antibodies should be formed. However, if it is injected into an A × B F_1 animal or a B animal, it should be possible to create anti-idiotypic antibodies, since such antiself-idiotypes should be absent from these strains. (This argument is somewhat weakened by the experimental finding [32] that, in some circumstances, it *is* possible to raise anti-idiotypic antibodies in rabbits against an antibody molecule that the individual has previously produced.)

Other theoretical tolerance models where responsiveness is dominant have been explored [33]. For example, if an immune response gene codes for a *repressor* molecule that *inhibits* production of a self-component, only the homozygote (which does *not* possess the repressor) will make the relevant self-component, and response to this antigen will be dominant. Similarly, dominant tolerance models can be made by proposing enzymes which "mask" or degrade self-components.

The rate of antigen degradation, a vital parameter in the immune response, must frequently depend on the presence or absence of suitable enzymes. One of the characteristics of the so-called thymus-independent antigens is their poor degradation and persistence in the body (see Chap. 6). It would seem likely that even in the absence of an immune system, considerable "self-nonself" discrimination could occur, perhaps via enzymes that break down components not normally present in the individual. Even single cell organisms, such as the ameba, appear to be capable of some self-nonself discrimination.

There are several examples of the importance of genetic factors in the phagocytic system. In mice infected with arbovirus B, a recessive allele in phagocytic cells of susceptible mice allows viral replication and continuing invasion. Certain strains of mice infected with hepatitis virus show a similar genetic influence or susceptibility that is determined by the selective destruction of macrophages that normally prevent viremia. Resistance appears to be controlled by a single dominant gene, possibly a lysosomal enzyme [34,35]. The defect in genetic nonresponder mice at the Ir-3 locus can be overcome by the administration of syngeneic peritoneal exudate cells ("macrophages") [36]. Marked differences attributed to macrophage activity were noted in strains of mice selected and bred for high or low response to sheep red blood cells [37,275]. The high-responder strain had a relatively slow clearance of antigen, whereas clearance was rapid in the low-responder strain.

It would seem quite likely that genetic polymorphisms in the structure of membrane proteins might influence their ability to act as receptor sites for attachment of viruses [38]. At present, there is little evidence for this possibility, although one gene (Fv-2) [39] in the complex series of events related to *susceptibility* to murine leukemia virus is dominant, consistent with a receptor role or tolerance to the virus due to "molecular mimicry" [40]. The Fv-2 gene is not linked to the MHC. On the other hand, the Rgv-1 gene, which controls *resistance* to Gross virus leukemogenesis in the mouse [41], is also dominant. This gene has been mapped to the K end of the MHC. However, the situation is rather complex, since the F_1 hybrid between two susceptible strains was highly *resistant*. The genetic control of specific immune responses to certain viral infections has recently been reviewed [42].

There is strong evidence that some instances of genetic control of immune responsiveness are at the level of structural genes for antibody variable region (see Sec. VI. A), and there is also some circumstantial evidence for control at the combining sites for antigen on B, and possibly T, cells [3]. *It would be expected, however, that recognition of most antigens could occur via many different determinants and that a single mutation that alters the affinity of a single receptor would not be detectable.* These topics will be discussed in more detail in a later section.

Genetic factors might also play a role in determining the degree of clonal expansion after triggering of lymphocytes. The role of accessory, or "amplifying," factors, such as histamine, lymphokines, or complement, is uncertain. Few genetic deficiencies in complement components have any deleterious effects on immune competence [43], although there are marked differences in complement levels among various inbred strains of mice [43-46]. Female mice, in general, have lower complement levels than do males. Genetic aspects of the complement system have been reviewed by Alper and Rosen [43].

Yet another series of points where genetic influences could act is in the deficiencies of immunocytic differentiation, as discussed in Sec. II. These defects are, in general, not antigen specific, although there may be broad differences in responses to the thymus-dependent and thymus-independent antigens. They may shed considerable light on the pathways of immunocytic differentiation.

III. Immune Deficiency States

A. B-cell Defects

The known B-cell defects are associated, in general, with marked defects in immunoglobulin synthesis. Most information comes from study of humans, and no mouse counterpart has yet been described. The classic "Bruton" type [47] is known to be genetic in origin, and the gene involved lies on the

X chromosome. The defect is recessive, and therefore only expressed in males, who experience recurrent infections with pyogenic organisms. Since the known immunoglobulin structural genes are not located on the X chromosome, it is reasonable to postulate that the defect lies in some form of B-cell differentiation or regulation rather than in immunoglobulin structure or control. In the few well-documented cases that have been studied, it was found that there was a marked deficiency of lymphocytes in "B areas" and grossly diminished numbers of recirculating lymphocytes with high-density surface immunoglobulin [48]. The considerable number of subclasses of this disorder have been discussed by Cooper et al. [49].

B. T-cell Defects

The first well-documented instance of an isolated T-cell defect was described by DiGeorge [50]. There are defects in the differentiation of the third and fourth pharyngeal pouches and corresponding defects in the differentiation of thymus and parathyroid tissue. Such children have apparently normal B-cell development, and the "B-cell areas" of lymph node, spleen, and Peyer's patches are not depleted. Their antibody levels are normal, and most of the circulating lymphocytes bear large amounts of surface immunoglobulin and are therefore probably B cells. Evidence for a genetic cause is not very satisfactory, although one family [51] has been described where the illness occurred in related individuals.

A similar deficiency disease exists in the congenitally athymic ("nude") mouse [52]. These mice have a deficiency in body hair and a marked abnormality of thymic development. The thymic anlage develops initially, but by the 14th day of development, it is found to be abnormal, and it subsequently stops developing. Such mice are rather susceptible to a variety of infections, but with meticulous attention to their environment, they can be maintained in good health. Nude mice have greatly impaired graft rejection and, in fact, appear to accept indefinitely skin grafts from such widely differing phylogenetic sources as frogs, birds, and cats [53]. The "nude" mouse almost totally lacks functional T cells, although some debate continues about the completeness of the defect [55,55]. Under some circumstances, lymphocytes from such mice can be induced to display typical T-cell markers, such as Thy-1 or Tla [56]. These mice have proven extremely useful as a research tool.

C. Combined Immune Deficiency

Deficiencies of this type are extremely rare. They have been most extensively studied in humans, although only about 100 cases have been reported. Both T and B cells are affected, and the unfortunate children afflicted are very susceptible to all kinds of infection, most notably by organisms that are not usually pathogenic to normal individuals, such as *Pneumocystis carinii* [57]. The thymus is very small and almost devoid of lymphoid cells and Hassal's corpuscles, although epithelial cells are still present. There are very few circulating lymphocytes, and the peripheral lymphoid organs, such as lymph node, spleen, and Peyer's patches, are greatly depleted in both T and B areas. The exact defect is unknown but would appear to be at the level of differentiation from a primitive stem cell to a cell that is a precursor for all lymphoid cells. Various subgroups, and even more serious defects, which involve both the lymphoid and granulocytic series, have been described [49]. The survival of these children is extremely short.

IV. Antigen-specific Genetic Control

A. Early Studies

The study of antigen-specific genetic factors in immune responses began with the demonstration by Bernstein that the ABO blood groups are determined by three allelic genes. In the next few years, perhaps the most significant work was that of Landsteiner, whose brilliant studies on human blood groups ultimately made safe blood transfusion a clinical reality. Other early studies include those of Smith [58], who in 1905 demonstrated familial differences in the susceptibility of guinea pigs to the lethal effect of diphtheria toxin, and Cook and Van der Veer [59], who showed that inheritance plays a major role in the development of a variety of diseases for which an immunologic component is likely, namely, hay fever, bronchial asthma, and other forms of human allergy. Differences in the susceptibility to tuberculosis [60] and *Salmonella* infections [61] were attributed to genetic causes. Other particulate antigens, such as xenogeneic erythrocytes, have also been studied. Marked differences were found in the level of natural antibodies [62] and response after immunization [63] in various strains of inbred mice. More recently, Biozzi et al. [37] were able to produce high- and low-responder strains by selectively breeding outbred mice for high and low response to sheep erythrocytes. The effect of genetic differences on the response to protein antigens, such as tetanus or diphtheria toxoids [64,65], and carbohydrate antigens, such as pneumococcal polysaccharide [66], have also been explored. A detailed account of studies of this type has been given by Gasser and Silvers [24].

These early studies, in general, showed only a definite *correlation* between responses of parent and offspring, without any clear-cut pattern of inheritance. This result was probably due to the type and dosage of antigen and may have reflected multigenic control. Over the last 10 years, studies have been considerably refined and simplified by careful attention to the nature and dose of antigen used, and by the use of various inbred strains of animals with well-defined genetic characteristics. By the use of these techniques, it has frequently been possible to demonstrate *single* loci which determine the immune response in a given situation. These loci have been termed "immune regulatory" or "immune response" (Ir) genes.

B. Choice of Antigen

The first mentioned technique (choice of antigen and dosage) probably depends mainly on production of an immunization regimen that stimulates only a very small number of clones. In this way, it would be hoped that any genetic differences among individuals in clone size or responsiveness for a particular determinant would be emphasized. There are several possible ways of tackling such a problem. First, one may use very low doses of antigen to stimulate only those (presumably rare) clones which have high affinity for the immunodominant groups on the antigen. By this technique, genetic differences in response to complex antigens have been shown [67,68]. Similarly, the *type* of antigen may be chosen such that the number of differences between the corresponding "self"-protein and the antigen in question are small. For example, Arquilla and Finn [69] showed that strain-2 guinea pigs made antibody to the amino terminal end of the A and B chains of porcine insulin, whereas strain 13 only made antibody to the carboxy terminal determinants.

Antigens with even more limited variation from "self" can be produced by use of myeloma allotypes [70]. These antigens are genetic variants of immunoglobulin amino acid sequences for a given class, which usually involve only one or two amino acids and usually in the constant region of the light or heavy chains. Yet another way of limiting the effective heterogeneity of antigen is by the use of synthetic polypeptides, which have been extensively explored by Sela and Fuchs [72]. Such antigens are usually randomly linear or branched copolymers of a limited number of amino acids, often on a well-defined "backbone," such as poly-L-lysine. *Despite these restrictions, such antigens are by no means rigorously defined chemically and may vary greatly in molecular weight and immunogenicity from batch to batch.*

C. Inbred Animals

A second major factor in the current explosion of knowledge about the genetics of the immune response has been the use of inbred animals. Due to the work of Snell, Stimpfling, Klein, Shreffler, Amos, and others, a large stock of inbred strains of mice with well-defined genetic characteristics has been produced. The convenience of the mouse as a laboratory animal and the ready availability of a wide variety of strains has made it the animal of choice for many studies. Although the mouse is by far the best characterized mammal with respect to immunologic characteristics, inbred guinea pigs have also been extensively studied.

Of particular interest are the "congenic" strains of mice (i.e., pairs of strains that differ at only one locus or one small group of linked genes), which were extensively studied by Snell [73]. Such mice are produced by crossing two inbred lines, repeatedly backcrossing the progeny to one of the parental lines, and selecting progeny with the desired genotype. By prolonged backcrossing over 15 to 20 generations, mice are produced which are genetically identical to one parental strain, except for the desired chromosomal segment of the other parent. For example, C57Bl/10 mice (abbreviated B10) were crossed with strain A. The resultant F_1 hybrids were backcrossed to strain B10, and the progeny were selected for the major histocompatibility locus (H-2) of strain A (H-2^a). These progeny were then repeatedly backcrossed to B10 (H-2^b), with selection of the progeny for H-2^a. Eventually, a new strain was produced which was identical to B10, except for the H-2 region. The new strain is designated B10.A, and the pair B10 and B10.A are said to be congenically *resistant*, because they reject tumors from the partner strain.

By an analogous process, it has been possible to transfer en bloc the structural genes for the immunoglobulin heavy chains (which are all closely linked) from one strain to another, producing mice congenic for immunoglobulin heavy-chain allotype. Similarly, the "nude" mutation (Sec. III.B), which arose in outbred mice, has been transferred to standard inbred lines. Any desired gene may be transferred onto a given background by this process.

The congenic mice have played a central role in localization of certain immune response genes to the major histocompatibility locus and will be referred to frequently in the rest of this chapter. A further technique that promises to be useful for rapid screening of linkage of newly defined genes is the "recombinant inbred mice" of Bailey [74].

V. Immune Response Genes in the Guinea Pig

A. The PLL and Related Genes

One of the earliest examples of immune response genes to be studied in detail was in guinea pigs. When randomly bred Hartley guinea pigs were immunized with hapten conjugated poly-L-lysine (PLL), it was found that the conjugates were only immunogenic in some animals [75]. This discovery arose partly from a chance observation [15] made during attempts to produce anti-dinitrophenyl (anti-DNP) antibodies of restricted heterogeneity by coupling DNP to a presumed nonimmunogenic carrier (PLL). The antibodies were, in fact, highly heterogeneous, but the incidental observation of differences in response to PLL marked the beginning of an important new line of work.

It was also found [75] that the immune response to 2,4-dinitrophenyl-glutamic acid-lysine copolymer (DNP-GL) or GL alone showed a similar variation among outbred Hartley guinea pigs. Responder animals made large amounts of anti-DNP antibodies and showed delayed-type hypersensitivity (DTH) to the relevant antigens. The nonresponders produced negligible quantities of specific antibodies and did not show DTH to these antigens.

When inbred guinea pigs were studied, it was found that all strain-2 animals were responders to DNP-PLL and DNP-GL, whereas all strain-13 guinea pigs were nonresponders. F_1 hybrids (2 × 13) were responders [23]. Studies of backcross animals showed that a single gene was involved. There was no sex linkage. Thus, the ability of guinea pigs to respond to DNP-PLL is controlled by a single, autosomal, dominant gene (the "PLL gene").

So far, the PLL gene and the gene that controls the response to DNP-GL have not been separated. More recently, specific genes have been described that control the response of guinea pigs to other amino acid copolymers, such as a copolymer of glutamic acid and tyrosine (GT) and glutamic acid and alanine (GA). Strain-13 guinea pigs are responders to GT and nonresponders to GA, whereas strain-2 animals are responders to GA but not to GT [76-78]. So far, test matings have revealed few, if any, recombinational events that separate these genes. Whether they are alternative alleles at the same locus or very closely linked but distinct genes ("pseudo-alleles") has not yet been unequivocally established. In outbred guinea pigs, some individuals are responders to GA but nonresponders to PLL, which suggests that the genes responsible, in this case at least, may be separate. It is not entirely clear, though, whether the GA genes in the inbred and outbred guinea pigs are the same [79]. The poorly defined genetics of the guinea pig has been a considerable problem in this type of work.

B. Linkage to the Major Histocompatibility System

In 1968, McDevitt and Tyan [17] found that the Ir-1 locus in mice, which controls the immune response to the synthetic polypeptide (H,G)-A–L, was linked to the major histocompatibility locus (see Sec. VI.A).

This finding prompted examination of the linkage of the PLL and related genes. It was found [80] that in the progeny of $F_1 \times 2$ backcross animals, only individuals with type-2 histocompatibility (H) determinants (as assessed by lysis of lymphocytes by 13 anti-2 serum) were responders. Similarly, only lymphocytes from responder individuals provoked proliferation when cultured with strain-13 lymphocytes, which implied that the responders had inherited the strain-2 H antigens.

C. Other H-linked Ir Genes

Several other examples of H-linked specific immune response genes have been found in guinea pigs. When guinea pigs were immunized with *limiting doses* of bovine serum albumin (BSA) emulsified in complete Freund's adjuvant (CFA), the responder status segregated in parallel to responsiveness to PLL [67]. Another intriguing example is that of an immune response gene to dinitrophenylated guinea pig albumin (i.e., a slightly modified "self"-antigen) [81]. However, if larger doses are given, the genetic control to these antigens can be overridden, and all individuals become responders. Presumably, in the limiting cases, only clones of very high affinity for the antigen concerned are triggered.

D. Cellular Expression of the H-linked Ir Genes

By the technique of adoptive transfer, similar genes in the mouse were shown to be expressed in lymphoid cells [17]. Thus, the question of whether these genes are expressed in T lymphocytes, B lymphocytes, and/or macrophages became of central importance in understanding their action. This issue has been approached from several directions.

Green and coworkers [82] showed that nonresponder animals could be made to produce specific anti-DNP antibodies by immunization with DNP-PLL coupled to a recognizable foreign "carrier" protein, such as BSA or ovalbumin (OVA). However, this maneuver did *not* restore DTH in the nonresponders. This important experiment implied that the nonresponder animals possessed the necessary anti-DNP antibody-forming cell precursors (AFCP) and immunoglobulin structural genes but that these cells were not being triggered due to lack of recognition of the PLL "carrier" moiety.

It had previously been shown [83] that for a strong anti-DNP antibody titer in a secondary response, DNP had to be coupled to the *same* carrier molecule in the booster dose as in the original priming dose (the "carrier effect"). This phenomenon, a puzzle for many years, was eventually shown to be due to a need for "cooperation" between T cells, which recognized the carrier protein but did not secrete classic antibody, and B cells, which, upon triggering, produced anti-DNP antibody [84]. Thus, the defect in carrier recognition in the nonresponders was at the level of T-cell triggering or T-B cooperation. Moreover, the lack of DTH (for which there is good evidence that T-cell rather than B-cell recognition is crucial [85]) in the nonresponders pointed to a *defect in T-cell triggering.*

These and many other experiments with haptenated antigens demonstrate an apparent difference in the *specificity* of T- and B-cell recognition. It might have been expected that by priming with a hapten-carrier complex, both *antihapten* and anticarrier helper T cells would be induced. However, the carrier effect would seem to imply that there were no hapten-reactive T cells. This implication would, in turn, suggest that recognition of antigen by T cells differs in some fundamental way to that of B cells [3] and is an argument used in support of the notion of a *nonimmunoglobulin* receptor for antigen on T cells.

However, the situation of differing specificity of T- and B-cell antigen recognition is far from clear. Humoral immune responses are very frequently studied by measurement of *antihapten* rather than anticarrier antibody, for technical convenience. Thus, the impression might be gained, for largely methodologic reasons, that B cells recognize haptens or small antigenic determinants, whereas T cells recognize "carriers" or "overall configuration" of antigen.

There are many possible explanations for the carrier effect that do not invoke differing receptor specificity between B and T cells. The haptens used, such as DNP, are frequently very hydrophobic, and simple differences in antigen presentation due to this or other physicochemical properties of the hapten may influence the as yet unknown molecular events among T cells, B cells, macrophages, and antigen which lead to triggering. Similarly, if there are large amounts of natural anti-DNP antibody, this antibody will compete for antigen much more effectively against T cells (which have few receptors) than against B cells [86]. There are several reports in the literature of T cells reactive to very small antigenic determinants [86-89]. Indeed, the carrier effect is by no means an "all or none" situation. It should be borne in mind, however, that, under some circumstances, a "helper" effect can be produced by antihapten antibody [90,91]. The literature is frequently confused by a failure to distinguish between receptor specificity and other requirements for T-cell activation.

If the "holes" in the immune response exemplified by the nonresponders are due to a lack of appropriate receptor genes, this lack would imply that T-cell diversity is less than that of B cells. It is clear that T cells are capable of exquisitely fine antigen recognition, and, in some circumstances, this recognition may be even finer than B-cell recognition. In mice, the synthetic polypeptides (T,G)-A–L, (Phe,G)-A–L and (H,G)-A–L cross react very extensively at the B-cell level but not at the T-cell level [167]. Any attempt to understand the mechanism of the H-linked Ir genes must deal with this fine antigenic discrimination of T cells.

As an alternative approach to the question of the cellular locus of action of the H-linked Ir genes in the guinea pig, Levin and colleagues studies the specificity of antibodies to DNP-oligolysine conjugates in guinea pigs [92]. Guinea pigs were immunized with DNP coupled to short chains of PLL, given in complete Freund's adjuvant. Both responders and nonresponders produced anti-DNP antibody, probably because of the provision of a "carrier" function by formation of complexes with the adjuvant. However, only the responders exhibited DTH to these antigens. The anti-DNP antibodies were tested for their binding energy (as assessed by fluorescence quenching) against a panel of DNP-oligolysine conjugates of varying chain length. It was found that only antibody produced by the *responder* animals was able to distinguish (by differences in binding energy) between chains of oligolysine that differed in length by only one amino acid. The highest binding energy was seen when the antibodies were tested against the same chain length as was used for immunization. The authors concluded that "the antibody forming cell possesses a highly specific recognition system for carrier conformation," and that "the polylysine gene exerts its control at the antihapten antibody-forming cell."

Another approach in the study of heterogeneity of specific antibody is the technique of isoelectric focusing (IEF) [93], in which the antibodies are subjected to electrophoresis in a continuous pH gradient and thus migrate to the position where the pH is precisely equal to their isoelectric point. They then cease migration, since their net charge is zero at that point. IEF is capable of exquisite resolution of minor differences in amino acid content of proteins and allows the identification (with reasonable certainty) of products of single clones (and therefore single variable-region genes) in different individuals. In a later series of experiments that employed this technique, Schlossman [94] found no evidence for significant differences in heterogeneity of anti-DNP-oligolysine antibodies between responders and nonresponders, and many clones of specific antibody were shared between the two. Similar results were reported in mice by Melchers et al. [95], who used the B subunit of lactic dehydrogenase (LDH_B) as the antigen. These results, which are in apparent contradiction to the fluorescence quenching studies [92], suggest that the differences between responders and nonresponders do *not* lie at the antibody (and therefore B-cell) level.

E. Effects of Alloantisera on Antigen-induced Proliferation

As mentioned earlier, the PLL gene was found to be closely linked to the H genes in the guinea pig. To define more closely the gene product responsible for such effects, attempts were made to inhibit genetically controlled immune responses in inbred guinea pigs by the use of antisera directed against the histocompatibility and/or immune response gene products. Strain-2 guinea pigs are responders to DNP-GL, whereas strain 13 are nonresponders. On the other hand, strain-2 animals are nonresponders to GT, whereas strain-13 guinea pigs are responders. Shevach et al. [96] showed that the proliferative response of peritoneal exudate cells to these antigens (which depends on the presence of reactive T cells) was inhibited by such antisera. F_1 hybrids (2 × 13) were immunized with both DNP-GL and GT. It was found that anti-2 antibodies inhibited the response to DNP-GL but had no effect on the response to GT. Conversely, the response to GT was blocked by anti-13 serum but not by anti-2 serum. Such results gave considerable support to the concept that these antibodies were directed against the products of the MHC-linked Ir genes and implied that such products might represent receptor for antigen, the inhibition of alloantisera being due to blockage of antigen-receptor interaction (but see Ref. 315).

However, such inhibition follows the *histocompatibility* gene status rather than the *responder* status in animals where these have been separated [97,274]. One possible explanation for this finding could be that the immune response gene product is the "variable region" for an antigen receptor, while the constant region of the receptor is the H antigen. In this case, the products of these two linked genes would also have to be physically linked on the cell surface, much in the same way as for B-cell surface immunoglobulin [97].

The inhibition of antigen-induced proliferation by alloantisera in the guinea pig is only effective when $F_{(ab)2}$ or whole antisera are used. $F_{(ab)1}$ fragments cause no inhibition, even when the reduced avidity of binding of monomeric fragments is taken into account [98]. These results suggest that the blocking caused by alloantisera is not due to interference with antigen-receptor interaction. Inhibition is effective, even if the cells are exposed to the alloantisera several hours after contact with antigen [98], which indicates that the antisera may act at a point in lymphocyte activation subsequent to antigen/receptor interaction.

In an attempt to determine the nature of the relevant antigens recognized by strain-2 anti-13 and strain-13 anti-2 sera, the antibodies were absorbed with a variety of cell populations [99]. Surprisingly, perhaps, the antigens appeared to be present in much larger amounts on B cells (such as L_2C leukemia) than on T cells. *The antigens were not present on nonlymphoid cells* [101]. The antigens recognized by these antisera have been partially characterized [110]. They are *not* immunoglobulin in nature and have a molecular weight of about 25,000. Their predominant expression in B cells, molecular weight, and association with histocompatibility and immune responses all indicate a striking similarity to the Ia (immune response gene-associated) antigens in mice (see Sec. VI.D).

These findings cast some doubt on whether the antigens concerned are histocompatibility antigens in the general sense of the word. Further, they imply that a structural product on B cells influences T-cell triggering. It is generally thought, however, that optimal B-cell activation depends on T-cell "help" but that the converse is not true (see discussion of T-B asymmetry by Cohn [31]). The defect in antibody production in the nonresponders might be explained by a B-cell defect or a defect in T-B collaboration, but the findings from studies of DTH cannot easily be fitted into such a model.

A requirement for identity at the major histocompatibility complex for effective interaction between T cells and macrophages has been shown for guinea pigs [101]. In the mouse, there is evidence that suggests a need for histocompatibility for effective interaction between cooperating T and B cells [172] and between killer T cells and virus-infected cells [102,103]. The significance of these findings is unknown, but the data suggest that the histocompatibility genes, or closely linked genes, may be important in cell-cell interactions (see Sec. VI.C).

F. Summary

The evidence presented so far strongly suggests that the PLL gene is expressed in T cells but not in B cells, since the defect in the nonresponders is at the carrier recognition level; the nonresponders are unable to mount DTH to the antigen in question; B cells in the nonresponders are able to make antibodies to DNP-PLL when this antigen is coupled to an immunogenic carrier; and since isoelectric focusing data suggest that the antibodies in question have a similar heterogeneity, and many clones are shared between responders and nonresponders.

The guinea pig studies have provided many important clues to the action of the H-linked Ir genes, perhaps the most important of which are the availability of a technically satisfactory in vitro assay for antigen-induced proliferation of lymphocytes, which allows the study of the effects of anti-H antisera on functional Ir gene effects, and the availability of a satisfactory assay for DTH as a direct measure of T-cell function. The measurement of DTH in the mouse is fraught with technical difficulties, although some new approaches are promising [104].

Some of the studies that show inhibition of specific immune responses by alloantisera in the guinea pig support the receptor hypothesis, whereas others do not. It is not absolutely certain whether the targets for such antisera are T cells, B cells, or macrophages. It should be stressed that *the exact nature of the target antigens is also unclear because of lack of truly congenic strains of guinea pig.* The guinea pig studies have been held back by serious deficiencies in two main areas, namely, the poorly defined genetics of the available strains and the lack of good markers for T and B lymphocytes.* The last two factors constitute the major strengths of the mouse as an experimental model, as will be apparent in Sec. VI.

VI. Immune Response Genes in the Mouse

A. Introduction

1. History: the Ir-1 Locus

Progress in murine immunogenetics was greatly accelerated by the finding in 1965 of McDevitt and Sela [16] that the ability of inbred mice to make antibodies to certain synthetic polypeptides, such as (T,G)-A–L [a long backbone of PLL with side chains of poly-D-L-alanine coupled to the ϵ amino groups and with random sequences of tyrosine and glutamic acid coupled to the side chains (Fig. 2)] was under genetic control. This finding was prompted by the chance discovery of marked differences in the immune response to (T,G)-A–L in Sandylops and Himalayan rabbits. The gene that controls responsiveness in mice was shown to be inherited as a Mendelian dominant and was designated Ir-1. C57 mice were found to be high responders, whereas CBA mice responded poorly. F_1 hybrids between the two were intermediate to high responders.

The genetic control was subsequently shown to be transferable by immunocompetent cells, but there was no association of responder or nonresponder status with immunoglobulin allotype or class. These cell transfer experiments were sometimes complicated by graft-versus-host disease (when transferring allogeneic cells to irradiated recipients), and to circumvent this problem, studies were undertaken with pairs of "congenic" mice (see Sec. IV.C) which had the same major histocompatibility (H-2) type but on a different background genotype. The totally unexpected result obtained was

Note added in proof: The genetics of the guinea pig MHC are now much better understood [293].

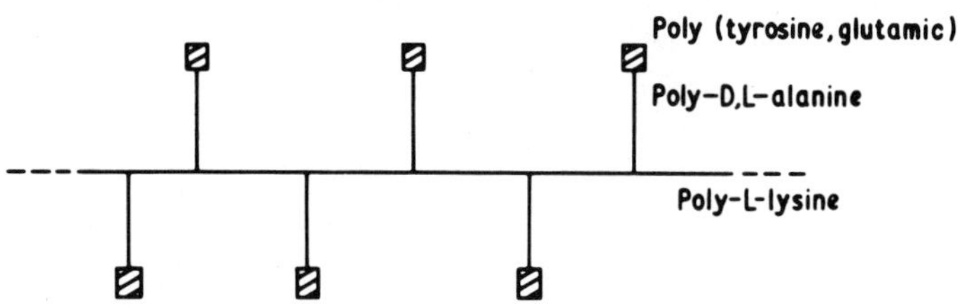

FIG. 2. The synthetic copolymer (T,G)-A–L

that the responder/nonresponder status was controlled by genes in the H-2 chromosomal segment. Animals with H-2^k (e.g., C3H) were low responders, whereas those which were H-2^b (e.g., C3H.SW, which differs from C3H only at H-2) were high responders [17]. The gene locus responsible will be discussed in detail in subsequent sections. In the years that followed, the immune response to dozens of antigens has been shown to be controlled by genes linked to H-2 [106]. The antigens used have generally consisted of synthetic polypeptides, proteins which differ from self by only small changes (e.g., myeloma allotypes), and *low doses* of other proteins. *These antigens are all "thymus dependent" (i.e., depend on T-B cooperation for optimal responses).*

2. *Linkage Relationships of Immunoglobulin Structural Genes*

The linkage relationships of immunoglobulin structural genes may be summarized as follows. The light (κ and λ) -chain genes are not linked to each other, nor are they linked to the heavy-chain genes. However, where data are available, the genes for all heavy-chain classes are very closely linked [14]. Thus, the situation is analogous to the hemoglobin structural genes, where the β-, γ-, and δ-chain genes are closely linked but are not linked to the α-chain genes [107]. The immunoglobulin (Ig) variable-region genes, which contain the genes for antibody (and presumably receptor) -combining site, are known to be very closely linked to the constant-region genes in all cases where data are available, and there are probably good theoretical reasons why this might be a general rule [14].

One of the ways of determining linkage of Ig structural genes depends on the use of Ig allotypes (genetically controlled antigenic determinants on Ig molecules of a given class in individuals of the same species, usually but not always on the constant portion of the molecule) as markers. In view of the apparent specificity of the MHC-linked immune response genes, it was of considerable interest to determine whether these genes code for immunoglobulin variable regions. Such a finding would have considerable importance. At present, there is no known linkage between the MHC-linked Ir genes and any immunoglobulin subclass [3]. In the mouse, the γ-chain allotypes (i.e., presumably the structural genes for the constant portion of the γ-heavy chains) are known to be *not* linked to the MHC. Unfortunately, there are no known allotypes for the light (κ or λ) chains in the mouse, so the linkage of these genes is unknown. However, in man, the InV allotypic marker (for κ-light chains) is known to be *not* linked to the MHC, and there are reasons for supposing that the MHC in the mouse and man are homologous [108]. The possibility that the murine MHC-linked Ir genes code for the K chain or a new and unique class of immunoglobulin, perhaps restricted to the surface receptors of lymphocytes, has been discussed by Cohn [31]. Recent work has allowed this possibility to be examined directly (see Sec. VI.D).

3. *Allotype-linked Immune Response Genes*

A second major class of "immune response" genes in the mouse has been characterized. These genes are linked to the loci known to control immunoglobulin allotypes. These genes are not as clearly defined in terms of response/nonresponse as those previously mentioned and are frequently understood more in terms of the ability to produce an antibody of a given idiotype (variable-region determinant that may be related to antigen-binding specificity) or particular fine specificity.

Several such genes have been described. For example, mice which are high responders to α-1,3-dextran, which is a "thymus-independent" antigen, make a particular idiotype that is lacking in the low-responder strains. The locus responsible is probably a structural gene for the variable region at the immunoglobulin heavy chain [109]. Other examples are the linkage of the strain A/J heavy-chain constant-region allotype (Ig-1e) with genes that control the idiotypic specificity of anti-*p*-azophenylarsonate antibodies (ARS idiotype) [110] and genes that control idiotypic specificity of certain antistreptococcal carbohydrate antibodies (A5A idiotype) [111]. The T15 idiotype of an antiphosphorylcholine antibody has also been linked to allotypic markers [112]. The strains of mice selected by Biozzi for high or low responsiveness to heterologous erythrocytes have been shown to differ in immunoglobulin allotype [113]. Of particular interest has been the recent demonstration [114] that the genes that control the ARS and A5A idiotypes are both linked to the Ig-1e allotype structural gene and that ARS and A5A genes can be separated by crossing over. This is the first recorded instance of recombination between immunoglobulin variable-region genes. Another example of allotype-linked genes that control specific immune responsiveness comes from the work of Imanishi and Mäkelä [115], who demonstrated that a gene that controls the ability to produce antibody of a particularly fine specificity (a heteroclitic antihapten antibody) was linked to immunoglobulin allotype.

Unfortunately, the extensive data on immunoglobulin amino acid sequences [14] and the data on DNA/RNA hybridization [116-118] have not yet allowed agreement on whether *all* V-region genes are carried in the germ line or whether some, or perhaps most, diversity is somatically generated [5-7]. The data on inheritability of idiotypes and antibody fine specificity imply that at least some diversity is carried in the germ line, although these data obviously do not rule out further somatic diversification. It is clear that the allotype-linked immune response genes are expressed in B cells, but their expression in T cells is still uncertain, largely due to lack of a well-defined humoral T-cell product.

4. *The Ir-2 Locus*

This locus, which was originally described by Gasser [119], controls the response in mice to Ea-1, an antigen present on the erythrocytes of most wild mice but few of the standard inbred strains. Strain-YBR mice are responders, while CBA or BALB/c are nonresponders. When YBR animals are crossed with BALB/c or CBA, the ability to respond to Ea-1 antigens is transmitted as a *recessive* trait controlled by a single gene, which was designated Ir-2. At first, it appeared to be due to a single genetic factor linked to agouti (a coat color) and to the minor histocompatibility loci H-3 and H-6 in the fifth linkage group (chromosome 2). Neither linkage was particularly close. However, in crosses between YBR and C57B1 (low-responder) mice, responsiveness is transmitted as a multigenic *dominant* trait [120]. Subsequent work [121] has suggested that several genes are involved, one of which is linked to H-2 (the major histocompatibility locus), in the ninth linkage group (chromosome 17). The Ir-2 gene has not been studied as widely as the other immune response genes, and its exact nature is still undergoing evaluation.

5. The Ir-3 Locus

This locus was first described by Mozes et al. [122]. It controls the antibody response to the *polyproline region* of two related synthetic polypeptides, (T,G)-Pro–L, and (Phe,G)-Pro–L, and is not linked to H-2 or to known immunoglobulin allotypes. Responsiveness is dominant. SJL mice are high responders, whereas DBA/1 mice are low responders. (The response to the *(Phe,G)* determinant of (Phe,G)-A–L, on the other hand, is controlled by a separate gene linked to H-2.)

Experiments that involved syngeneic transfer of graded numbers of bone marrow or thymus cells, together with an excess of the collaborating cell type, have suggested that the defect in the DBA/1 low responders lies in the bone marrow population. However, this type of experiment is based on several assumptions, and its design has been criticized [31]. Interactions between T and B lymphocytes are not "symmetric" (i.e., T cells are needed for optimal B-cell response, but the converse is not true). Further, it is not entirely clear whether there was a true excess of collaborating cells. *The experimental design assumes that the response after transfer of a given number of cells will accurately reflect the frequency of precursor cells for the antigen in question.* However, not all transfer curves resulted in the expected Poisson distribution. The adoptive transfer system is very complex, especially in its dose-response kinetics, and the necessary assumptions may not always be valid [123].

Recently, data have been obtained that suggest that the defect in the low-responder mice at the Ir-3 locus may be corrected by the transfer of an excess of syngeneic peritoneal exudate cells. The active cell was probably a macrophage. Evidence was presented to show that the correction did *not* involve more efficient "antigen processing" but rather was related to some interaction between macrophages and marrow-derived immunocompetent cells [36].

B. The Major Histocompatibility Complex in the Mouse

The rejection of tissue grafts from individuals of the same species is under genetic control and is determined by multiple genes. In each species, however, there appears to be a major *histocompatibility complex* which is of predominant importance. These genes code for antigenic molecules on the cell surface, but the biologic function of these molecules is as yet unknown. Differences between graft and recipient at the major histocompatibility complex often cause rapid graft rejection, while differences at the minor loci may cause rejection after prolonged periods or, in some cases, not at all [124]. The genes in the complex appear to be unusually polymorphic (i.e., have many alleles in a given species). The reason for such polymorphism is unknown and has provoked considerable speculation [8,125,126,270,272,273].

It is well established that in the mouse [106] and in man [127] the major histocompatibility complex consists of at least two, and possibly three or more, distinct loci, each of which may have many alleles in an outbred population. There is also evidence for a two-locus structure in the rhesus monkey [128]. The biologic role of the complex is not understood and has been the subject of much speculation [8,125,129]. One possibility is that it could prevent cancer from being a contagious disease. At least two examples of contagious tumors have been described, where the tumor cells themselves rather than their etiologic agent appear to be responsible. One was in dogs [130], and the other was in hamsters [131]. However, outbreaks of contagious cancer are not commonly seen in laboratories where there are large numbers of genetically identical mice. The complex has also been postulated to be important in the generation of antibody diversity [125], surveillance against cancer [129], or as "differentiation antigens" [132] needed for cell-cell recognition and tissue development.

The structure and function of the murine histocompatibility (H-2) complex has recently been extensively reviewed [106].

1. *The K and D Regions*

The H-2 complex consists of several tightly linked genes, as shown in Fig. 3. The K and D loci, which may be homologous to the FOUR (second) and LA (first) loci, respectively, in the human HL-A complex [108], are separated by a map distance of about one unit (i.e., crossovers between the two are detected in about 1% of matings). The K and D loci are defined serologically, and differences at these loci lead to rapid graft rejection and production of cytotoxic antibodies. However, it is not yet absolutely certain whether these genes, or very closely linked genes, or a combination of the two, are primarily responsible for graft rejection. The K and D loci code for separate polypeptide chains of a molecular weight of about 45,000 [133], and these chains move

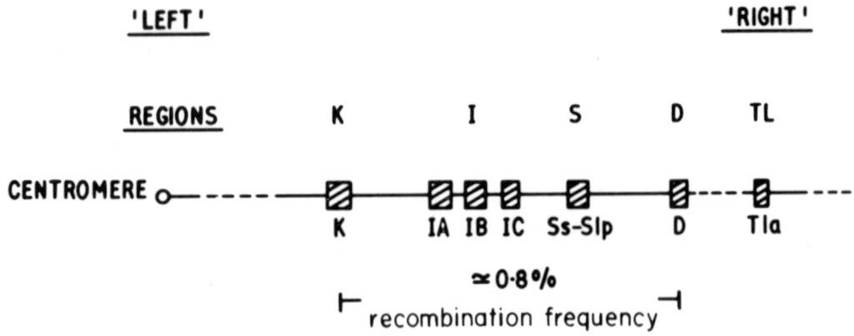

FIG. 3. The major histocompatibility (H-2) complex in the mouse

independently on the surface of the cell [134]. There is room for several hundred genes between K and D, assuming that all of the DNA in the region is active [8,106].

Of considerable interest in this field has been the discovery of β_2 microglobulin (reviewed in Ref. 135), a protein of molecular weight 11,000, which was first found in the urine of patients with certain renal tubular defects. This molecule is intimately associated with, but *not* covalently linked to, the major histocompatibility locus products in man and mouse [135]. Interestingly, it has an amino acid sequence that shows remarkable similarity to the third domain of the constant region of the γ-immunoglobulin chain, which suggests a possible functional or evolutionary relationship between immunoglobulin and histocompatibility gene products. Its biologic role is quite unknown, although in view of the uncertainty of the nature of the T-cell receptor, and the association of many T-cell functions with histocompatibility products, it is undergoing intensive study. The structural genes for β_2 microglobulin in man are *not* linked to the major histocompatibility locus. Antisera against human β_2 microglobulin are mitogenic for murine B lymphocytes [136].

2. *The S Region*

The S region of the H-2 complex (Fig. 2) controls the Ss and Slp serum protein traits [106]. The Ss (serum serologic variant) trait involves variations in the *amount* of a serum β-globulin detected by a specific rabbit antiserum. The Slp (sex-limited protein) trait controls production of a serum protein that normally only occurs in males and is detected by alloantisera. So far, the Ss and Slp loci have not been separated by recombination, but there is strong evidence that at least two proteins are involved [106]. The Ss locus maps between H-2K and H-2D and thus provides a very convenient genetic marker.

The function of these proteins is unknown. However, they may be associated with the Hom-1 locus, which is an H-2-linked gene that maps in the

K or I region and is associated with differences in weights of seminal vesicles, testes, and thymus, plasma testosterone levels, and testosterone-binding protein [137]. Variations in the level of hemolytic complement associated with different S-region haplotypes have also been described [12], but so far the Ss-Slp proteins have not been identified with any of the known complement components [106]. Recent reports have demonstrated linkage of genes that control levels of the second component of complement to HL-A in man [138] and the third component of complement to H-2 in the mouse [276] (see addendum).

There is no evidence for involvement of the S region in specific immune response gene phenomena, and antigens controlled by the region are not expressed on lymphoid cells.

3. *The I Region*

The availability of intra H-2 recombinant mouse strains allowed McDevitt et al. [139] to map the Ir-1 gene (Sec. VI.A) to the chromosomal region between K and the S loci, thus defining a new H-2 region. This region was initially known as the Ir region, but the nomenclature has been changed to the "I" region [140]. Genes that control apparently specific immune responses to well over 20 antigens have now been mapped to this region [106]. The antigens concerned include synthetic polypeptides [16], myeloma proteins [70], other native antigens, such as lactic dehydrogenase [95], thyroglobulin [141], and ovalbumin [142], ragweed extract [143], and a histocompatibility antigen controlled by the Y chromosome [144]. The H-2 region is also associated with susceptibility or resistance to autoimmune disease [11] and virus-induced neoplasia [10]. Though the latter effects may be a reflection of a more physiologically relevant result of Ir genes, this notion is by no means proven. The genes concerned have not been as accurately mapped as have some of the immune response genes. A detailed list of antigens, strains, and responses has been given by Shreffler and David [106].

It is of particular interest to note that each of the "independent" (i.e., not recombinant from known H-2 types) H-2 haplotypes shows a different pattern of responses to such a panel of antigens [106]. Whether this difference is due to a few loci with many different alleles, or many loci, is not yet known, although the latter possibility is probably favored by most workers at the present time. In attempts to directly determine whether there might be several distinct Ir genes in the I region, a search for crossovers that dissociate specific immune responses was made in the area. So far, extremely few such crossovers have been found [70,71]. This could indicate that there are very few genes responsible or that if there are multiple genes, they are very tightly linked. A search for further recombinants is underway in several laboratories, but since recombinants between the K and D ends of the complex only occur in about 1% of matings, one might anticipate that many thousands

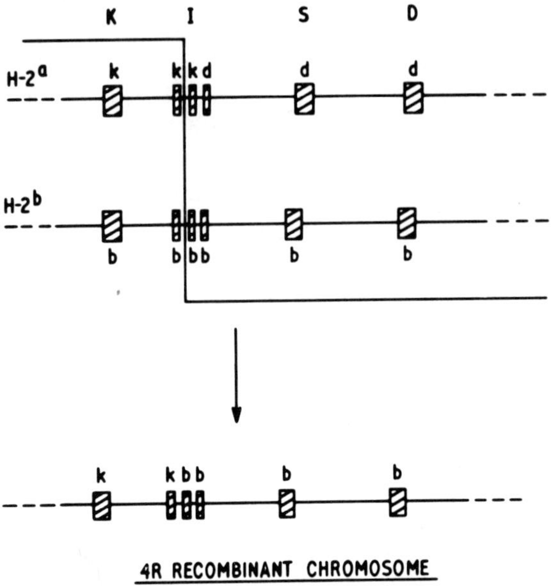

FIG. 4. Evidence for distinct Ir genes separable by recombination, an intra-I region crossover in the B10.A(4R) mouse strain.

of mice will have to be screened to find a few intra-I region recombinants.

One of the few strains of mouse where such a crossover has occurred is BIO.A (4R) (Fig. 4). The work of Liebermann et al. [70] established that in this mouse, there was probably a crossover within the I region, since the responses to IgA and IgG myeloma allotypes were separated by this recombination. The I region was thus divided into Ir-IgA, which controls responses to IgA myeloma allotypes, and Ir-IgG, which controls responses to IgG myeloma allotypes. The locus that controls the response to (T,G)-A–L has so far not been separated from Ir-IgA. Ir-IgA is now known as the IA region, and Ir-IgG as the IB region [106]. A third I region (IC) has recently been described [106] on the basis of surface antigens on lymphocytes, but so far no specific immune responses have been shown to be controlled by it. A second strain (D2.GD) which may have had an intra-I region recombination has also recently been described [71].

The I region is also associated with several other immunologic phenomena. It is of major importance in determining proliferation in the mixed lymphocyte culture (MLC or MLR) [145,146] and has been shown [147] to be associated with quite strong histocompatibility effects. Further, the I region has been shown to control serologically detectable antigens on the surface of lymphocytes and other cells [148-151]. Whether the various I-region properties are related is as yet uncertain. *The antigens detected by antisera against the I region (Ia antigens) and/or those detected by the MLC may represent products of the immune response genes.* This possibility has provoked a great deal of recent work and will be explored in detail in Sec. VI.D.

4. The TL Region

This region is located about 1 centimorgan to the right of H-2D and is marked by the Tla locus [106]. The Tla antigens are expressed on thymocytes [106], but so far there is no evidence for their expression on peripheral lymphoid cells. The TL region is also associated with histocompatibility effects [152,153]. The Tla antigens are expressed in some leukemias, not necessarily in the same pattern as thymocytes. Tl-positive leukemias may arise in T1-negative hosts [154]. It is important to note that TL differences frequently accompany H-2 differences and may complicate interpretation of experiments that involve the region [155].

Tl-positive cells may become phenotypically Tl negative after treatment with anti-Tl antibody ("antigenic modulation"). This change is probably due to capping [156,157] and endocytosis or shedding of Tl antigens.

C. Cellular Expression of Murine Histocompatibility-linked Ir Genes

Much of the available evidence points to the exclusive expression of the H-2-linked Ir genes in T lymphocytes, although most such evidence is indirect. The observed effects could occur at any point in the triggering of the T lymphocyte, although the specificity of the Ir gene effects point to antigen-receptor interaction in T cells or tolerance induction as the site of action. On the other hand, most of the available methods for assessment of murine T-cell responses to well-defined antigens involve "helper" function. Thus, a defect in low responders due to *failure of collaboration* rather than T-cell activation might account for much of the data. The H-linked Ir genes in the mouse and guinea pig probably function in a similar manner. The following sections will explore some of the more informative approaches that have been used in the mouse.

1. Bypass of T-cell Requirements: Interconversions of Responders and Nonresponders

As for the PLL gene in the guinea pig (see Sec. V), mice of nonresponder strains to (T,G)-A–L (Fig. 2) can be converted into responders by coupling (T,G)-A–L onto a recognizable carrier, such as methylated BSA [158]. Similarly, nonresponders can be converted into responders by a "graft-versus-host" reaction against the nonresponder lymphocytes (the "allogeneic effect") [105,159]. The allogeneic effect is known to allow bypass of the need for carrier recognition (i.e., T-cell help) under some circumstances [159]. Further, it has been shown that the defect in the nonresponders lies in the secondary IgG responses, which are highly T dependent, while the primary IgM responses are similar in "responders" and "nonresponders" [160]. Responders can be converted into nonresponders by neonatal thymectomy [161]. Recent work by Lonai and McDevitt suggests that only *responder* T cells proliferate when cultured with antigen in secondary responses [162]. However, this approach has not yet been widely used in the mouse and presents considerable technical difficulties.

The immune response to the synthetic copolymer GAT_{10} is under genetic control in the mouse. In this system, there is evidence for the induction of the so-called suppressor T cells in the nonresponders [163-164]. This would imply that *T-cell recognition of GAT can occur in the nonresponders but that the pathway of activation, or the type of T cell triggered, is different.*

2. *Limiting Dilution Experiments*

In a series of experiments designed to determine the cell type involved in the Ir-1 locus, Shearer and colleagues transferred syngeneic bone marrow or thymus cells into irradiated syngeneic recipients in graded numbers, along with an excess of the collaborating cell type [165]. The results suggested that the defect in the nonresponders to (T,G)-A–L was at the B-cell level in most cases, although there was also evidence for a T-cell defect in SJL ($H\text{-}2^s$) mice. However, this type of experiment is subject to criticism on several grounds (see Sec. VI.A.5), and interpretation is not simple.

3. *Antibody Specificity*

The possible differences in antibody specificity between the responder and nonresponder guinea pigs immunized with DNP-PLL have already been mentioned (Sec. V). In the mouse, there is little evidence for differences in the specificity of antibody production between high and low responders. Melchers and associates [95] found no marked differences in the isoelectric focusing patterns of anti-LDH_B antibodies in high-responder and low-responder mice, which implied that the specificity of antibodies against this antigen was similar in both cases. It is interesting to note that although the responses to the synthetic polypeptides (T,G)-A–L, (H,G)-A–L, and (Phe,G)-A–L may be under distinct Ir gene control at the T-cell level, they cross react extensively at the B-cell level [167].

4. Antigen-binding Experiments

It has been known for some time that the number of B cells that bind radioiodinated (T,G)-A–L is similar in responder and nonresponder mice [166]. However, due to the substantial difficulties in demonstrating antigen-binding T cells, it was not until comparatively recently that similar studies were published for T cells. The results [167-169] suggested approximately equal numbers of binding cells in responders and nonresponders. After immunization, however, only the *responders* showed an increase in binding cells. This finding indicates either that the defect in the nonresponders is a step other than binding to receptor or that the cells capable of being *triggered* by antigen are only a small subset (of high-affinity binding) of the measured set of binding cells, and this subset is absent in the nonresponders.

Binding was partially inhibited by anti-Ig and anti-Thy-1 (an antigen only present on T lymphocytes) sera and was strongly inhibited by an anti-H-2 sera. However, the anti-Ig sera were absorbed against thymocytes prior to the experiment, so that if T-cell Ig has only weak cross reactivity with B-cell Ig, and only a minor subset of anti-Ig molecules reacted with T-cell Ig, a negative result would have been guaranteed by such an absorption. Of the anti-H-2 sera, both anti-"K end" (including the I region) and anti-"D end" (*not* including the I region) produced strong inhibition, which suggests that inhibition of antigen binding by these sera was *not* related to the Ir gene product.

Perhaps the most revealing experiment was one which showed that anti-H-2 sera directed against *either* responder or nonresponder parental haplotype completely inhibited binding of antigen to F_1 cells. This finding suggested that the histocompatibility antigens are physically close to the receptor for antigen on T cells but are not the receptor itself. If the latter were the case, it would be expected that inhibition would be only partial. In a later paper, the authors showed that antisera against product of the I region (Ia antigens) did not inhibit binding of antigen to T cells [169].

5. The Histocompatibility System and Interactions Among T Lymphocytes, B Lymphocytes, and Macrophages

As a further approach to the question of the cellular site of action of the H-linked Ir genes, numerous studies of T-B collaboration between various populations of genetic responder and nonresponder mice have been undertaken. A large range of well-defined strains congenic for H-2 or heavy-chain structural genes are available. It was hoped that such studies might pinpoint the site of the defect in the nonresponders.

These types of experiments are always complicated by the possibility of "allogeneic effects" due to the mixing of allogeneic lymphocytes. Such effects can either enhance or inhibit concurrent immune responses. In particular, they can override the carrier effect and may provide a T cell-replacing factor ("allogeneic effect factor") [171]. A wide variety of ingenious approaches have been used to circumvent these problems. It should be stressed that *all such systems are highly artificial* and depend on many assumptions, especially concerning the effects of irradiation on cells. What they reveal about *normal* physiology is not yet clear.

While studies of cooperation between allogeneic lymphocytes have not yet unequivocally determined the site of the defect in the nonresponders, a second intertwined concept has emerged: the apparent *need for histocompatibility* for certain cell-cell interactions. Such a requirement has no precedent in terms of hormone-receptor interactions and has certain conceptual difficulties. If there are frequent variations of a given histocompatibility factor concerned with cell-cell interaction, and these variant factors can only interact effectively with individuals with a shared H genotype, it would seem that there would have to be an equally large number of exactly parallel variations in the *receptor* for that factor (presumably controlled by a different gene). On the other hand, the biologic role of the MHC is quite unknown, and such data may point to a form of cell-cell interaction based on molecular *similarity* rather than *complementarity* (see addendum).

Kindred and Shreffler [170] investigated T-B collaboration in backcrosses of nude and BALB/c mice and found that effective T-cell help was only obtained when the T cells were from H-2-compatible donors. In this case, the nude mice are incapable of causing allogeneic effects, since they lack functional T cells. Similarly, Benacerraf and Katz, in a large series of experiments, showed a similar requirement for histocompatibility for optimal T-B collaboration (reviewed in Ref. 172). The experimental design depended on transfer of carrier$_A$-primed spleen cells from one parent into a normal unprimed F_1 recipient. Twenty-four hours later, the recipient was irradiated and injected with hapten-carrier$_B$ spleen cells from the other parent. The second inoculum of cells had been treated with anti-Thy-1 serum and complement to remove T cells, which would have caused graft-versus-host and allogeneic effects. The mice were then challenged with hapten-carrier$_A$. Details of the rationale and assumptions behind this type of approach have been reviewed by Benacerraf and Katz [172]. It was found that optimal T-B collaboration only occurred when the T and B cells shared an H-2 determinant controlled by the K or I region. It was subsequently shown [173] that identity at the I region was crucial for T-B interactions, even if the antigens concerned were not under Ir gene control.

When one parent was a nonresponder, however, it was found that F_1 T cells could provide help for responder B cells but not for nonresponder B cells [174]. It would appear, then, that, under these circumstances, a difference in Ir genes for the carrier antigen prevented cooperation and/or that the Ir genes are also expressed in B cells. In a subsequent paper, it was found that nonresponder B cells could cooperate in vitro with F_1 T cells only if small amounts of the antigen were presented on macrophages [175].

On the other hand, Katz and Unanue found that allogeneic macrophages were just as effective as syngeneic macrophages in mice [176]. These data appear to be in conflict with those of Shevach and Rosenthal [101], who found that in the guinea pig, identity between macrophages and lymphocytes was required for optimal antigen-induced proliferation in vitro. The apparent conflict may be a reflection of the different parameters measured (helper effect versus antigen-induced proliferation).

Another approach to the question of T-B collaboration across major histocompatibility barriers has used allophenic ("tetraparental") mice produced by artificial fusion of embryos at the eight-cell stage. It is assumed that such mice are tolerant to the antigens of all parents, although some debate about this assumption continues [177-180]. Some of the confusion regarding tolerance in allophenic mice stems from the use of immunologically abnormal parental mice, such as NZB and SJI. NZB mice have a very high incidence of autoimmune disease. When more conventional strains are used, the majority of the evidence suggests that the allophenic mice are completely tolerant to all parental strains.

Bechtol et al. [181] created allophenes between responder mice of one immunoglobulin allotype and nonresponders of another allotype. When challenged with an antigen under Ir gene control, large quantities of specific antibody of the nonresponder allotype were produced, which implied that collaboration could occur across H-2 differences. The data also indicate that there is no defect in B cells in the nonresponders. These results are in direct conflict with those of Katz et al., and there is at present no way of rationalizing such differences. The allophenic mice have the important advantages that no irradiation or cell transfer is needed to perform collaboration experiments. It is my personal prejudice to favor the results from the allophenic mice rather than those that employed irradiated and transferred cells.

Taussig and coworkers have developed yet another model to study T-B collaboration across H-2 differences [182-184]. T cells are activated in vivo to (T,G)-A–L and then cultured *in vitro* with the same antigen. Supernatants from the cultures contain a factor which can replace the need for specific T cells in a collaborative system. The use of supernatants rather than cells appears to avoid the allogeneic effect. The factor is produced by both responder and nonresponder T cells (with the exception of nonresponder strain SJL, which is unable to produce the factor) but is only capable of activating *responder* B cells. Thus, the defect in the nonresponders is at the B-cell level. The factor is antigen specific and bears H-2 determinants but is not immunoglobulin [184]. These findings are inconsistent with those that involve the allophenic mice, the antigen-binding data, the guinea pig data, and the demonstration [162] that only responder T cells proliferate *in vitro* in response to antigen. On the other hand, the data are consistent with the limiting dilution data and make more sense of the finding that lymphocyte surface antigens controlled by genes in the "immune response" segment are predominantly on B cells (see next section). It is conceivable that non-response could involve several categories, some involving a block at the T-cell level and others a block in collaboration or at the B-cell level. Table 1 summarizes the currently available data on cellular expression of H-linked Ir genes.

Yet another requirement for histocompatibility for cell interactions has been described by Zinkernagel and Doherty [102], who studies lysis by specifically sensitized T cells of target cells infected with lymphocytic choriomeningitis or ectromelia virus. It was found that H-2 identity was needed for optimal killing. Similar results with cytotoxic T cells and trinitrophenylated target cells have been reported by Shearer [185].

6. *Are the MHC-linked Ir Gene Effects Due to Tolerance?*

There is a very considerable body of evidence to indicate that nonresponse in the case of the MHC-linked Ir genes is *not* due to cross reaction of the relevant antigens with "self"-components, although there is one report [186] in the literature of weak cross reaction between histocompatibility antigens and (T,G)-A–L. However, such an explanation would have some attractions, in that the set of *all* clones with receptors capable of reacting to a given antigen would be involved, rather than merely those of a given variable-region structure, as in the receptor hypothesis.

Responder cells in a nonresponder environment (and stem cells of responder genotype that mature in a nonresponder environment) remain responders [187,188]. The F_1 hybrids between responders and nonresponders are intermediate to high responders (see Sec. VII). The half-life of anti-lactate dehydrogenase antibodies in rats is the same in responder and nonresponder strains [189], as is the half-life of anti-(T,G)-A–L antibodies in mice [198]. On the other hand, "suppressor T cells" have been shown in nonresponders to GAT but not in other Ir gene systems [163,164]. Whether the GAT system is atypical is not yet known, but T-cell suppression in the nonresponders would not seem to apply in the allophenic mice, where nonresponder B cells are clearly capable of making specific antibody (see above).

Taken as a whole, the data do not really support a tolerance model. It is a little farfetched to suppose that genes for a large series of antigens that cross react with antigens under Ir gene control lie in one tiny cluster in the

TABLE 1

Is the Defect in Histocompatibility-linked Ir Gene Nonresponders in B or T Cells?

Evidence That Supports Expression in B Cells	Evidence That Supports Expression in T Cells
Limiting dilution experiments [165]	Thymectomy data [161]
Taussig experiments [182-184]	Conversion of nonresponders into responders by coupling antigen to an immunogenic carrier [82,158]
F_1 T cells only collaborate with responder B cells [174]	Conversion of nonresponders into responders by the "allogeneic effect" [105]
Ia antigens predominantly expressed on B cells [19,20,193,194]	Defect in low responders most evident in secondary IgG responses [160]
Fluorescence quenching data [92]	Allophenic mice experiments [181]
	Delayed-type hypersensitivity only occurs in responder guinea pigs [75]
	Isoelectric focusing data [94,95]
	Antigen-induced proliferation only in responder cells [162]

middle of the H-2 complex and are separable from the major histocompatibility antigens by recombination. One might expect Ir genes due to self-tolerance to be scattered throughout the entire genome. However, some form of tolerization in the nonresponders has not been entirely ruled out.

D. The Ia Antigens

1. Discovery

The I region is known to be associated with strong stimulation in the MLC, but until recently, I-region products were not detected serologically. This led Bach et al. [191] to postulate the existence of two distinct groups of lymphocyte antigens, which were defined either *serologically* (SD) or by ability to stimulate in the MLC (*"lymphocyte defined,"* or LD). However, for many years, it has been known that some alloantisera in mice contain antibodies which do not kill 100% of lymphocytes in cytotoxicity tests. These antibodies were largely ignored and were thought to represent "cross reactions" or "weak" reactions [106]. Moreover, with the production of congenic pairs of mice that differ only in the I and S regions, it rapidly became clear that *high-titer* antibodies could be raised against products of the I region but that such antibodies only killed a subpopulation of lymphocytes [148-151]. By appropriate selection of target cells, similar antibodies were also demonstrated in mice immunized against cells from partner strains which were not fully congenic at the I region [106]. It is now clear that many anti-H-2 sera also contain antibodies against I-region products [106] (see chapter 11). These antigens were initially known as β [149], Lna (lymph node antigen) [148], or Ir 1.1 [151], but it has now been agreed that they be designated Ia (antigens associated with the I region), with no assumptions as to their cellular localization or functions [140].

2. *Cellular Localization*

Since the bulk of the evidence suggests that the H-2-linked Ir genes are expressed in T cells, it was expected that the corresponding antisera against I-region products would also react exclusively with T cells. Indeed, several early papers claimed such a result [150,151]. However, it is now very clear that the predominant activity of such antisera is directed against B cells [20,149,192,193]. During the last year or two, the pendulum has swung all the way from exclusive T-cell localization [150,151] to exclusive B-cell localization [20,149] and back to localization predominantly in B cells but with definite, though weaker, T-cell activity [193,194].

Radioautographic studies in our laboratory [193], where binding of radioiodinated anti-Ia sera were used to study the cellular localization of Ia antigens, have shown that

1. Only lymphoid cells were significantly labeled, and these could be divided into discrete populations of very heavily labeled cells and cells with virtually no detectable labeling.
2. There was a bimodal distribution of grains in lymph node and spleen, a unimodal distribution in thymus, and a heterogeneous distribution in bone marrow (Fig. 5).
3. The heavily labeled cells were B cells.
4. There was a slight, but highly significant, degree of labeling of at least a subpopulation of T cells.

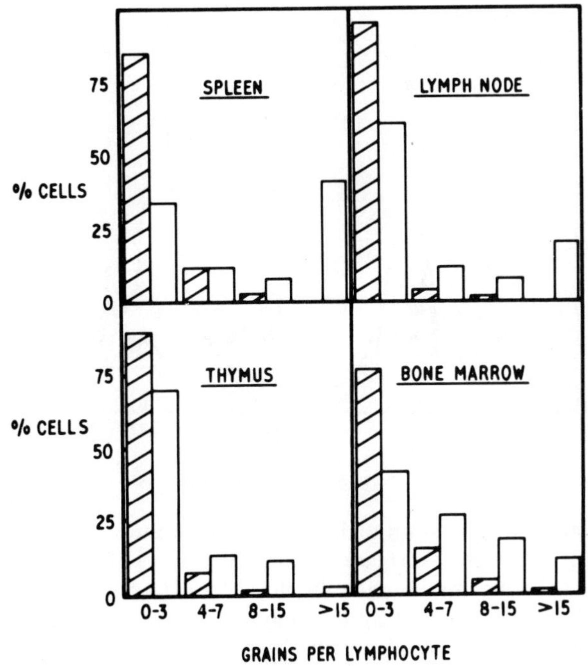

FIG. 5. Tissue distribution of Ia antigens on lymphocytes. Cells were held with ^{125}I-labeled A.TH anti-A.TL serum, washed, and processed for radio-autography. Shaded A.TH cells (control); open columns, A.TL cells.

5. The Ia antigens and immunoglobulin move independently on the cell surface.

Ia antigens are also present on antibody-forming cells [20,193,194], possibly in smaller amounts than on other B cells. They are also expressed on epidermal cells, macrophages, spermatozoa, and fetal liver cells [195,196], but it is not yet clear whether the antigens on the various tissues are coded for by the same genes.

3. *Structure*

Ia antigens have been partially characterized by biosynthetic labeling [197,198] or surface radioiodination [193,196,199], followed by detergent extraction, immunologic precipitation, and analysis by polyacrylamide gel electrophoresis in the presence of sodium dodecyl sulfate. They have a fundamental monomeric molecular weight of approximately 30,000 (Fig. 6). Similar procedures

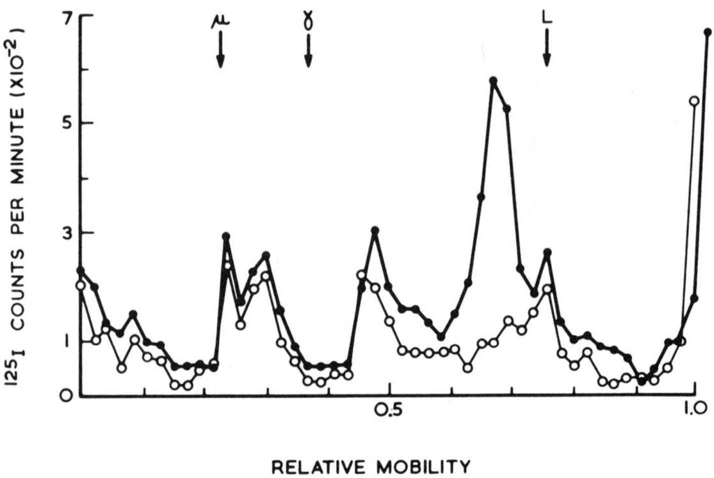

FIG. 6. Partial characterization of Ia antigens. The outer cytoplasmic membrane of A.TL spleen cells was labeled with ^{125}I by the lactoperoxidase technique, and the membrane was solubilized by detergent. Surface immunoglobulin was partially removed by immunoadsorption, and Ia antigens were precipitated by A.TH anti-A.TL serum, followed by rabbit antimouse γ-globulin. Precipitates were then reduced by mercaptoethanol and analyzed by polyacrylamide gel electrophoresis in the presence of sodium dodecyl sulfate. This procedure separates molecules on the basis of molecular weight: those of lower molecular weight migrate further into the gel. A peak of radioactivity that corresponds in mobility to a molecular weight of 30,000 and migrates just behind the light chains is seen in the experimental (A.TH anti-A.TL, filled circles) but not in the control (normal A.TH, open circles) precipitates. In addition, small peaks of radioactivity that correspond in mobility to μ and light chains, and a third Ig chain with a mobility slightly faster than the μ-chain standard, are observed. The peak which migrates a little faster than the γ standard is not immunoglobulin, because it is precipitable by a noncross-reacting fowl γ-globulin/antifowl γ-globulin system. It may represent a cell surface component with affinity for antigen-antibody complexes [193].

reveal a molecular weight of 45,000 for the K and D antigens. The Ia antigens may dimerize into units of 60,000 molecular weight which appear to be held together by disulfide bonds [197]. They are probably glycoproteins that contain fucose, mannose, and galactose [197]. By the use of more specific antisera or sequential precipitation, it has been shown that there are at least two separable Ia molecules [197]. Ia antigens are not immunoglobulin, because they move independently from Ig on the cell membrane [193,200] and are distinct from any known immunoglobulin chain in molecular weight.

4. *Functional Role*

No definite functional role has yet been established for the Ia antigens, and their relationship (if any) to the IR gene effects is unknown. It seems very likely that they will be found to consist of several different entities, which possibly have different functions. It is clear that the Ia antigens are not immunoglobulin and are therefore *not* the receptor for antigen on B cells. (It might be mentioned that extremely few cell surface antigens have been associated with a clear biologic function. One notable exception is an antigen on the surface of sheep erythrocytes which may represent a component of the sodium pump [201]). It was hoped that the discovery of the Ia antigens might have enabled a definitive answer to the puzzle of the T-cell receptor. Such hopes have not yet been realized. Anti-Ia sera do not inhibit the binding of antigen to T lymphocytes [169] and, indeed, appear to react mainly with B cells. On the other hand, if the Ir gene products are *clonally expressed* on T lymphocytes, they might not easily be detected by anti-Ia sera.

It seems quite likely that the Ia antigens, as detected serologically, are the predominant stimulating antigens in the MLC [202-204]. Proliferation can be blocked when anti-Ia antisera are directed against the stimulator cells. This is also true for parent-F_1 situations, where the antisera only block if directed against the *stimulating haplotype* of the F_1 cells [204]. In these experiments, there was no significant blocking of proliferation when the antisera were directed toward the *responder* cells, which suggests that such antisera did not have anti-T cell receptor activity. The physiologic meaning, if any, of the MLC is unknown. It is of interest, however, that two recent reports have shown that the predominant MLC-stimulating activity in the mouse [205] and man [206] lies in B cells, although there are reports that T cells are capable of stimulation [207,208]. Anti-H-2 sera against "killer" T cells do *not* abolish killing [214].

Originally, it appeared that "killer" T cells could not be produced against I-region differences (e.g., Ref. 209). However, most of these studies involved the use of blast cells transformed by phytohemagglutinin as targets. Such targets would be almost exclusively T cells. In view of the predominant expression of Ia antigens on B cells, it might be expected that the use of B-cell blasts (stimulated by lipopolysaccharide) as targets would allow killing to be domonstrated. This appears to be the case [210]. Evidence has also been presented [211,212] that proliferation in the MLC is a necessary prerequisite for development of killer T cells. It is known that the antigens concerned in MLC and killer activity are different and that different cell populations are involved in these activities [213]. These results have led to a postulate of T-T synergy [211]. Nabholz et al. [214] have shown, on the other hand, that killing *can* occur in the absence of significant MLC activity. The whole question of T-T synergy and SD/LD differences is still undergoing evaluation.

Anti-Ia sera have been shown to block the binding of aggregated IgG to B lymphocytes, and it has been proposed that the Ia antigens represent polymorphisms of the receptor on B cells for the Fc portion of IgG [215]. However, such effects may be due to steric hindrance by binding to a molecule which is physically close to, but not identical with, the Fc receptor, since potent inhibition of binding was also seen when the antisera were directed at only one parental haplotype of F_1 hybrid cells. In addition, "capping" the Fc receptor on B lymphocytes leaves the Ia antigens uniformly distributed over the cell surface [216,217], which indicates that either the Ia antigens are not the Fc receptor or that the Fc receptor represents only a minor subcomponent of Ia antigens.

An attractive possibility is that the *Ia antigens represent polymorphisms of a receptor on B cells for a T-cell product* [218]. Other possibilities for function of the Ia antigens come from work that suggests that "allogeneic effect factor" (AEF) has Ia determinants [171]. This factor, which is released into the supernatant of MLCs, may represent "collaborative factor" or the "second signal" (in addition to antigen) for activation of B cells. AEF is said to be nonantigen specific [219]. In contrast, the *specific* collaborative factor recently described by Taussig (see earlier) has been shown to express H-2 determinants but not Ig determinants. In this model, the Ir gene product might be equated with the Ia antigens on B cells. Collaboration would then involve an antigen-specific T-cell factor which is for some reason unable to interact with nonresponder B cells. On the other hand, Feldmann (Chap. 8) has described an antigen-specific T-cell collaborative factor which has Ig determinants. Thus, just about every possibility has some data to support it.

Very recently, studies of the effects of anti-Ia serum on collaborative T-B interactions in vitro have been undertaken [220,221]. Considerable blocking of IgG responses was reported. However, such experiments have many technical difficulties, such as "capping" and resynthesis of Ia antigens after exposure to anti-Ia serum. Normal mouse serum often has powerful inhibitory effects on cultured murine cells. Such studies may well provide important clues about the relationship between Ia antigens and Ir gene products, but they are in a very early stage at present, and it would be premature to draw conclusions from them. Whether the MLC-stimulating antigens, Ir products, and Ia antigens are related is still an open question, but one may anticipate rapid progress in this field.

VII. Association of Disease Susceptibility with Certain HL-A Types in Man

A. Evidence for Homology of H-2 and HL-A

It is likely that the major histocompatibility locus is a universal entity in mammals and birds. There is evidence for such a structure in man [127],

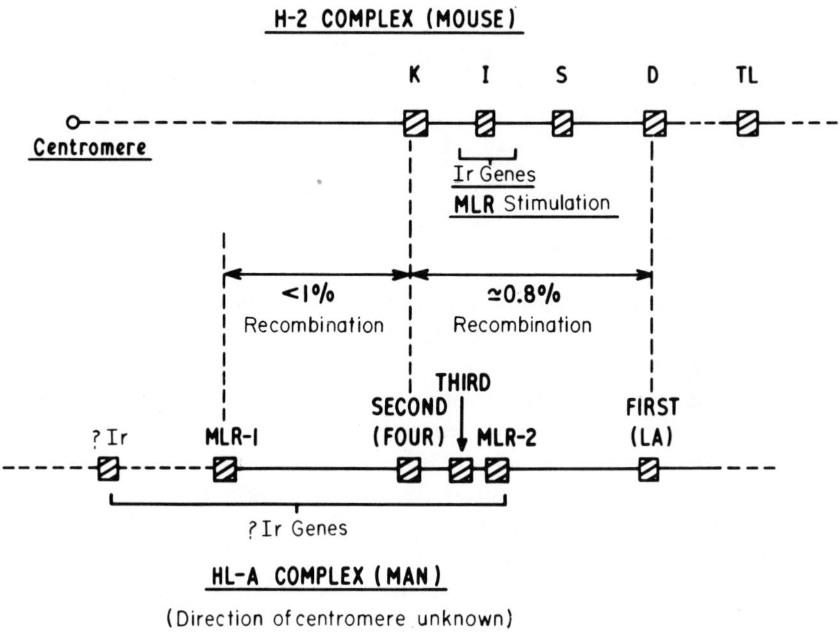

FIG. 7. Comparison of the murine (H-2) and human (HL-A) major histocompatibility complexes. Note that the homology is rather imperfect. When more precise information on the location of the third human locus becomes available, it may be possible to demonstrate a more exact homology.

mouse [106], dog [223], rat [222], monkey [128], and fowls [224]. In man, mouse, and monkey, the major antigens involved lie in two closely linked loci, although there are several other histocompatibility loci in this region, such as the "third" locus of man [127] and the I region and TL region histocompatibility genes in the mouse [147,152,153].

There is reason to believe that the major histocompatibility systems in man (HL-A) and mouse (H-2) are homologous [108,234] (Fig. 7). Both consist of two major loci: LA (first) and FOUR (second) in man and D and K, respectively, in the mouse. Both systems have a closely linked but distinct locus which determines strong stimulation in the MLC. One point where the two systems differ, however, is that the major MLC locus maps *within* the complex in the mouse [145,146] but just outside it (closely linked to the second sublocus) in man [225]. *So far, there has been no unequivocal evidence for HL-A-linked Ir genes in man,* although an Ir gene to ragweed pollen seems to be a likely candidate [226,227]. MHC-linked Ir genes have been demonstrated in the rhesus monkey [228].

It is of interest that the MHC-linked Ir genes and the major MLC locus maps in the same area (the "K end") of the murine MHC. It is not known whether the same genes are responsible for these two phenomena, but it is of interest that most associations of disease with HL-A types, and possibly human MHC-linked Ir genes, appear to be associated with the second sublocus, which is also closely linked to the locus that controls strong MLC stimulation.

B. HL-A-associated Disease

After the initial associations of duodenal ulcer with blood group O, and carcinoma of the stomach with blood group A [107], it was logical to look for similar associations with HL-A types. A further logical basis for such studies came from the known associations between murine H-2 types and resistance to Gross virus-induced leukemogenesis [229] and susceptibility to Tennant virus-induced leukemias [230]. There is also an association between H-2 and susceptibility to the Bittner virus, which causes mammary tumors in mice [231]. Similarly, the initial observations that linked Ir-1 to H-2 in the mouse, and the subsequent demonstration that the PLL gene was linked to the MHC in guinea pigs, suggested that HL-A-linked Ir genes might exist in man. These genes might then be associated with clinical disease of an immunologic nature.

Certain HL-A types have been associated with neoplastic, autoimmune, inflammatory, and allergic diseases. Such associations have been the subject of many excellent reviews [232-234]. The review of Morris [233] is particularly recommended. These studies have many pitfalls, and great care is needed to establish that a putative association is truly significant [233]. One particular problem arises from the possibility of taking selected rare events and comparing their incidence with a control group. The probability of finding a fortuitous association increases with the number of specificities compared, and to test the null hypothesis (i.e., that there was no difference between groups), *the computed probability values must be multiplied by the number of specificities compared.* Such a correction often eliminates seemingly significant associations, and its application may clarify many conflicting data. Other difficulties include cross reactivity between specificities of each series and the problem that "few truly identical antisera exist for most specificities" [233]. In addition, the diseases themselves may well be heterogeneous in etiology. This is particularly likely for Hodgkin's disease and the leukemias.

The correlation between murine H-2 types and resistance to Gross leukemia virus [229] prompted detailed examination of HL-A types in human leukemia patients. Conflicting results emerged, with some groups reporting normal profiles for acute lymphoblastic leukemia [235], but an excess of

HL-A2 and HL-A12 was reported by others [236]. The situation is not yet resolved, although the evidence for an increased incidence of HL-A2 appears particularly strong [237]. For chronic lymphatic leukemia, excesses of HL-A3, HL-A11 [239], and W27* [240] have been reported in small groups of patients, although, once again, normal profiles have been found by other groups [241,242].

An early report by Amiel [243] showed an increase of HL-A4c in Hodgkin's disease. Since then, a profusion of reports has appeared, but the data have been inconsistent (see Ref. 232 for additional references). HL-A4c has now been split into HL-A5, W5, and W18, and cross reaction also occurs between these types and W15. Of the truly significant studies, most with positive results showed an increase in these antigens [233]. During the Fifth Histocompatibility Workshop [244], several hundred patients were typed for HL-A by use of same antisera, and the histology was blindly classified by an expert team of pathologists. A significant percentage of the patients did not appear to have Hodgkin's disease. Increases were noted in HL-A1, HL-A8, and W18. There was a marginal increase in HL-A10 in patients over the age of 45. Other neoplastic diseases where associations have been reported include increases in HL-A2 and decreases in HL-A13 in nasopharyngeal carcinoma in the Chinese living in Hong Kong and Singapore [247].

Associations of HL-A antigens with a variety of non-neoplastic diseases have also been reported. Many of these diseases are suspected of having an immunologic component in their causation. HL-A1 and/or HL-A8 have been associated with gluten enteropathy [248,249], dermatitis herpetiformis [250], systemic lupus erythematosus [251,252], myasthenia gravis [251-253], chronic active hepatitis [253], autoimmune thyroiditis [255], and possibly thyrotoxicosis [254]. Factors that predispose to autoimmune thyroiditis have been linked to the major histocompatibility complex in the mouse [11]. HL-A13 has been associated with psoriasis [256-258] and pemphigus [259]. Multiple sclerosis and paralytic poliomyelitis have been associated with HL-A3 and HL-A7 [260,261]. Recently, it has been reported that there is a strong association between multiple sclerosis and LD-7 and HL-A-linked specificity that controls MLC stimulation [262]. W15 has been associated with systemic lupus erythematosus [252] and insulin-dependent diabetes mellitus [263].

A strong association has been shown between W27 and psoriatic arthritis [264], Reiter's disease [265,266,271], and especially ankylosing spondylitis [256,257,267]. In the last case, the association is particularly striking; W27 is present in about 90% of those afflicted but only in 5 to 8% of normal controls. In each of these diseases, joint inflammation is a feature. There has been no association found, however, between W27 and rheumatoid arthritis [232].

---

*W signifies "workshop" specificity.

Of considerable interest in connection with the possibility of HL-A linked Ir genes has been the finding of segregation of ragweed pollen allergy with an HL-A haplotype in a family [238] and an association of sensitivity to ragweed antigen Ra5 with HL-A7 [226]. Recently, evidence was presented for linkage of an Ir gene that controls IgE production of a ragweed extract to the second sublocus in man [227]. In this case, the gene responsible mapped about 7 to 22 centimorgans from the second sublocus (i.e., *well outside the entire HL-A complex*). An H-2-linked Ir gene to ragweed antigens has also been described in mice [143].

C. Mechanisms of Association

The reason for such associations is unknown. They might be due to the serologically defined HL-A antigens themselves or, alternatively, due to closely linked but distinct genes. The latter proposition depends on certain assumptions. In an outbred population, such as man, even very closely linked genes are very likely to become "scrambled" by recombination over thousands of years, and one might not expect particular alleles of one locus to be associated with particular alleles of an adjacent locus any more than due to chance. However, such associations (termed *linkage disequilibrium,* or Δ) have been found in the HL-A system [234] (also see Refs. 272,273). The reasons for linkage disequilibrium are not well understood.

There are several examples of linkage disequilibrium between serologically defined HL-A antigens of the two subloci. Linkage disequilibrium is particularly striking between HL-A1 and HL-A8 [8], and, interestingly, this particular combination shows a very strong disease association. A similar situation probably applies to HL-A3, HL-A7, and an MLC allele which is associated with multiple sclerosis [262]. The important question of whether there might be linkage disequilibrium between certain HL-A antigens and specific Ir genes remains unanswered.

Many possible reasons for linkage disequilibrium in the HL-A system have been proposed [8]. Most of these hypotheses are very speculative. Linkage disequilibrium could occur because:

1. There has been insufficient time since the formation of the complex (or a mutation within the complex) for dissociation of linked traits.

2. There may have been an interaction between two linked loci such that certain combinations are favored [8]. Reasons for such interactions are not clear, although there is a possibility that some gene products in the region are associated physically on the cell membrane. It should be emphasized that the known diseases associated with certain HL-A types are rare and generally occur after the reproductive age, so that their selective influence is likely to

be small. The associations with disease may represent unfavorable byproducts of an otherwise favorable selection ("balanced polymorphisms"), such as the relationship between malaria and thalassemia, sickle cell anemia, and glucose 6-phosphate dehydrogenase deficiency [107]. Piazza et al. [268] studied Sardinian populations of common origin but who lived either in the highlands, where malaria was rare, or in the lowlands, where it was common. They found that the red blood cell abnormalities were far more common in those who lived in the lowlands and that there were considerable differences at the HL-A *second* sublocus but not for 22 other genetic markers.

3. The observed differences may have been due to migration and fusion of populations [232,269]. When two populations, one of which has a high frequency of two linked genes (e.g., HL-A1 and HL-A8) fuse, transient linkage disequilibrium will occur and will slowly disappear in future generations due to crossing-over [269]. A particular Ir gene (or even a *non-Ir gene that controls a given disease susceptibility*) may be associated with a particular HL-A type in such cases.

If HL-A-linked *Ir genes* are the explanation, they could act via a variety of mechanisms. They could perhaps produce an exaggerated tendency to autoimmunity, decreased surveillance against cancer, or decreased defense against (possible oncogenic) viruses. The mode of inheritance of the disease susceptibility (whether dominant or recessive) would thus depend on the manner of pathogenesis.

Alternatively, the HL-A products *themselves* may be responsible for the observed associations. In this case, there is a possibility that the antigens act as receptors for viruses (for which there is little evidence at present). If a pathogenic agent shared determinants with a given HL-A antigen, it might escape the host defenses due to self-tolerance ("molecular mimicry") [40]. Most of the available data indicate that *susceptibility* is dominant, perhaps suggesting autoimmune processes or "molecular mimicry." The almost absolute association of W27 with ankylosing spondylitis suggests that it is the W27 antigen itself, rather than a closely linked gene, that is responsible.

The study of the histocompatibility systems thus extends into receptor physiology, T-B collaboration, and tissue typing for clinical transplantation (although its value when donor and recipient are unrelated is quesitonable). It has proven to be a useful tool in anthropology. In the future, such studies may be relevant to diagnosis, eugenics, and genetic counseling, although the therapeutic implications of the finding of HL-A-associated diseases are somewhat bleak.

What are the biologic functions of the histocompatibility antigens? Surely they are not present just to keep immunologists employed. Indeed, *while a locus may be detected serologically, this does not necessarily imply that its function is immunologic*. The histocompatibility antigens may be concerned with cell differentiation. Indeed, genes in the H-2 complex in the mouse code for "differentiation antigens" [132] that are predominantly expressed on individual cell types, such as Ia (predominantly expressed in B cells; see Sec. VI) or Tla (expressed in thymocytes). The differentiation antigens might function as receptors for cell-cell interactions.

Alternatively, the great polymorphism in HL-A genes has been explained on the basis of avoidance of parasitic infestation [270]. By ensuring great variability in the histocompatibility antigens, at least some individuals might survive an infestation by rejecting the parasite. Yet another theory has been put forward by Burnet [129], who proposed that the HL-A system would prevent "contagious cancer" or invasion by foreign cells, such as maternal cells during gestation. However, highly inbred laboratory mice do not seem to suffer from these problems. Jerne [125] has proposed the ingenious theory that histocompatibility genes are concerned with both morphogenesis and cell-cell recognition, and that individuals are born with a library of antigen receptors that code for "antiself." Selection of mutant genes for receptors that do *not* react with self is, then, the basis of generation of diversity. The theory appears to require strict parallel evolution of histocompatibility genes and antigen receptors, which is unlikely [8].

Thus, the biologic function of the histocompatibility antigens remains a puzzle. However, rapid progress is being made in this field, and it is to be hoped that data that allow a choice between some of the alternatives will soon be available.

VIII. Summary

Genetic controls operate at virtually every stage in the immune response. They are known to regulate the level of natural antibodies, self-tolerance, processing of antigen by macrophages, immunoglobulin structure, differentiation of cell lines, and the expression of "immune response" genes linked to the major histocompatibility complex. There is strong evidence that the histocompatibility-linked immune response genes influence recognition of antigen by T lymphocytes. The proposal that they code for the T-cell receptor for antigen is still undergoing evaluation.

In the mouse, the "immune response" (I) chromosomal region contains genes that code for antigens expressed predominantly on B lymphocytes. These antigens are not immunoglobulins. In their monomeric form, they have a molecular weight of about 30,000. It is likely that the Ia antigens play an important role in T-B collaboration, but their relationship to specific immune response effects is not yet clear.

In man, there are associations between several diseases and certain histocompatibility (HL-A) types. Most of these diseases appear to have an immunologic component in their causation. The reason for such associations are under intensive investigation; in particular, the role of immune response genes linked to the HL-A region is being assessed. Because there is evidence for linkage disequilibrium in the region, certain HL-A types may be associated with specific immune response genes, even in an outbred population, such as man. In addition, even more meaningful associations with lymphocyte antigens detected by the MLC may emerge.

The major histocompatibility complex is held to represent a cluster of functionally and evolutionarily related genes, although the precise relationship between the various associated phenomena still requires investigation. While the initial impetus to the study of the HL-A complex was the need to understand and control rejection of human allografts, the ramifications of immunogenetics have now extended into such disease fields as receptor physiology, epidemiology, clinical diagnosis, and anthropology. In the future, a greater understanding of immune response genes and their effects is likely to have widespread practical consequences.

Acknowledgments

Original work in this chapter was supported by grants from The National Health and Medical Research Council and The Australian Research Grants Committee, Canberra, Australia; by Grants AI-0-3958 and AI-10886 from the National Institutes of Health, United States Public Health Service and by Contract NO1-CB-23889 with The National Cancer Institute, National Institutes of Health, United States Department of Health, Education, and Welfare; and by Volkswagen Foundation Grant 112147.

Addendum

Since this chapter was written, many important findings have been reported. The following is a brief and selective account of areas in which progress has been particularly rapid.

Immunoglobulin Genetics

Opinion seems to be moving more toward the idea that there are relatively few structural genes for immunoglobulin in the germ line. When DNA complementary to light-chain messenger RNA (synthesized via reverse transcriptase) was hybridized with nuclear DNA, the reaction kinetics indicated that the K-chain constant region was only represented two to four times her haploid genome [277,278]. While the data concerning the K-variable region were less clear-cut, the bulk of the evidence indicated that relatively few genes were involved.

Of particular interest concerning the possible role of immunoglobulin in recognition of antigen by T cells is the demonstration by Binz and Wigzell [279] that similar or identical idiotypes can be detected on IgG molecules and on T-cell receptors with specificity for the same alloantigens. The anti-idiotypic antibodies bound to 5 to 7% of T cells and were capable of inhibiting proliferation in the MLC [280,281].

Antibodies to murine IgD and IgM were found to be present in many non-congenic anti-H-2 sera. These antibodies were shown to reflect genetic polymorphisms in murine IgD and IgM, and permitted the mapping of the respective structural genes (named Ig-5 and Ig-6) to the heavy chain linkage group [289, 290]. The availability of these antisera allowed the demonstration that most B cells possess both IgM and IgD receptors [291]. These receptors share the same variable region [291] and always come from the same chromosome on individual cells (haplotype exclusion) [292].

Structure and Function of the Major Histocompatibility Complex

For a detailed overview of the murine H-2 complex, the recent book by Klein [282] is highly recommended. An extensive review of the B-antigen system in chickens [283] has appeared. HL-A nomenclature has been changed [284]. The relationships between HL-A and disease are discussed in a recent volume of *Transplantation Reviews* (Vol. 22). In the guinea pig, it now seems very likely that the 2 and 13 antigens are closely linked to, but distinct from, the B (major histocompatibility) locus [285]. This adds support to the notion that the 2 and 13 antigens are homologous to the Ia antigens in mice [286,293]. Recent evidence suggests that the antigens associated with strong proliferation in the human MLC are serologically detectable and are selectively represented on B lymphocytes [287,288].

The murine Ss protein has been shown to be the fourth component of complement [294-296]. Preliminary amino acid sequences of H-2 and HL-A antigens indicate homology with each other; but not with immunoglobulin [317].

The biochemical nature of Ia antigens on murine thymocytes has recently been partially characterized in our laboratory [297]. These antigens have an apparent molecular weight of about 30,000, as assessed by sodium dodecyl sulfate-polyacrylamide gel electrophoresis (i.e., similar to B-cell Ia antigens) and appear to have limited heterogeneity with regard to molecular weight. Further evidence for the presence of I-region antigens on T cells was obtained by studying the transplantation properties of a series of T-cell lymphomas [298,299]. When these tumors were transplanted into mice which differed at the I region, they were rapidly rejected, although they possessed only very low amounts of serologically detectable Ia.

The possibility of a unique association between Ia antigens and the receptor for the Fc portion of IgG on B cells [300] now appears rather less attractive, because antisera to several other H-2 components also block this receptor [301,302].

Mechanism of Action of the Murine Histocompatibility-linked Immune Response Genes

It seems rather likely that the H-linked Ir genes represent a special and limiting case of a physiologically important mechanism in T-B collaboration and/or T-cell activation, but the precise mechanisms remain elusive.

Kapp et al. [303] have presented data that show that helper T cells to GAT can be generated in "nonresponder" mice. The fraction of thymocytes that binds GAT in responders and nonresponders was equal [304]. These data would appear to rule out the possibility that nonresponse to GAT is due to lack of structural genes for the T-cell receptor. Recent work has also cast doubt on the interpretation of the effects of alloantisera on T-cell proliferation [315].

A great deal of work has appeared on the need for identity at various H-2 regions for certain effects to be seen when using allogeneic cell combinations. Identity at the K or D ends is both necessary and sufficient for maximal cell-mediated lysis of target cells infected with lymphocytic choriomeningitis virus [305]. Similarly, spleen cells sensitized against trinitrophenylated syngeneic cells were only capable of lysing trinitrophenylated target cells which were identical at K or D. I-region identity was apparently not crucial, although Ir gene effects may occur [306,307]. These results suggest that, in these systems, the killer cells were generated against "altered self"-determinants.

In contrast, transfer of DTH was only successful when donor and recipient shared one I-region haplotype [308], a finding which is analogous to previous work that indicates a need for I-region identity for optimal T-B collaboration [309]. It should be noted, however, that *when the allogeneic cells are fully tolerant to each other* (as in the allophenic mice or radiation chimeras), identity at the I region is *not* needed for optimal T-B collaboration (see Refs. 310,311). Erb and Feldmann have found evidence that identity at the I-A region was essential for optimal interaction between macrophages and T cells [312]. This finding raises the possibility that antigen is presented to T cells via macrophages as "altered self," and suggests possible mechanisms for the action of the H-2 linked Ir genes. Shevach [316] has provided evidence for Ir gene expression in macrophages.

Other recent work has indicated that, under some circumstances, the combined action of two H-linked genes may be needed for optimal immune responses [313,314]. Dorf et al. [313] found that certain F_1 hybrids, derived from parental strains which were nonresponders to the synthetic copolymer GLϕ, were responders. Similarly, Munro and Taussig have presented evidence that indicates that nonresponse to (T,G)-A–L may be due to a defect at either the T- or B-cell level, depending on the mouse strain. In some cases, T-cell recognition occurred, but B cells were apparently unable to "accept" an antigen-specific "collaborative factor" [314]. If confirmed, these rather controversial experiments would appear to clarify many problems concerning T-cell recognition and the nature of collaboration. However, they have not yet gained widespread acceptance.

References

1. J. D. Watson and F. H. C. Crick, Nature (London) **171**, 737 (1973).
2. F. M. Burnet, *The Clonal Selection Theory of Acquired Immunity,* Vanderbilt University Press, Nashville, Tenn., 1959.
3. H. O. McDevitt and M. Landy (eds.), *Genetic Control of Immune Responsiveness,* Academic Press, New York, 1972.
4. L. Hood and D. W. Talmage, Science **163**, 325 (1970).
5. H. Wigzell, Scand. J. Immunol. 2, 199 (1973).
6. J. D. Capra and J. M. Kehoe, Scand. J. Immunol. **3**, 1 (1974).
7. A. J. Cunningham and L. M. Pilarski, Scand. J. Immunol. **3**, 5 (1974).
8. W. F. Bodmer, Nature (London) **237**, 139 (1972).
9. G. Möller (ed.), Transplant. Rev. **15**, 3-200 (1973).
10. F. Lilly, Transplant. Proc. **3**, 1239 (1971).
11. A. O. Vladutiu and N. R. Rose, Science **174**, 1137 (1971).
12. P. Demant, J. Capkova, E. Hinzova, and B. Voracova, Proc. Nat. Acad. Sci. USA **70**, 863 (1973).
13. B. Benacerraf and H. O. McDevitt, Science **175**, 273 (1972).
14. J. A. Gally and G. M. Edelman, Annu. Rev. Genet. **6**, 1 (1972).
15. B. Benacerraf, J. Immunol. **113**, 431 (1974).
16. H. O. McDevitt and M. Sela, J. Exp. Med. **122**, 517 (1965).
17. H. O. McDevitt and M. L. Tyan, J. Exp. Med. **128**, 1 (1968).
18. H. O. McDevitt and A. Chinitz, Science **163**, 1207 (1969).
19. D. H. Sachs and J. L. Cone, J. Exp. Med. **138**, 1289 (1973).
20. G. J. Hammerling, B. D. Deak, G. Mauve, U. Hammerling, and H. O. McDevitt, Immunogenetics **1**, 68 (1974).

21. E. Gunther, Transplant. Proc. **5**, 1315 (1973).
22. W. H. Hildemann, Annu. Rev. Genet, **7**, 19 (1973).
23. I. Green, Immunogenetics **1**, 4 (1974).
24. D. L. Gasser and W. K. Silvers, Advan. Immunol. **18**, 1 (1974).
25. B. Benacerraf, Scand. J. Immunol. **3**, 381 (1974).
26. E. Mozes and G. M. Shearer, Curr. Topics Microbiol. Immunol. **59**, 168 (1972).
27. B. Cinader, S. W. Kogh, and D. Naylor, Int. Arch. Allergy Appl. Immunol. **35**, 150 (1969).
28. H. H. Fudenberg, Amer. J. Med. **51**, 295 (1971).
29. A. C. Allison, Contemp. Topics Immunobiol. **3**, 227 (1974).
30. J. A. Clagett and W. O. Weigle, J. Exp. Med. **139**, 643 (1974).
31. M. Cohn, in *Genetic Control of Immune Responsiveness* (H. O. McDevitt and M. Landy, eds.), Academic Press, New York, pp. 370-448, 1972.
32. L. S. Rodkey, J. Exp. Med. **139**, 712 (1974).
33. J. J. Marchalonis, P. J. Morris, and A. W. Harris, J. Immunogenet. **1**, 63 (1974).
34. G. T. Goodman and H. Koprowski, J. Cell. Comp. Physiol. **59**, 333 (1962).
35. R. Gallily, A. Warwick, and F. B. Bang, J. Exp. Med. **125**, 537 (1967).
36. F. W. Falkenberg, A. Sulica, G. M. Shearer, E. Mozes, and M. Sela, Cell. Immunol. **12**, 271 (1974).
37. G. Biozzi, C. Stiffel, D. Mouton, Y. Bouthillier, and C. Decreusefond, Ann. Immunol. (Inst. Pasteur) **125C**, 107 (1974).
38. L. B. Crittenden and W. E. Briles, Transpl. Proc. **3**, 1259 (1971).
39. F. Lilly, in *Genetic Control of Immune Responsiveness* (H. O. McDevitt and M. Landy, eds.), Academic Press, New York, pp. 279-288, 1973.
40. G. D. Snell, Folia Biol. (Prague) **14**, 335 (1968).
41. F. Lilly, Transplant. Proc. **3**, 1239 (1971).
42. H. O. McDevitt, M. B. A. Oldstone, and T. Pincus, Transplant. Rev. **19**, 209 (1974).
43. C. A. Alper and F. S. Rosen, Advan. Immunol. **14**, 252 (1971).
44. U. R. Nilsson and H. J. Müller-Eberhard, J. Exp. Med. **125**, 1 (1967).
45. W. D. Terry, T. Borsos, and H. J. Rapp, J. Immunol. **92**, 576 (1964).
46. R. P. Erickson, D. D. K. Tachibana, L. A. Herzenberg, and L. T. Rosenberg, Fed. Proc. **22**, 612 (1963).
47. O. C. Bruton, in *Immunologic Deficiency Diseases in Man* (D. Bergsma and R. A. Good, eds.), The National Foundation, New York, p. 2, 1968.
48. M. D. Cooper and R. A. Lawton, Amer. J. Pathol. **69**, 513 (1972).
49. M. D. Cooper, R. G. Keightley, L. F. Wu, and A. R. Lawton, Transplant. Rev. **16**, 51 (1973).
50. A. M. DiGeorge, in *Immunologic Deficiency Diseases in Man* (D. Bergsma and R. A. Good, eds.), The National Foundation, New York, p. 116, 1968.
51. R. W. Steele, C. Lumas, G. B. Thurman, M. Schuelein, H. Bauer, and J. A. Bellanti, N. Engl. J. Med. **287**, 787 (1972).

52. E. M. Pantelouris, Immunology **20**, 247 (1971).
53. D. D. Manning, N. D. Reed, and C. F. Shaffer, J. Exp. Med. **138**, 488 (1973).
54. F. Loor and G. E. Roelants, in *The Immune System: Genes, Receptors, Signals* (E. E. Sercarz, A. R. Williamson, and C. F. Fox, eds.), Academic Press, New York, pp. 201-216, 1974.
55. F. Loor and G. E. Roelants, Nature (London) **251**, 229 (1974).
56. M. P. Scheid, M. K. Hoffmann, K. Komuro, U. Hammerling, J. Abbott, E. A. Boyse, G. H. Cohen, J. A. Hooper, R. S. Schulof, and A. L. Goldstein, J. Exp. Med. **138**, 1027 (1973).
57. M. D. Cooper, A. E. Gabrielsen, and R. A. Good, Annu. Rev. Med. **18**, 113 (1967).
58. T. Smith, J. Med. **13**, 341 (1905).
59. R. A. Cooke and A. Van der Veer, J. Immunol. **1**, 201 (1916).
60. S. Wright and P. A. Lewis, *Amer. Naturalist* **55**, 636 (1921).
61. P. A. Gorer, and H. Schütze, J. Hyg. **38**, 647 (1938).
62. K. Stern, K. S. Brown, and J. DAvidson, Genetics **41**, 517 (1956).
63. J. K. Dineen, Nature (London) **202**, 101 (1964).
64. J. Ipsen, J. Immunol. **83**, 448 (1959).
65. I. F. Scheibel, Acta Pathol. Microbiol. Scand. **20**, 464 (1943).
66. M. A. Fink and U. A. Quinn, J. Immunol. **70**, 61 (1953).
67. I. Green, J. K. Inman, and B. Benacerraf, Proc. Nat. Acad. Sci. USA **66**, 1267 (1970).
68. N. M. Vaz, J. M. Philips-Quagliata, B. B. Levine, and E. Vaz, J. Exp. Med. **134**, 1335 (1971).
69. E. R. Arquilla and J. Finn, J. Exp. Med. **122**, 771 (1965).
70. R. Liebermann, W. E. Paul, W. Humphrey, J. H. Stimpfling, J. Exp. Med. **136**, 1231 (1972).
71. M. E. Dorf, F. Lilly, and B. Benacerraf, J. Exp. Med. **140**, 859 (1974).
72. M. Sela and S. Fuchs, in *Handbook of Experimental Immunology* (D. M. Weir, ed.), Blackwell Scientific Publications, Oxford, Vol. 1, p. 1.1, 1973.
73. G. D. Snell, J. Nat. Cancer Inst. **21**, 843 (1958).
74. D. W. Bailey, Transplantation **11**, 325 (1971).
75. F. S. Kantor, A. Ojeda, and B. Benacerraf, J. Exp. Med. **117**, 55 (1963).
76. H. Bluestein, I. Green, and B. Benacerraf, J. Exp. Med. **134**, 458 (1971).
77. H. Bluestein, I. Green, and B. Benacerraf, J. Exp. Med. **134**, 471 (1971).
78. H. Bluestein, I. Green, and B. Benacerraf, J. Exp. Med. **134**, 1529 (1971).
79. H. G. Bluestein, Fed. Proc. **32**, 985 (1973).
80. L. Ellman, I. Green, J. Martin, and B. Benacerraf, Proc. Nat. Acad. Sci. USA **66**, 322 (1970).
81. I. Green, W. E. Paul, and B. Benacerraf, J. Immunol. **109**, 457 (1972).
82. I. Green, W. E. Paul, and B. Benacerraf, J. Exp. Med. **123**, 859 (1966).
83. Z. Ovary and B. Benacerraf, Proc. Soc. Exp. Biol. Med. **114**, 72 (1963).
84. N. A. Mitchison, Eur. J. Immunol. **1**, 10 (1971).
85. J. F. A. P. Miller and D. Osoba, Physiol. Rev. **47**, 437 (1967).
86. M. J. Becker, A. Ray, L. C. Andersson, and O. Mäkelä, Immunochemistry, in press (1975).

87. M. E. Bush, S. S. Alkan, D. E. Nitecki, and J. W. Goodman, J. Exp. Med. **136**, 1478 (1972).
88. B. Rubin and H. Wigzell, Nature (London) **242**, 467 (1973).
89. C. Henry and P. E. Trefts, Eur. J. Immunol. **4**, 824 (1974).
90. C. A. Janeway, J. Immunol. **111**, 1250 (1973).
91. C. A. Janeway and W. E. Paul, Eur. J. Immunol. **3**, 340 (1973).
92. H. A. Levin, H. Levine, and S. F. Schlossman, J. Exp. Med. **133**, 1199 (1971).
93. A. R. Williamson, in *Handbook of Experimental Immunology* (D. M. Weir, ed.), Blackwell Scientific Publications, Oxford, Vol. 1, p. 8.1, 1973.
94. S. Schlossman, in *Genetic Control of Immune Responsiveness* (H. O. McDevitt and M. Landy, eds.), Academic Press, New York, p. 60, 1972.
95. I. Melchers, K. Rajewski, and D. C. Shreffler, Eur. J. Immunol. **3**, 754 (1973).
96. E. Shevach, W. E. Paul, and I. Green, J. Exp. Med. **136**, 1207 (1972).
97. E. M. Shevach, I. Green, and W. E. Paul, J. Exp. Med. **139**, 679 (1974).
98. H. G. Bluestein, J. Exp. Med. **140**, 481 (1974).
99. E. M. Shevach, W. E. Paul, and I. Green, J. Exp. Med. **139**, 661 (1973).
100. W. E. Paul, E. M. Shevach, S. Z. Ben-Sasson, F. Finkelman, and I. Green, in *The Immune System: Genes, Receptors, Signals* (E. E. Sercarz, A. R. Williamson, and C. F. Fox, eds.), Academic Press, New York, pp. 175-190, 1974.
101. E. M. Shevach and A. S. Rosenthal, J. Exp. Med. **138**, 1213 (1973).
102. R. M. Zinkernagle and P. C. Doherty, Nature (London) **248**, 701 (1974).
103. P. C. Doherty and R. M. Zinkernagle, Transplant. Rev. **18**, 89 (1974).
104. M. Vadas, J. F. A. P. Miller, J. Gamble, and A. Whitelaw, Int. Arch. Allergy Appl. Immunol. **49**, 670 (1975).
105. J. C. Ordal and F. C. Grumet, J. Exp. Med. **136**, 1195 (1972).
106. D. C. Shreffler and C. S. David, Advan. Immunol. **20**, 125 (1975).
107. L. L. Cavalli-Sforza and W. F. Bodmer, *The Genetics of Human Populations,* W. H. Freeman, San Francisco, 1971.
108. G. D. Snell, M. Cherry, and P. Demant, Transplant. Rev. **15**, 3 (1973).
109. B. Blomberg, W. R. Geckeler, and M. Weigert, Science **177**, 178 (1972).
110. L. L. Pawlak, E. B. Mushinski, A. Nisonoff, and M. Potter, J. Exp. Med. **137**, 209 (1973).
111. K. Eichmann and C. Berek, Eur. J. Immunol. **3**, 599 (1973).
112. R. Lieberman, M. Potter, E. B. Mushinski, W. Humphrey, and S. Rudikoff, J. Exp. Med. **139**, 983 (1974).
113. R. Lieberman, C. Stiffel, R. Asofsky, D. Mouton, G. Biozzi, and B. Benacerraf, J. Exp. Med. **136**, 790 (1972).
114. K. Eichmann, A. S. Tung, and A. Nisonoff, Nature (London) **250**, 509 (1974).
115. T. Imanishi and O. Mäkelä, J. Exp. Med. **140**, 1498 (1974).
116. E. Premkumar, M. Shoyab, and A. R. Williamson, Proc. Nat. Acad. Sci. USA **71**, 99 (1974).

117. S. Tonegawa, C. Steinberg, S. Dube, and A. Bernardini, Proc. Nat. Acad. Sci. USA **71**, 4027 (1974).
118. T. Delovitch and C. Baglioni, Cold Spring Harbor Symp. Quant. Biol. **38**, 739 (1973).
119. D. L. Gasser, J. Immunol. **103**, 66 (1969).
120. D. L. Gasser, J. Immunol. **105**, 908 (1970).
121. D. L. Gasser and D. C. Shreffler, Immunogenetics **1**, 133 (1974).
122. E. Mozes, H. O. McDevitt, J. C. Jaton, and M. Sela, J. Exp. Med. **130**, 1263 (1969).
123. J. W. Stocker, D. G. Osmond, and G. J. V. Nossal, Immunology **27**, 795 (1974).
124. R. J. Graff and D. W. Bailey, Transplant. Rev. **15**, 26 (1973).
125. N. K. Jerne, Eur. J. Immunol. **1**, 1 (1971).
126. J. Klein, Annu. Rev. Genet. **8**, 63 (1974).
127. E. Thorsby, Transplant. Rev. **18**, 51 (1974).
128. H. Balner, Transplant. Rev. **15**, 50 (1973).
129. F. M. Burnet, Nature (London) **226**, 123 (1970).
130. D. Cohen, Transplantation **17**, 8 (1974).
131. H. L. Cooper, C. M. Mackay, and W. G. Banfield, J. Nat. Cancer Inst. **33**, 691 (1964).
132. E. A. Boyse and L. J. Old, Annu. Rev. Genet. **3**, 269 (1969).
133. S. G. Nathenson, Annu. Rev. Genet. **4**, 69 (1970).
134. C. Neuport-Sautes, F. Lilly, D. Silvestre, and F. M. Kourilsky, J. Exp. Med. **137**, 511 (1973).
135. G. Möller (ed.), Transplant. Rev. **21**, 3-143 (1974).
136. G. Möller and U. Persson, Scand. J. Immunol. **3**, 445 (1974).
137. P. Ivanyi, R. Hampl, L. Starka, and M. Mickova, Nature [New Biol.] **238**, 280 (1972).
138. S. M. Fu, H. G. Kunkel, H. P. Brusman, F. H. Allen, and M. Fotino, J. Exp. Med. **140**, 1108 (1974).
139. H. O. McDevitt, B. D. Deak, D. C. Shreffler, J. Klein, J. H. Stimpfling, and G. D. Snell, J. Exp. Med. **135**, 1259 (1972).
140. D. Shreffler, C. David, D. Gotze, J. Klein, H. McDevitt, and D. Sachs, Immunogenetics **1**, 189 (1974).
141. V. Tomazic, N. R. Rose, and D. C. Shreffler, J. Immunol. **112**, 965 (1974).
142. E. K. Dunham, M. E. Dorf, D. C. Shreffler, and B. Benacerraf, J. Immunol. **111**, 1621 (1973).
143. M. E. Dorf, P. E. Newburger, T. Hamaoka, D. H. Katz, and B. Benacerraf, Eur. J. Immunol. **4**, 346 (1974).
144. J. H. Stimpfling and A. E. Reichert, Transplantation **12**, 527 (1971).
145. T. Meo, J. Vives, V. Miggiano, and D. Shreffler, Transplant. Proc. **5**, 377 (1973).
146. F. H. Bach, M. B. Widmer, M. L. Bach, and J. Klein, J. Exp. Med. **136**, 1430 (1972).

147. J. Klein, M. Hauptfeld, and V. Hauptfeld, Immunogenetics **1**, 45 (1974).
148. C. S. David, D. C. Shreffler, and J. A. Frelinger, Proc. Nat. Acad. Sci. USA **70**, 2509 (1973).
149. D. H. Sachs and J. L. Cone, J. Exp. Med. **138**, 1289 (1973).
150. D. Gotze, R. A. Reisfeld, and J. Klein, J. Exp. Med. **138**, 1003 (1973).
151. V. Hauptfeld, D. Klein, and J. Klein, Science **181**, 167 (1973).
152. E. A. Boyse, L. Flaherty, E. Stockert, and L. J. Old, Transplantation **13**, 431 (1972).
153. L. Flaherty and S. S. Wachtel, Proc. Vth Int. Congr. Transplant. Abstr. p. 19 (1974).
154. E. A. Boyse and L. J. Old, Annu. Rev. Genet. **3**, 269 (1969).
155. J. A. Frelinger, D. B. Murphy, and J. F. McCormick, Transplantation **18**, 292 (1974).
156. R. B. Taylor, P. H. Duffus, M. C. Raff, and S. de Petris, Nature [New Biol.] **233**, 225 (1971).
157. E. A. Boyse, E. Stockert, and L. J. Old, J. Exp. Med. **128**, 85 (1968).
158. H. O. McDevitt, J. Immunol. **100**, 485 (1968).
159. D. H. Katz, Transplant. Rev. **12**, 141 (1972).
160. F. C. Grumet, J. Exp. Med. **135**, 110 (1972).
161. G. F. Mitchell, F. C. Grumet, and H. O. McDevitt, J. Exp. Med. **135**, 126 (1972).
162. P. Lonai and H. O. McDevitt, J. Exp. Med. **140**, 977 (1974).
163. R. K. Gershon, P. H. Maurer, and C. F. Merryman, Proc. Nat. Acad. Sci. USA **70**, 250 (1973).
164. J. A. Kapp, C. W. Pierce, S. Schlossman, and B. Benacerraf, J. Exp. Med. **140**, 648 (1974).
165. G. M. Shearer, E. Mozes, and M. Sela, J. Exp. Med. **135**, 1009 (1972).
166. G. J. Hämmerling, T. Masuda, and H. O. McDevitt, J. Exp. Med. **137**, 1180 (1973).
167. G. J. Hämmerling and H. O. McDevitt, J. Immunol. **112**, 1726 (1974).
168. G. J. Hämmerling and H. O. McDevitt, J. Immunol. **112**, 1734 (1974).
169. G. J. Hämmerling and H. O. McDevitt, J. Exp. Med. **140**, 1180 (1974).
170. B. Kindred and D. C. Shreffler, J. Immunol. **109**, 940 (1972).
171. D. Armerding, D. H. Sachs, and D. H. Katz, J. Exp. Med. **140**, 1717 (1974).
172. B. Benacerraf and D. H. Katz, Advan. Cancer Res. **21**, 121 (1975).
173. D. H. Katz, M. Graves, M. E. Dorf, H. Dimuzio, and B. Benacerraf, J. Exp. Med. **141**, 269 (1975).
174. D. H. Katz, T. Hamaoka, M. E. Dorf, P. H. Maurer, and B. Benacerraf, J. Exp. Med. **138**, 734 (1973).
175. B. Benacerraf, J. A. Kapp, C. W. Pierce, and D. H. Katz, J. Exp. Med. **140**, 185 (1974).
176. D. H. Katz and E. R. Unanue, J. Exp. Med. **137**, 967 (1973).
177. B. Mintz and J. Palm, J. Exp. Med. **129**, 1013 (1969).
178. T. G. Wegmann, I. Hellström, and K. E. Hellström, Proc. Nat. Acad. Sci. USA **68**, 1644 (1971).

179. R. D. Barnes, M. Tuffrey, C. F. Graham, J. Holliday, and C. Thornton, Scand. J. Immunol. **3**, 789 (1974).
180. T. Meo, T. Matsunaga and A. M. Rijnbeek, in *Immunobiology of Transplantation: The Histocompatibility Systems* (F. H. Bach, ed.), Grune and Stratton, New York, p. 109, 1973.
181. K. B. Bechtol, T. G. Wegmann, J. H. Freed, F. C. Grumet, B. W. Cheseboro, L. A. Herzenberg, and H. O. McDevitt, Cell. Immunol. **13**, 264 (1974).
182. M. J. Taussig, Nature (London) **248**, 234 (1974).
183. M. J. Taussig, E. Mozes, and R. Isac, J. Exp. Med. **140**, 301 (1974).
184. M. J. Taussig and A. J. Munro, Nature (London) **251**, 63 (1974).
185. G. M. Shearer, Eur. J. Immunol. **4**, 527 (1974).
186. A. Ebringer and D. A. L. Davies, Nature [New Biol.] **241**, 144 (1973).
187. M. L. Tyan and H. O. McDevitt, J. Immunol. **105**, 1190 (1970).
188. B. W. Cheseboro, G. F. Mitchell, F. C. Grumet, L. A. Herzenberg, H. O. McDevitt, and T. G. Wegmann, Eur. J. Immunol. **2**, 243 (1972).
189. U. Wurzburg, H. Schutt-Gerowitt, and K. Rajewsky, Eur. J. Immunol. **3**, 762 (1973).
190. G. F. Mitchell, Personal communication (1974).
191. F. H. Bach, M. B. Widmer, M. Segall, M. L. Bach, and J. Klein, Science **176**, 1024 (1975).
192. V. Hauptfeld, M. Hauptfeld, and J. Klein, J. Immunol. **113**, 181 (1974).
193. J. W. Goding, G. J. V. Nossal, D. C. Shreffler, and J. J. Marchalonis J. Immunogenet. **2**, 9 (1975).
194. J. A. Frelinger, J. E. Niederhuber, C. S. David, and D. C. Shreffler, J. Exp. Med. **140**, 1273 (1974).
195. T. L. Delovitch and H. O. McDevitt, submitted for publication (1974).
196. H. O. McDevitt, K. B. Bechtol, G. J. Hämmerling, P. Lonai, and H. O. McDevitt, in *The Immune System: Genes, Receptors, Signals* (E. E. Sercarz, A. R. Williamson, and C. F. Fox, eds.), Academic Press, New York, p. 597, 1974.
197. S. E. Cullen, C. S. David, D. C. Shreffler, and S. G. Nathenson, Proc. Nat. Acad. Sci. USA **71**, 648 (1974).
198. S. E. Cullen and S. G. Nathenson, in *The Immune System: Genes, Receptors, Signals* (E. E. Sercarz, A. R. Williamson, and C. F. Fox, eds.), Academic Press, New York, p. 191, 1974.
199. E. S. Vitetta, J. Klein, and J. W. Uhr, Immunogenetics **1**, 82 (1974).
200. E. R. Unanue, M. E. Dorf, C. S. David, and B. Benacerraf, Proc. Nat. Acad. Sci. USA **71**, 5014 (1974).
201. D. L. Kropp and J. R. Sachs, Nature (London) **252**, 244 (1974).
202. C. G. Fathman, B. S. Handwerger, and D. H. Sachs, J. Exp. Med. **140**, 853 (1974).
203. E. Lozner, D. Sachs, G. Shearer, and W. Terry, Science **183**, 757 (1974).
204. T. Meo, C. S. David, A. M. Rinjbeek, M. Nabholz, V. Miggiano, and D. C. Shreffler, Transplant. Proc. **7**, 127, Supplement 1 (1975).
205. J. M. D. Plate and I. F. C. McKenzie, Nature [New Biol.] **245**, 247 (1973).

206. H. P. Lohrmann, L. Novikovs, and R. G. Graw, Nature (London) **250**, 144 (1974).
207. H. von Boehmer, J. Immunol. **112**, 70 (1974).
208. P. Lonai and H. O. McDevitt, J. Exp. Med. **140**, 1317 (1974).
209. B. J. Alter, D. J. Schendel, M. L. Bach, F. H. Bach, J. Klein, and J. H. Stimpfling, J. Exp. Med. **137**, 1303 (1973).
210. M. Nabholz, H. Young, A. M. Rinjbeek, R. Boccardo, C. S. David, T. Meo, V. Maggiano, and D. C. Shreffler, Eur. J. Immunol. **5**, 594 (1975).
211. D. J. Schendel and F. H. Bach, J. Exp. Med. **140**, 1534 (1974).
212. V. P. Eijsvoogel, R. du Bois, C. J. M. Melief, W. P. Zeylemaker, L. Raat-Koning, and L. De Groot-Koov, Transpl. Proc. **5**, 415 (1973).
213. F. H. Bach, M. Segall, K. S. Zier, P. M. Sondel, B. Alter, and M. L. Bach, Science **180**, 403 (1973).
214. M. Nabholz, J. Vives, H. M. Young, T. Meo, V. Miggiano, A. Rijnbeek, and D. C. Shreffler, Eur. J. Immunol. **4**, 378 (1974).
215. H. B. Dickler and D. H. Sachs, J. Exp. Med. **140**, 779 (1974).
216. B. Pernis, Personal communication (1974).
217. A. Basten, J. F. A. P. Miller, R. Abraham, J. Gamble, and E. Chia, Int. Arch. Allergy Appl. Immunol. **50**, 309 (1976).
218. D. H. Katz and B. Benacerraf, Transplant. Rev. **22**, 175 (1974).
219. D. Armerding and D. H. Katz, J. Exp. Med. **140**, 19 (1974).
220. C. W. Pierce, J. A. Kapp, S. M. Solliday, M. E. Dorf, and B. Benacerraf, J. Exp. Med. **140**, 921 (1974).
221. J. A. Frelinger, J. E. Niederhuber, and D. C. Shreffler, Science **188**, 268 (1975).
222. W. K. Silvers, D. B. Wilson, and J. Palm, Transplantation **5**, 1053 (1967).
223. H. M. Vriesendorp, R. B. Epstein, J. D'Amaro, D. L. Westbroek, and J. J. van Rood, Transplantation **14**, 299 (1972).
224. P. Ivanyi, Curr. Topics Microbiol. Immunol. **53**, 8 (1970).
225. F. H. Bach, M. L. Bach, P. M. Sondel, and G. Sundharadas, Transplant. Rev. **12**, 30 (1972).
226. D. G. Marsh, W. B. Bias, and S. H. Hsu, Science **179**, 691 (1973).
227. M. N. Blumenthal, D. B. Amos, H. Noreen, N. R. Mendell, and E. J. Yunis, Science **184**, 1301 (1974).
228. M. E. Dorf, H. Balner, M. L. de Groot, and B. Benacerraf, Transplant. Proc. **6**, 119 (1974).
229. F. Lilly, E. A. Boyse, and L. J. Old, Lancet **(ii)**, 1207 (1964).
230. J. R. Tannant, in *Advances in Transplantation* (J. Dausset, G. Mathe, and J. Hamburger, eds.), Munksgaard, Copenhagen, p. 507, 1968.
231. S. Nandi, Proc. Nat. Acad. Sci. USA **58**, 485 (1967).
232. J. Dausset, L. Degos, and J. Hors, Clin. Immunol. Immunopathol. **3**, 127 (1974).
233. P. J. Morris, Contemp. Topics Immunobiol. **3**, 141 (1974).
234. H. O. McDevitt and W. F. Bodmer, Lancet **(i)**, 1269 (1974).
235. S. D. Lawler, P. T. Klouda, R. M. Hardesty, and M. M. Till, Brit. J. Haematol. **21**, 595 (1971).
236. R. L. Walford, S. Finkelstein, R. Neerhout, P. Konrad, and E. Shanbrom, Nature (London) **225**, 461 (1970).

237. G. N. Rogentine, R. A. Yankee, J. J. Gart, J. Nam, and R. J. Trapani, J. Clin. Invest. **51**, 2420 (1972).
238. B. Levine, R. Stember, and M. Fotino, Science **178**, 1201 (1972).
239. G. D. Pegrum, I. C. Balfour, C. A. Evans, and V. L. Middleton, Brit. J. Haematol. **19**, 493 (1970).
240. R. L. Walford, R. Zeller, L. Coombs, and P. Konrad, Transplant. Proc. **3**, 1297 (1971).
241. L. Degos, Y. Drolet, and J. Dausset, Transplant. Proc. **3**, 1309 (1971).
242. M. Schlesinger and B. Amos, in *Human Transplantation* (F. T. Rapaport and J. Dausset, eds.), Grune and Stratton, New York, p. 601, 1968.
243. J. L. Amiel in *Histocompatibility Testing, 1967* (E. S. Curtoni, P. L. Mattiuz, and R. M. Tosi, eds.), Munksgaard, Copenhagen, p. 79, 1967.
244. J. Dausset and W. Bodmer (eds.), *Histocompatibility Testing, 1972,* Munksgaard, Copenhagen, 1973.
245. J. Bertrams, E. Kuvert, U. Boohme, H. E. Reis, W. M. Gallmeier, O. Wetter, and C. G. Schmidt, Tissue Antigens **2**, 41 (1972).
246. J. Bertrams, P. Schildberg, W. Hopping, U. Böhme, and E. Albert, Tissue Antigens **3**, 78 (1973).
247. M. J. Simons, G. B. Wee, N. E. Day, P. J. Morris, K. Shanmugaratnam, and G. B. de The, Int. J. Cancer **13**, 122 (1974).
248. P. L. Stokes, P. Asquith, G. K. T. Holmes, P. Mackintosh, and W. T. Cooke, Lancet **(ii)**, 162 (1972).
249. Z. M. Falchuk, G. N. Rogentine, and W. STrober, J. Clin. Invest. **51**, 1601 (1972).
250. A. G. White, R. St. C. Barnetson, J. A. Da Costa, and D. B. McClelland, Lancet **(i)**, 108 (1973).
251. H. Waters, P. Konrad, and R. L. Walford, Tissue Antigens **1**, 68 (1971).
252. F. C. Grumet, A. Coukell, J. G. Bodmer, W. F. Bodmer, and H. O. McDevitt, N. Engl. J. Med. **285**, 193 (1971).
253. I. R. Mackay and P. J. Morris, Lancet **(ii)**, 793 (1972).
254. S. Whittingham, P. J. Morris, and F. I. R. Martin, Tissue Antigens, **6**, 23 (1975).
255. F. C. Grumet, J. Konishi, R. D. Payne, and J. P. Kriss, Clin. Res. **21**, 493 (1973).
256. T. J. Russell, L. M. Schultes, and P. Kuban, N. Engl. J. Med. **287**, 738 (1972).
257. S. H. White, V. D. Newcomer, M. R. Mickey, and P. I. Terasaki, N. Engl. J. Med. **287**, 740 (1972).
258. L. S. Krain, V. O. Newcomer, and P. I. Terasaki, N. Engl. J. Med. **288**, 1245 (1973).
259. S. J. Katz, M. V. Dahl, S. N. Penney, R. J. Trapani, and W. Rogentine, Arch. Dermatol. **108**, 53 (1973).
260. C. Jersild, A. Svejgaad, T. Fog, and T. Ammitzboll, Tissue Antigens **3**, 243 (1973).
261. M. Pietsch and P. J. Morris, Tissue Antigens **4**, 50 (1973).
262. J. Jersild, G. S. Hansen, A. Svejgaad, T. Fog, M. Thomsen, and B. Dupont, Lancet **(ii)**, 7840 (1973).

263. J. Nerup, P. Platz, O. O. Andersen, M. Christy, J. Lyngsoe, J. E. Poulson, L. P. Ryder, M. Thomsen, L. S. Nielsen, and A. Svejgaad, Lancet **(ii)**, 864 (1974).
264. A. Svejgaad, E. Svejgaad, L. Staub-Nielsen, and B. Jacobsen, Transplant. Proc. **5**, 1797 (1973).
265. K. Aho, P. Ahvonew, A. Lassus, K. Sievers, and A. Tilikainen, Lancet **(ii)**, 157 (1973).
266. J. C. Woodrow, Lancet **(ii)**, 671 (1973).
267. L. Schlosstein, P. I. Terasaki, R. Bluestone, and C. M. Pearson, N. Engl. J. Med. **228**, 704 (1973).
268. A. Piazza, M. C. Belvedere, D. Bernoco, C. Conighi, L. Conti, E. S. Curtoni, P. L. Mattiuz, W. Mayr, P. Richiardi, G. Scudeller, and R. Ceppelini, in *Histocompatibility Testing, 1972* (J. Dausset and W. Bodmer, eds.), Munksgaard, Copenhagen, p. 73, 1973.
269. L. Degos and J. Dausset, Immunogenetics **1**, 195 (1974).
270. J. Dausset, *Prog. Clin. Immunol.* **1**, 183 (1972).
271. J. C. Woodrow, B. Treanor, and N. Usher, Tissue Antigens, **4**, 533 (1974).
272. W. F. Bodmer, Israel J. Med. Sci. **9**, 1503 (1973).
273. J. Bodmer and W. F. Bodmer, Israel J. Med. Sci. **9**, 1257 (1973).
274. H. Bluestein, J. Immunol. **113**, 1410 (1974).
275. E. Wiener and A. Bandieri, Eur. J. Immunol. **4**, 457 (1974).
276. A. Ferreira and V. Nussenzweig, J. Exp. Med. **141**, 513 (1975).
277. J. Stavnezer, R. C. C. Huang, E. Stavnezer, and J. M. Bishop, J. Mol. Biol. **88**, 43 (1974).
278. P. Leder, T. Honjo, S. Packman, D. Swan, M. Nau, and B. Norman, Proc. Nat. Acad. Sci. USA **71**, 5109 (1974).
279. H. Binz and H. Wigzell, J. Exp. Med. **142**, 197 (1975).
280. H. Binz, T. Bachi, H. Wigzell, H. Ramseier, and J. Lindenmann, Proc. Nat. Acad. Sci. USA **72**, 3210 (1975).
281. H. Binz and B. A. Askonas, Eur. J. Immunol. **5**, 618 (1975).
282. J. Klein, *Biology of the Mouse Histocompatibility-2 Complex. Principles of Immunogenetics Applied to a Single System,* Springer-Verlag, New York, 1975.
283. F. Pazderka, B. M. Longenecker, G. R. J. Law, and R. F. Ruth, Immunogenetics 2, 101 (1975).
284. WHO-IUIS Terminology Committee, Transplant. Proc. **8**, 109 (1976).
285. E. Shevach, S. Z. Ben-Sasson, F. Finkelman, W. E. Paul, and I. Green, Transplant. Proc. **7**, 141 (1975).
286. F. D. Finkelman, E. M. Shevach, E. S. Vitetta, I. Green, and W. E. Paul, J. Exp. Med. **141**, 27 (1975).
287. R. J. Winchester, S. M. Fu, P. Wernet, H. G. Kunkel, B. Dupont, and C. Jersild, J. Exp. Med. **141**, 924 (1975).
288. P. Wernet, R. Winchester, H. G. Kunkel, D. Wernet, M. Giphart, A. Van Leeuwen, and J. J. van Rood, Transplant. Proc. in press (1975).
289. J. W. Goding, G. W. Warr, and N. L. Warner, Proc. Nat. Acad. Sci. USA **73**, 1305 (1976).

290. N. L. Warner, J. W. Goding, G. A. Gutman, G. W. Warr, L. A. Herzenberg, W. v. d. Loo, S. J. Black, and M. R. Loken, Nature (London) submitted for publication (1976).
291. J. W. Goding and J. E. Layton, J. Exp. Med. **144**, in press (1976).
292. L. A. Herzenberg, L. A. Herzenberg, S. J. Black, M. R. Loken, K. Okumura, W. v. d. Loo, B. A. Osborne, D. Hewgill, J. W. Goding, G. Gutman, and N. L. Warner, Cold Spring Harbor Symp. Quant. Biol. **41**, in press (1976).
293. B. D. Schwartz, W. E. Paul, and E. M. Shevach, Transplant. Rev. **30**, 174 (1976).
294. P. J. Lachman, D. Grennan, A. Martin, and P. Demant, Nature (London) **258**, 242 (1975).
295. B. Curman, L. Ostberg, L. Sandberg, I. Malmheden-Eriksson, G. Stalenheim, L. Rask, and P. Peterson, Nature (London) **258**, 243 (1975).
296. T. Meo, T. Krasteff, and D. C. Shreffler, Proc. Nat. Acad. Sci. USA **72**, 4536 (1975).
297. J. W. Goding, E. White, and J. J. Marchalonis, Nature (London) **257**, 230 (1975).
298. J. W. Goding and N. L. Warner, J. Exp. Med. **142**, 536 (1975).
299. N. L. Warner and J. W. Goding in *Membrane Receptors of Lymphocytes* (M. Seligmann, J. L. Preud'homme, and F. M. Kourilsky, eds.), North-Holland Publishing Company, Amsterdam, p. 287, 1975.
300. H. Dickler and D. Sachs, J. Exp. Med. **140**, 779 (1974).
301. V. Schirrmacher, P. Halloran, and C. S. David, J. Exp. Med. **141**, 1201 (1975).
302. P. Halloran, V. Schirrmacher, and C. S. David, J. Immunogenet. **2**, 349 (1975).
303. J. A. Kapp, C. W. Pierce, and B. Benacerraf, J. Exp. Med. **142**, 50 (1975).
304. L. J. Kennedy, M. E. Dorf, E. R. Unanue and B. Benacerraf, J. Immunol. **114**, 1670 (1975).
305. P. C. Doherty and R. M. Zinkernagle, J. Exp. Med. **141**, 502 (1975).
306. G. M. Shearer, T. G. Rehn, and C. A. Garbarino, J. Exp. Med. **141**, 1348 (1975).
307. J. Forman, J. Exp. Med. **142**, 403 (1975).
308. J. F. A. P. Miller, M. A. Vadas, A. Whitelaw, and J. Gamble, Proc. Nat. Acad. Sci. USA **72**, 5095 (1975).
309. D. H. Katz, M. Graves, M. E. Dorf, H. Dimuzio, and B. Benacerraf, J. Exp. Med. **141**, 263 (1975).
310. H. von Boehmer, J. Sprent, and M. Nabholz, J. Exp. Med. **141**, 322 (1975).
311. H. von Boehmer, L. Hudson, and J. Sprent, J. Exp. Med. **142**, 989 (1975).
312. P. Erb and M. Feldmann, J. Exp. Med. **142**, 460 (1975).
313. M. E. Dorf, J. H. Stimpfling, and B. Benacerraf, J. Exp. Med. **141**, 1459 (1975).
314. A. J. Munro and M. J. Taussig, Nature (London) **256**, 103 (1975).
315. H. Ruhl and E. M. Shevach, J. Immunol. **115**, 1493 (1975).
316. E. M. Shevach, J. Immunol. **116**, 1482 (1976).
317. J. Silver and L. Hood, Cont. Topics Molec. Immunol., in press (1976).

Glossary of Abbreviations

ABC	Antigen-binding cells
AFC	Antibody-forming cells
ALL	Acute lymphoblastic leukemia (man)
α-LMG	α-Methyl-D-glucopyranoside
ALS	Antilymphocyte serum
ASRL	Antigen-induced selective recruitment of recirculating lymphocytes
ATC	Activated T cell
ATxBM	Adult thymectomized, irradiated, bone marrow-protected mice (B mice)
B cell	Bone-marrow or bursa-derived lymphocyte
B^{γ} cell	B-cell precursor of IgG-secreting cell
B^{μ} cell	B-cell precursor of IgM-secreting cell
B_m lymphocyte	Memory B cell
B_v lymphocyte	Virgin B cell
B mice	Mice depleted of T cells but not of B cells
BCG	*Mycobacterium* Calmette-Guérin

BGG	Bovine γ-globulin
BSA	Bovine serum albumin
C′	Complement
C3	Third component of complement
cAMP	Cyclic adenosine 3′,5′-monophosphate
cGMP	Cyclic guanosine 3′,5′-monophosphate
CBP	Colchicine-binding proteins
CFU	Colony-forming unit
CL	Cytotoxic lymphocytes
CLL	Chronic lymphocytic leukemia (man)
C region	Ig constant region or domain
con A	Concanvalin A
CRL	Lymphocytes bearing receptors for complement
CS	Corticosteroid
CTDD	Chronic thoracic duct drainage
D-B cell	T cell-dependent B cell (i.e., B cell which requires T-cell influence for expression of its antibody-secreting potential)
DNP	2,4-Dinitrophenyl
D-TGA	A synthetic polypeptide, *p* (D-Tyr, D-Glu, D-Ala)
DTH	Delayed-type hypersensitivity
Fab	Antigen-binding fragment of Ig
Fc	Complement-fixing fragment of Ig
Fc receptor	Cell surface component with binding affinity for Fc fragment of IgG
FγG	Fowl γ-globulin (CGG, chicken γ-globulin; IgY)
GALT	Gut-associated lymphatic tissue
GLT	A synthetic terpolymer, poly α-(L-Glu^{57}, L-Lys^{38}, L-Tyr^{5})

GVHR	Graft-versus-host reaction
H-2	Murine major histocompatibility antigen
Hgb	Hemoglobin
HL-A	Human leukocyte antigen
HMR	High-mobility (electrophoretic) region
HRBC	Horse red blood cell
$[^3H]$ TdR	Tritiated thymidine
I-B cell	T cell-independent B cell (i.e., B cell not requiring T-cell influence for expression of its antibody-secreting potential)
Ig	Immunoglobulin
IgT	T-cell immunoglobulin (also IgM^T)
KLH	Keyhole limpet hemocyanin
LCM	Lymphocytic choriomeningitis
LD	Lymphocyte defined
LMR	Low-mobility (electrophoretic) region
LN	Lymph node
LPS	Bacterial lipopolysaccharide
LT	Lymphotoxin
LY	Murine lymphocyte antigens
MIF	Migration-inhibitory
MHC	Major histocompatibility complex
MLN	Mesenteric lymph node
MLR	Mixed leucocyte reaction
MON	Monomeric subunit of *Salmonella* flagellin
MSH	*Maia squinada* hemocyanin

NAGAL	*N*-acetyl-D-galactosamine
NAD	New antigenic determinant
NIP	4-Hydroxy-3-iodo-*t*-nitrophenylacetic acid
NNP	3,5-Dinitro-4-hydroxyphenylacetic acid
NSF	T-cell factor which is not specific for antigen
NTx	Neonatally thymectomized
PALS	Periarteriolar lymphocyte sheath
PB cell	B-cell precursor
PBL	Peripheral blood lymphocytes
Pca	Plasma cell antigen (murine)
PCV	Postcapillary venule
PFC	Hemolytic plaque-forming cells
PHA	Phytohemagglutinin
POL	Polymerized *Salmonella* flagellin
POX	Horseradish peroxidase
poly(A,U)	Polyadenylic acid-polyuridylic acid complex
PPD	Purified protein derivative of BCG
PVP	Polyvinylpyrrolidone
PWN	Pokeweed nitrogen
RBC	Red blood cell
RER	Rough endoplasmic reticulum
RES	Reticuloendothelial system
RFC	Rosette-forming cell (binds to RBC)
RLP	Recirculating lymphocyte pool
RPcV	Receptor on lymphocyte for postcapillary venule
SIII	Type-III polysaccharide from *Streptococcus pneumoniae*
SD	Serologically defined
SF	Antigen-specific factor (from T cell)
sRBC	Sheep red blood cell

T cell	Thymus-derived lymphocyte
T_1 and T_2	Differentiation stages in the T-cell lineage
TDL	Thoracic duct lymphocytes
Thy-1 or θ	Murine thymus and T-cell alloantigen
TIGAL	(Tyr, Glu)-Ala–Lys
TL	Thymus leukemia antigen
T_M lymphocyte	Memory T cell
TMVP	Tobacco mosaic virus protein
TNP	2,4,6-Trinitrophenyl
T-TDL	Thymus-derived thoracic duct lymphocytes (activated to H-2 antigen)
T_v lymphocyte	Virgin T cell
TxBM	Thymectomized, irradiated, and bone marrow-protected mice
V region	Ig variable region